PENNSYLVANIA COLLE

5 0608 0

MW01435580

DISCARDED

Date Due

BRODART, CO.   Cat. No. 23-233-003   Printed in U.S.A.

E. W. Morscher (Ed.)
Endoprosthetics

Springer
*Berlin
Heidelberg
New York
Barcelona
Budapest
Hong Kong
London
Mailand
Paris
Tokyo*

E. W. Morscher (Ed.)

Endoprosthetics

With a Preface by M. E. Müller

With 196 Figures and 32 Tables

Springer

ISBN 3-540-58499-4 Springer-Verlag, Berlin Heidelberg NewYork
ISBN 0-387-58499-4 Springer-Verlag, Berlin Heidelberg NewYork

Library of Congress Cataloging-in-Publication Data

Endoprosthetics: with 32 tables; [commemorative volume for Dr. med. h. c. Otto Frey-Zünd] / E. W. Morscher (ed.) – Berlin; Heidelberg; New York; Barcelona; Budapest; Hong Kong; London; Milano; Paris; Tokyo: Springer, 1995
  Dt. Ausg. u.d.T.: Endoprothetik
  ISBN 3-540-58499-4 (Berlin...)
  ISBN 0-387-58499-4 (New York...)
NE: Morscher, Erwin [Hrsg.]; Frey-Zünd, Otto: Gedenkschrift

This work is subject to copyright. All rights are reserved, wether the whole or part of the material is concerned, specifically the rights of translation, reprinting, reuse of illustrations, recitation, broadcasting, reproduction on microfilm or in other way, and storage in data banks. Duplication of this publication or parts thereof is permitted only under the provisions of the German Copyright Law of September 9, 1965, in its current version, and permission for use must always be obtained from Springer-Verlag. Violations are liable for prosecution under the German copyright law.

© Springer-Verlag Berlin Heidelberg 1995
Printed in Germany

The use of general descriptive names, registered names, trademarks, etc. in this publication does not imply, even in the absence of a specific statement, that such names are exempt from the relevant protective laws and regulations and therefore free for general use.

Product liability: The publisher cannot guarantee the accuracy of any information about dosage and application contained in this book. In every individual case the user must check such information by consulting the relevant literature.

Production: PRODUserv Springer Produktions-Gesellschaft, Berlin;
Cover-layout: Erich Kirchner, Heidelberg;
Typesetting: Graphische Werkstätten Lehne GmbH, Grevenbroich-Kapellen
SPIN 10677760   24/320 – 5 4 3 2 1 – Printed on acid-free paper

Commemorative volume
for

OTTO FREY-ZÜND

Dr. med. h. c.

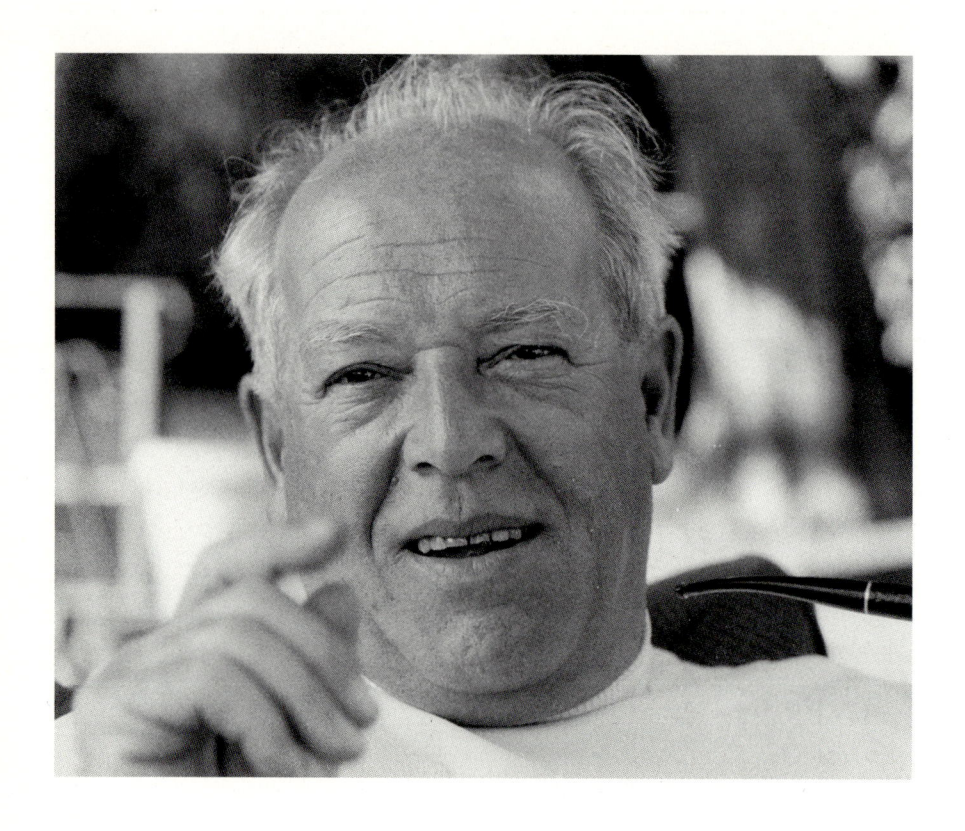

Dr. med. h. c. Otto Frey-Zünd
* July 1, 1925
† December 19, 1992

This book was written to honour the memory of
Dr. Otto Frey-Zünd, known as the "father of the
Sulzerjoints", by orthopaedic surgeons and engineers
of Sulzer Medical Technology, with whom he developed
artificial joints.

For these achievements, Otto Frey
was awarded an honorary doctorate of
medicine by the University of Basel in 1988.

Foreword

SULZERmedica, a subsidiary of the international company Gebrüder Sulzer, has been intensively involved in the production of joint implants for the locomotor apparatus. The foundry technologist Dr. Otto Frey contributed decisively to the development of Sulzer Medizinaltechnik between 1965 and the end of the 1980s. Prof. Erwin Morscher was the first to honor Otto Frey's work in medicine and since his death has spared no effort, in collaboration with fellow workers at Sulzer and renowened authors from the firms PROTEK and ALLO PRO, in putting together this commemorative volume. Erwin Morscher has asked me to write this foreword and to make critical remarks and express my personal opinion.

Authors from SULZERmedica such as E. Morscher, P.Schuster, L. Spotorno, H. Wagner, B. G. Weber, D. Weill, H. G. Willert, and K. Zweymüller have written on the hip prosthesis. Other chapters deal with prostheses for the knee joint (N. Gschwend, M. A. R. Freeman, W. Schwägerl, and N. Böhler) and upper extremities (N. Gschwend and H. C. Meuli) or implants still in the experimental stages. Not to be forgotten is A. H. Huggler, the first medical advisor of Sulzer Medizinaltechnik, who in 1965 developed a prosthesis similar to the McKee prosthesis but with better congruence. Here he presents his interesting pressure disk prosthesis.

The influence that Sulzer Medizinaltechnkik has had on its authors is best seen in their willingness to incorporate the three characteristic new developments at Sulzer, at least in part, into *their* prosthesis components: *Protasul-100*, Sulzers's titanium-niobium alloy used in prosthesis shafts; *Sulmesh*, the poyethylene coating with pure titanium wires (less than 1 mm thick, multilayered); and *Metasul*, using metal for both of the gliding parts. All three brand names are patented by Sulzer.

Protasul-100 is used by all the authors for noncemented shafts ("cement-free" seems linguistically questionable to me!). According to the histologist Schenk, the experimental surgeon Bereiter, and the clinician Morscher, Sulmesh is a guarantee for osseointegration, that is, direct ossification between bone and implant. According to Morscher there is evidence of osseointegration in over 95 % of his press-fit acetabula. Zweymüller prefers osseointegration with a microstructured (3–5 μm) acetabular surface. Gschwend, Weber, Weill, and Willert follow indictions for using Sulmesh to coat the artificial acetabula that differ in part from Morscher's. Metasul has captured worldwide interest and in the course of the past 3 years has been used at least experimentally by all the authors mentioned.

Knowing the critical attitude that surgeons have towards all new, untried and untested products, this agreement can be considered a great success for the scientific staff working with M. Semlitsch and R. Streicher and the technical team at Sulzer Medizinaltechnik in Wintherthur, Switzerland. In an important contribution examining the raw materials used in hip endoprostheses, M. Semlitsch and H. C. Willert discuss the advantages of utilizing the titanium alloy for noncemented prosthesis components and the disadvantages of the formerly used titanium-polyethylene combination. The numerous corrosion defects after cementing of the titanium shafts, which got me and other orthopedic surgeons into difficulties during the years 1989–1991, is a topic that unfortunately is not covered.

"Fixation with or without cement?" Willert asks in his introduction, "what has 30 years of experience taught us?" Reading the chapters by Zweymüller, Wagner, and Weill one might think that only noncemented implants are "up to date." Fortunately, Weber – who uncompromisingly uses cement – presents excellent results using high-pressure cementing techniques, priving that cementing should not be neglected under any circumstances. I can personally look back on numerous cases of cemented primary prostheses which are still absolutely stable after 25–30 years. If polyethylene could be replaced by the metal/metal combination, the number of abrasion particles would be so greatly reduced that one could reckon with 30 or more years of stability. Morscher, Schuster, Spotorno, and Willert believe more in the future of the so-called hybrid prostheses. These require, however, that the shafts be centered exactly in the marrow cavity so that a regular cement coat develops which precludes all contact between bone and metal. Is this always possible?

All of the chapters on hip prostheses are of uniformly high quality. Lucid explanations of the principles and aims of the individual implants are provided, including details on their respective advantages and disadvantages. Zweymüller, for example, is quite frank regarding the difficulties in extracting his prosthesis. Every chapter is backed up by an extensive list of references, in Morscher's case stretching to over 320 publications.

The influence of the innovative developments at SULZERmedica can also be seen in prostheses for other joints. The GSB knee joint introduced by N. Gschwend had its day 20 years ago, but this "old" third-generation prosthesis still should not be forgotten in the case of severe deformity or in patients over 75 years of age. The knee replacement procedure developed by M. A. R. Freeman and K. M. Samuelson has been modified so often in the past 25 years that it has played a crucial part in forming many technicians' views. The overall experience

Foreword

at SULZERmedica was decisive in the development of the APS knee joint by W. Schwägerl and P. Zenz. The noncemented monocondylar knee prothesis of N. Böhler et al. is also based on recent technical innovations at SULZERmedica. After several modifications, the GSB-III elbow prosthesis designed by N. Gschwend, B. Simmen, and H. Bloch is enjoying great success. H. C. Meuli's wrist joint prosthesis can now also be recommended following a 10-year trial period.

Otto Frey was a driving force behind the developments at Sulzer Medizinaltechnik and in the field of hip prosthesis design in general, and many of his porposals were outstanding. However, his decision to standardize the offset (the distance between the axis of the prosthesis and the center of movement) in all hip prosthesis systems was a dubious one; the preoperative graphical planning which is so vital if equal leg length is to be achieved became almost impossible with only one single template per system. In addition, all prostheses are modular, i. e., they featrue a cone on which various heads can be fit. I personally use a monoblock prosthesis in a third of my patients without the slightest adverse effects and believe that modular prostheses are gradually being abandoned. This is also true for gamma irradiation of polyethylene, which is currently recommended almost universally.

Dysplasia prostheses are not specifically discussed, although these are the prostheses which sometimes make so-called custom-made prostheses superfluous. Replacement procedures as a result of aseptic loosening combined with a high degree of bone loss have become a serious problem in total hip replacement. H. Wagner is the only one to devote a few sentences to this issue, although corrective surgery represents the future of prosthetic surgery.

As is well known, there is no consensus among orthopedic surgeons regarding the documentation and evaluation of the results of total prosthetic surgery. Very few surgeons maintain records with microcopies of the X-rays from all their patients; evaluation of standardized X-ray is not uniform; and the criteria once suggested by Merle d'Aubigné and Harris for the assessment of total prostheses are not sufficient anymore today. Looking at a continuous, closed series of operations, only 60 %–80 % of patients present for follow-up. Over 20 % are lost to follow-up because of death, corrective surgery, or change of address, because they do not wish to come to follow-up examination, or because they are being treated by another surgeon in the meantime. In addition, patients having undergone previous operations and those comprising special cases are frequently not taken into account, which explains why over 90 % of the published results are excellent.

Considering the high cost of any documentation it would be advantageous if the producers would jump in and help develop a reliable documentation system, at least for their own implants.

This valuable commemorative volume in honor of Otto Frey provides a guide to the concepts, procedures, and motives of the renowned SULZERmedica authors for improving endoprostheses. It presents the state of the art of prosthetic development in Switzerland in 1995. For this reason alone this volume can be consulted over and over again. The references which have been put together by the authors are an important source of information for scientists and practitioners in the field of total prostheses.

Bern   Maurice E. Müller[*]

---

[*] Prof. Dr. med., Hon. FRCS (Eng.), Dr. med. h. c. mult.
Founder and President of the International Hip Society 1979–1982
President of SICOT 1981–1984

Acknowledgements

The editor and the authors of this book would like to thank Professor M. E. Müller for agreeing to write the foreword. Professor Müller, who together with Sir John Charnley is the most important pioneer in the field, developed prostheses and instruments in close collaboration with Otto Frey. We would also like to extend our gratitude to SULZERmedica, PROTEK, and ALLO-PRO and to the M. E. Müller Foundation and the Otto-Frey-Zünd Foundation for their moral and financial support in assisting us to realize this Commemorative Volume dedicated to Otto Frey. I would also like to thank my secretary, Regina Brunner, for her untiring efforts and patience in compiling the manuscripts. Also of great assistance in the preparation of this volume were Joe Steiner (SULZER Medical Technology), Dr. Andrea Mumenthaler, and Dr. Willy Frick (PROTEK).

Basel, June 1995   Erwin Morscher

Authors

A. Bähler
Orthopädie-Technik, Consulting, Kapfsteig 44a, CH-8032 Zürich

Dr. med. H. Bereiter
Leitender Arzt Orthopädische Abteilung, Kantonsspital, CH-7000 Chur

Dr. med. H. Bloch
Viale Castagnola 21F, CH-6900 Lugano

Prim. Univ. Prof. N. Böhler
Vorstand Orthopädische Abteilung, Allgemeines Krankenhaus der Stadt Linz, Krankenhausstr. 9, A-4020 Linz

Dr. G. Böhm
Patholog.-Anatom. Institut, Allg. Krankenhaus der Stadt Wien, Währinger Gürtel 18–20, A-1090 Wien

P. A. Costigan, M. Sc.
Research Associate, Motion Laboratory Manager, Clinical Mechanics Group, Kingston General Hospital Kingston, Ontario, K7L 2V7/Canada

M. A. R. Freeman, FRCS
Consultant Orthopaedic Surgeon, 149, Harley Street, London W1N 2DE/UK

Dr. phil. II W. Frick
Protek AG, Erlenauweg 17, CH-3110 Münsingen

G. Grappiolo, M. D.
Ospedali Riuniti Finale e Pietra Ligure, I-17027 Pietra Ligure (SV)

Prof. N. Gschwend
Chefarzt Orthopädie, Wilhelm Schulthess Klinik, Neumünsterallee 3, CH-8008 Zürich

Prof. A. Huggler
Steigstr. 181A, CH-7304 Maienfeld

Dr. A. Infanger
Orthopädische Abteilung, AKH Linz, Krankenhausstr. 9, A-4020 Linz

Dr. H. A. C. Jacob
Leiter Institut für Biomechanik, Orthopädische Universitätsklinik Balgrist, CH-8008 Zürich

Dr. med. O. Knüsel
Chefarzt Rheumatologie, Klinik Valens, CH-7317 Valens

Dr. H. P. Köhler
Orthopädische Universitätsklinik, Robert Koch-Str. 40, D-37075 Göttingen

Dr. med. G. Köster
Oberarzt Orthopädische Universitätsklinik, Robert Koch-Str. 40, D-37075 Göttingen

Univ. Prof. Dr. F. Lintner
Vorstand Pathol.-Bakteriolog. Institut, Baumgartner Höhe 1, A-1145 Wien

Prof. H. Ch. Meuli
Lindenhofspital, Bremgartenstr. 117, CH-3012 Bern

Prof. E. Morscher
Felix Platter-Spital, Burgfelderstr. 101, CH-4012 Basel

Prof. M. E. Müller
Murtenstr. 35, CH-3008 Bern

Dr. med. A. Mumenthaler
Redingstr. 4, CH-9000 St. Gallen

Dr. K. Pastl
Oberarzt Orthopädische Abteilung, AKH Linz, Krankenhausstr. 9, A-4020 Linz

K. M. Samuelson, M. D.
Director Intermountain Bone and Joint Institute, Total Joint and Arthritis Surgery of the Hip, Knee and Foot, 370 Ninth Avenue, Suite 205, Salt Lake City, Utah 84103-2818/USA

Prof. Dr. H. G. Scheier
Chefarzt Orthopädie, Klinik W. Schulthess, Neumünsterallee 3, CH-8008 Zürich

Prof. R. Schenk
Pathophysiologisches Institut, Murtenstr. 35, CH-3010 Bern

Prof. Dr. E. Schneider
Technische Universität Hamburg Harburg, Denickestr. 15, D-21073 Hamburg

Dr. med. P. Schuster
Chirurgie Orthopédique, Clinique Saint Nabor, 5, rue de Maillane, F-57504 St. Avold Cedex

Univ.-Prof. W. Schwägerl
Vorstand Orthopädische Abteilung KAV-PZ, Ludwig-Boltzmann-Institut für Orthopädische Rheumachirurgie, Wien, Sanatoriumstr. 2, A-1145 Wien

Dr. phil. M. Semlitsch
Sulzer Medizinaltechnik AG, Entwicklung Implantat Werkstoffe, Postfach 65, CH-8404 Winterthur

Dr. med. H. Siegrist
Oberärztin Orthopädie, Klinik Wilhelm Schulthess, Neumünsterallee 3, CH-8008 Zürich

Dr. med. B. Simmen
Chefarzt Orthopädie, Klinik Wilhelm Schulthess, Neumünsterallee 3, CH-8008 Zürich

Dr. L. Spotorno
Ospedali Riuniti Finale e Pietra Ligure, I-17027 Pietra Ligure (SV)

Dr. phil. R. M. Streicher
Sulzer Medizinaltechnik AG, Entwicklung Implantat Werkstoffe, Postfach 65, CH-8404 Winterthur

Prof. Dr. Heinz Wagner
Chefarzt Orthopädische Klinik Wichernhaus, Ärztl. Direktor Krankenhaus Rummelsberg,
Postfach 1162, D-90588 Schwarzendruck/Nbg.

Dr. med., Dr. med. univ. M. Wagner
Oberarzt Orthopädische Klinik Wichernhaus, Brennerstr. 2, D-905921 Schwarzenbruck/Nbg.

Prof. B. G. Weber
Orthopädie am Rosenberg, Rorschacherstr. 150, CH-9006 St. Gallen

Prof. D. Weill
Chef de Clinique chirurgicale Hôpital „Belle Isle", 2, rue Belle Isle, F-57045 Metz Cedex 1

Dr. med. L. Wiedmer
Bürgerspital, CH-4500 Solothurn

Prof. H. G. Willert
Leiter der Orthopädischen Klinik, Postfach 3742, D-37070 Göttingen

Prof. U. P. Wyss
McLaughlin Hall, Queen's University, Kingston Ont. K7L 3N6/CDN

Dr. P. Zenz
Pulmologisches Zentrum der Stadt Wien, Sanatoriumstr. 2, A-1140 Wien

Prim. Prof. Karl Zweymüller
Ärztlicher Direktor 2. Orthopädische Abteilung, Orthopädisches Krankenhaus Gersthof,
Wielemansgasse 28, A-1180 Wien

Contents

Part I Basic Principles

H. G. Willert, M. Semlitsch
The Lessons from 30 Years of Success and Failure of Total Joint
Replacement 3

M. Semlitsch, H. G. Willert
The Importance of Remembering Past Mistakes When Considering
Implant Materials for Future Hip Endoprostheses 18

R. M. Streicher
Tribology of Artificial Joints 34

B. G. Weber
The Reactivation of the Metal-Metal Pairing for the Total Hip
Prosthesis 49

R. Schenk
Osseointegration of Sulmesh Coatings 60

H. Bereiter
Biomechanics of Osseointegration of a Cementless Hip Joint Cup in
Animal Experiments 72

E. Schneider
Primary Stability of Cemented and Noncemented Implants 85

U. P. Wyss, P. A. Costigan
Gait Analysis: A Biomechanical Tool in the Development of Artificial
Joints 103

O. Knüsel, L. Wiedmer
Gait Analysis of Normal Persons and Patients with Coxarthrosis Before
and After Conservative Therapy and After the Implantation of a Total
Hip Endoprosthesis 116

Part II Cemented Acetabular Fixation

B. G. Weber
The Cemented Hip Cup: The Weber Polyethylene-Ceramic and Metasul
Cups and the High-Pressure Cementing Technique 131

Part III Noncemented Acetabular Fixation

E. MORSCHER
Noncemented Acetabular Fixation in Primary Total Hip Replacement .. 143

P. SCHUSTER
The Saint Nabor Cup: 8 Years of Experience 180

E. MORSCHER
Rationale of the Press-Fit Cup 190

Part IV Cemented Femoral Stem

B. G WEBER
The Weber Stem and the High-Pressure Cementing Technique 203

E. MORSCHER, L. SPOTORNO, A. MUMENTHALER and W. FRICK
The Cemented MS-30 Stem 211

H.-G. WILLERT, G. KÖSTER and H.-P. KÖHLER
The Cement-Fixed Hip Replacement System 220

Part V Noncemented Femoral Stem

E. MORSCHER
The Cementless Femoral Stem 237

A. H. HUGGLER, H. A. C. JACOB
The Development of the Thrust Plate Prosthesis 248

H. WAGNER, M. WAGNER
Conical Stem Fixation for Cementless Hip Prostheses for Primary
Implantation and Revisions 258

Part VI Noncemented Endoprosthesis Systems

L. SPOTORNO, G. GRAPPIOLO, A. MUMENTHALER
The CLS System 271

D. WEILL
The Cementless CLW System 297

K. ZWEYMÜLLER, F. LINTNER, G. BÖHM
The Development of the Cementless Hip Endoprosthesis: 1979–1994 .. 309

Part VII Knee Joint Arthroplasty

N. GSCHWEND, H. SIEGRIST, H. G. SCHEIER, A. BÄHLER
The Gschwend-Scheier-Bähler Knee Prosthesis 329

M. A. R. Freeman, K. M. Samuelson
Total Knee Replacement at the Royal London Hospital: 25 Years'
Experience 342

W. Schwägerl, P. Zenz
The APS Cement-Free Knee Joint Prosthesis in Varus Osseoarthritis:
Treatment and Results 360

N. Böhler, K. Pastl, A. Infanger
Uncemented Unicompartmental Knee Arthroplasty 368

Part VIII Arthroplasty of the Upper Extremities

N. Gschwend, B. Simmen, H. Bloch
Elbow Arthroplasty, with Particular Regard to the Gschwend-Scheier-
Bähler III Elbow Joint Prosthesis 379

H. C. Meuli
Total Wrist Arthroplasty 393

Part I

Basic Principles

The Lessons from 30 Years of Success and Failure of Total Joint Replacement

H. G. WILLERT, M. SEMLITSCH

This article presents some personal views on failures and successes of artificial hip joint replacements, based on more than 25 years' experience in orthopedic clinics, pathology, and biomaterials research.

Strictly speaking, the title should read "Lessons from 100 Years of Success and Failure of Total Joint Replacement" since it was 100 years ago that Themistokles Gluck in Berlin designed and published the first attempts of hip and knee joint replacement [25, 26].

Beginning in the early 1930s many attempts were made to develop this field. Philip Wiles was one of the pioneers who designed and implanted the very first all metal total hip endoprosthesis in 1938 [90]. Wiles' prototype for the replacement of femoral head and acetabulum looked quite similar to the early versions of McKee and Watson-Farrar's prosthesis [50, 51], while the Judet brothers [37], Moore [54, 55], Thompson [82], Townley [83], Valls [84], and others were working on hemiarthroplasties. Since the implants in those days had to be fixed directly to the bone, they were already noncemented implants.

However, as early as in the fist half of the 1950s Kiaer [39] and Haboush [27] independently used acrylic bone cement to provide fixation of arthroplasty components to bone. Kiaer et al. [40] and Henrichsen et al. [30] reported then their experiments on tissue reaction to acrylic plastics. Wiltse and coworkers [104] investigated autopolymerizing polymethylmethacrylate (PMMA), which was known from dentistry and neurosurgery. They implanted it into bone in animal experiments and suggested its use as fixation agent for endoprosthetic components but did not apply it routinely to humans.

This step was taken by Charnley, who was apparently unaware of this research or of the use of PMMA materials manufactured by North Hill Plastics in London and called Surgical Simplex [86]. Instead, Charnley consulted with Smith, from the Materials Laboratory of the Turner Dental School, Manchester University [12]. In 1958 Smith recommended self-curing acrylic dental cement (Nu-Life) that Charnley sterilized with formaldehyde vapor. This material was tested in six hemiarthroplasty patients between 1958 and 1960 after successful laboratory tests [10]. Following a close collaboration between Charnley and the manufacturer Calculated Molecular Weight (CMW), bone cement was produced by their laboratories [2].

Charnley today receives the credit for this great contribution to artificial joint replacement. In the early days, however, many orthopedic surgeons simply did not anticipate a major success using bulky foreign material such as metals and polymers substituting for bones and joints. The innovations of Charnley and the other pioneers demonstrate that *newly discovered methods become widely applied only when their time has come.* From this follows a second lesson for orthopedic surgeons: The method of artificial joint replacement worked although it needed improvement. However, soon one had to learn another lesson, namely: *the whole subject is not as simple as it seemed at the beginning. This continues to be a lesson for those who have not learned from past experiences.*

How complex the subject really is may be understood more easily if one considers the factors which may influence results over the long run. There are at least three different fields which are closely interconnected and interdependent. These are:
– Technology (represented by the designer, materials engineer, construction and testing, and the manufacturer),
– Craftmenship (represented by the surgeon),
– Biology (represented by the patient).

The way in which the requirements of the individual factors are met determines the success or failure of the whole procedure. The factors include the following:

Technology

Design and construction. How to design the replacement?

Fixation. How to fix the endoprosthetic components to the bone, initially and permanently?

Biomaterials. What biomaterials are suitable for joint endoprostheses?

Manufacturing. What are the demands on the quality of joint endoprostheses as a product?

Craftsmenship

Planning. How are patients selected for artificial joint replacement?
Implanation:
– What approach is chosen?
– How are the implants put in?
– What is the quality of the primary fixation?

Experience. At what level is the surgeon's experience and how has he developed in his learning curve?

Biology

Anatomy. What is to be replaced?
Tissue reactions:
- How dos the implant bed react to the anchoring parts of the components?
- How is the permanent fixation created?
- How do degradation and wear products affect the surrounding tissues?

Loading. How are the implants stressed in the human body:
- At the anchoring site,
- At the articulating surfaces and
- within the endoprosthetic components itself?

Of these complex variables only the topics fixation and materials are discussed below.

Fixation

An implant works satisfactorily and painfree only if it is firmly fixed to tbe bone, and micromovements at the interface do not occur [11, 14, 19].

Regarding fixation of the endoprosthetic components to the bone one must distinguish between primary or initial fixation and secondary or permanent fixation.

Primary fixation must have been achieved by the end of the operation. However, preparation of the implant bed damages the surrounding tissues, causing microfractures of the bony trabeculae and necroses of the adjacent bone and bone marrow. Soon after the endoprosthetic components have been put in, repair of the tissue damage starts. The necrotic bone is removed and gradually replaced by living bone, which to some extend is built directly onto the implant's surface. The new formation of bone then secondarily creates the permanent fixation. This mechanism applies for both cemented and noncemented implants [94, 97, 98, 100].

Simultaneously the bone adapts to the change in load transfer, which is a consequence of replacing parts of the weight-bearing skeleton and of fixing the endoprosthetic components to other parts of the remaining bones. Bone is built up at places where the load transfer occurs, while it is taken away from places shielded from stress. As any normal bone, the restored bone surrounding the implant is also subjected to continuous remodeling.

The resorption of bone (mainly of the necrotic one) during repair and remodeling sacrifices bony anchors initially involved in the primary fixation. To guarantee stability, even during the process of reshaping the bone, the quality of primary fixation must be so good that the loss of some initial bone anchors does not jeopardize the overall implant fixation.

Furthermore, overloading of the bony anchors, even after the permanent implant bed has been established, may lead to bone resorption and to loss of fixation.

Regarding fixation with and without cement we must accept the following lesson:

The bone into which the endoprostheses are implanted is not the same bone which carries the implants over the long run. Repair of damage, adaptation, and ongoing remodeling must be recognized as normal events which create the permanent fixation and are part of the acceptance of the implants by the recipient tissues. Primary fixation must be good enough to guarantee stability even during the postoperative repair and reshaping processes occuring in the implant bed.

Overloading the bony anchors at any time may lead to bone resorption.

Some conclusions from this lesson have been drawn in the past. Many attempts have been made to improve the cementing technique, for example using medullary plugs and syringes, vacuum mixing, pressurizing the cement, and optimizing its composition to reduce its side effects.

It must by all means be considered as a lesson of success that *nowadays a much better primary cement fixation can be secured.*

Regarding fixation without cement the shape and the optimal condition of the anchoring surfaces of the components are still controversial.

With several designs one pinned great hopes on a porous surface where bone should grow into the voids [8, 15, 16, 17, 20, 21, 31, 38, 46, 47]. The pores were obtained either by adding beads or a mesh onto the surface or by creating a spongy structure of the material. This always requires special materials and a special manufacturing process which, again, may change the materials properties. Some types of endoprostheses seem to have very good successs with porous ingrowth, while others do not. Problems arise particularly if revision surgery is necessary since its removal might be extremely difficult [52]. Extensive porous coating and massive bone ingrowth may lead to marked atrophy due to stress shielding. Thus, not only the size and shape of the pores but also the extent of the porous coating of the implant is recognized as being quite important.

Removing the debris from the implant bed has again become controversial. While a thorough cleaning procedure is still strongly recommended [3], Hofmann et al. [33] favour to add autologous bone chips or leave the bone paste in the implant bed since the autologous bone serves as an osteoconductive and osteoinductive matrix and is therefore advantageous for the attachment of porous-coated devices to the host bone.

Another very important factor is the type of material from which the anchoring surfaces are constructed.

It has been shown (65, 66, 79) that titanium and its alloys have superior surface characteristics due to the hydroxylation of oxidized titanium and its reaction with amino acids, which seems to attract the ongrowth of bone.

We therefore prefer titanium or titanium alloys as material for the anchoring surfaces of our noncemented endoprostheses. Astonishingly, it turns out that even plane, nonporous, but rough shotpeened surfaces (Rz = 20–30 μm) offer excellent conditions to bone for ongrowth and building up a good permanent fixation, as long as the implant material is titanium or one of its alloys. [43, 63, 76, 87, 107].

Thus it appears that many details concerning successful non cemented fixation are still emerging.

Of course, fixation must withstand any possible loading of the endoprosthetic components in the human body.

Recent findings by Bergmann et al. who instrumented femoral ceramic heads in artificial hip joints have shown that the forces which act on the artificial joint and its anchorage depend particularly on walking speed and on muscle coordination; load increases with walking speed and with insufficient muscle coordination. Extreme loading peaks were measured as a result of "accidental forces," for example, due to stumbling while walking. This means, however, that weight bearing during slow and normal walking does not produce the highest stresses. Torsional moments leading to high bones stresses rise with decreasing anteversion angles. Therefore, implant anteversion must also be taken thoroughly into consideration [6].

The same authors have found that the amount of load reduction which the patient applies using crutches seems to depend more on the postoperative pain and walking ability than on the advice given by the physiotherapist. After a period of more than 4–6 weeks postoperatively load reduction by using crutches is only low; therefore refraining from weight bearing by using crutches for more than 6 weeks does not appear necessary [4, 5].

The lesson that we can learn from this is that *loading of the endoprosthesis may produce stresses in a quite different pattern to what has been assumed theoretically up to now.*

Since the greatest stresses applied to the anchoring mechanism are those due to rotational forces, primary fixation must secure the implant especially against torsional displacement. However, some of the presently available noncemented femoral components do not fulfill this requirement. For example, femoral stems with a rectangular cross-section [106, 107], possibly increased by fins [78], contribute much more to rotational stability than stems with a round cross-section.

As we have seen already, one cannot discuss artificial joint replacement without taking the materials into account. Therefore, out of the list of factors, mentioned at the beginning, the second topic shall be the performance of materials.

Materials

Demands on the materials differ according to the functions which they must fulfill. Basically, any material must be biocompatible and resistant to degradation. In addition, the bearing materials comprising the artificial joint surfaces should have low friction properties and must be wear resistant. As anchoring material they must resist the permanent and changing loads to which they are exposed and should neither release constituents nor corrode.

It is generally accepted today that materials used for artificial joint components must meet these basic requirements. However, this had to be learned by trial and error.

Materials for Bearing Surfaces

When Charnley established the low friction principle, he choose Teflon for the socket as bearing material against stainless steel of the femoral head. While the low-friction principle proved successful, the wear restistance of Teflon was poor.

At this point, the demands made with regard to wear resistance must be qualified insofar as any material is subjected to a certain amount of wear as soon as it moves in a bearing against other materials [91].

Loading of an endoprosthesis affects wear because the greater the muscle forces acting on the joint and the larger the number of moving cycles the higher is the wear rate. Very active and younger persons wear their artificial joint more and faster than less active and older persons.

The process of wear releases small particles. In an artificial joint these particles come into contact with the surrounding tissue, which is mostly the restored joint capsule. Macrophages and foreign body giant cells phagocytose the wear particles, store them, and transport them away, for example, via the perivascular lymphatics. If the extent of wear remains within certain limits, an equilibrium can be established between release and elimination of wear products.

However, if wear increases, the quantity of wear particles may exceed the eliminating capacity. Particles accumulate in the surrounding tissue, as do the phagocytes which store the material. The storing cells then form *granulomas*, and these finally occupy most of the joint capsule and other surrounding tissues and tend to become necrotic.

At this point the tissue reaction decompensates. The local tissues can no longer cope with the particles, and they now spread to remote tissues such as bone marrow and the bone/implant interface. Here, again, they cause the formation of foreign body granulomas. And, as with granulomas from other causes, they induce resorption of the adjacent bone, which means loss of bony anchors and consequently loss of fixation and loosening of the implant.

We detected this mechanism in the mid 1970s [95, 96], and it was confirmed by many other authors [13, 18, 24, 29, 35, 42, 49, 53, 59, 61, 64, 67, 85]. The lesson which we learned from this was that *accumulation of wear particles in the surrounding of artificial joint implants give raise to foreign body granulomas which, if they develop in the bone or at the bone/implant interface, induce osteolysis.*

Meanwhile, it was seen that *the biological reaction to particles, regardless of their origin, is generally the most important cause of loosening of joint replacements.*

We made these findings first with Teflon and similar materials in the late 1960s and early 1970s. Other polymer materials such as polyester, polyacetal, silicon rubber, PMMA and several kinds of metal were also subjected to high wear and produced the same bad results. We found similar granulomatous foreign body reactions to excessive release of wear particles, development of osteolysis, and implant loosening. Several innovations in the area of artificial joint replacement failed because of the poor wear restistance of these polymers [103].

Ultrahigh molecular weight (UHMW) polyethylene, introduced by Charnley as material for the socket after the Teflon disaster, is now the only polymer left that is fairly resistant to wear. It is therefore still used for joint bearings.

However, this is true only for concave bearing surfaces, while convex surfaces wear out fast [57, 58, 61, 62, 87, 89, 93, 103]. This is the reason why UHMW polyethylene should no longer be used for ball heads in the so-called "soft-top prostheses" (or convex joint surfaces in artificial knees).

The situation is made more complex by additional factors such as scratches in the metal partner, deterioration of the polymer with the passage of time (an inherent aging process), and entrapment of third bodies. Any of these factors accelerate the rate of wear. We have observed osteolysis and loosening due to excessive release of particles even with UHMW polyethylene [99, 103].

On the other hand, we do not believe that these phenomena justify abandoning polyethylene completely. It still is an acceptable bearing material as long as it is used properly.

The lesson drawn from these experiences is: *the use of biomaterials for endoprostheses must obey their properties.*

Quite recently this lesson has been confirmed by new experiences with titanium (aluminum-vanadium alloy) used for femoral heads, articulating with polyethylene sockets. In this case the non-surface-hardened titanium alloy was not sufficiently wear resistant. The heads produced considerable wear, which resulted in metallosis in the surrounding tissue and early loosening [1, 7, 45].

To prevent damage to and wear of wrought titanium alloy (Ti-6Al-7Nb) ballheads Sulzer recently developed a special oxygen-diffusion hardening (ODH) process which considerably increases the resistance of this alloy to wear and abrasion [81]. ODH-treated wrought Ti-6Al-7Nb alloy may now be considered a better bearing material for articulation against UHMW polyethylene [76]. This combination is now on clinical trial.

In the mid-1970s the search for improvements lead to the use of Al2O3 ceramic as bearing material. Sulzer introduced a combination of alumina-ceramic heads with UHMW polyethylene sockets [22, 73, 74]. Our measurements in Frankfurt and Göttingen confirmed the wear rate of this combination to be half that of metal/polyethylene [105].

Very recently a further innovation has been launched. The follow-up of the original all CoCrMo metal McKee – Watson – Farrar-, Huggler, and Müller types of joints show very low wear as long as the joint components are properly matched by 0.15–0.20 mm clearance betwenn ball and socket to allow a fluid interface. Once this was achieved several years ago, Sulzer decided in 1988 to revive the metal-to-metal combination in an modern design, called Metasul. The 5-year results are now available and are quite promising [75, 77, 80, 81].

Materials for Anchoring Parts

PMMA is the anchoring material in cemented endoprostheses. In the past cemented endoprostheses came loose over time. With prostheses from the early days this might have been attributed to poor cementing technique. However, one later had to learn that *acrylic bone cement may disintegrate mechanically into small particles.*

Originating either at the cement/bone or at the cement/implant, interface, the cement particles provoke the formation of granulomata which induce the osteolysis and loosening described above for wear particles of the bearing materials. Cement-induced osteolysis often develops at a site quite distant to the joint itself [13, 28, 35, 42, 64, 101]. Some authors call these phenomena "cement disease" [36]. This ignores the fact, however, that the same tissue reactions are found without cement. The common factor is particles [99]. We can therefore take the lesson on particles further by stating that: *the most important cause of aseptic loosening is the biologic reaction to particles produced by wear and degradation. There are no such conditions as cement disease, polyethylene or metal disease. These must all be attributed to particles and, if at all, might be called particle disease.*

In fact, the particle lesson has certainly not endet yet.

It has been shown, for example, by Carlsson and coworkers [9] and by Huddlestone [34] that defects in the bone cement mantle and direct contact of the endoprosthetic components to the bone accelerate disintegration of bone cement and determine the site at which osteolysis develops. As a result of these findings we believe that the cementing technique can be further improved by trying to guarantee an even thickness of the cement mantle (2–5 mm) and good centering of the anchoring parts within the cement [92].

UHMW polyethylene has been used not only as bearing but also as anchoring material. A few years ago we learned that *UHMW polyethylene and other polymers are also unsuitable for fixation direct to bone.*

If bone (or cartilage) grows onto the noncemented polyethylene implant, it rubs off particles from its relatively soft surface and starts the process of particle phagocytosis, granuloma formation, and bone resorption at the bone/implant interface. After a relatively short period of success [56] the result is again osteolysis and loosening of the implant. In most cases loosening becomes obvious after 4–8 years. In some cases the particles from the anchoring surface of the polyethylene cup spread to the bone/implant interface of the femoral shaft, inducing osteolysis there as well [23, 32, 41, 43, 60, 102].

Fatigue strength is another materials property that must be mentioned. We recall the unpleasant experiences from the 1960s and early 1970s when stems of cemented femoral components broke. This happened because they were made of cast CoCrMo alloy or soft-annealed stainless steel whose fatigue strength was inadequate for the dynamic loads to which they were subjected so that fatigue fractures could occur [48, 69, 72]. The lesson learned from this experience was that *low-fatigue strength alloys are less suitable for anchoring parts, especially of endoprosthetic stems, since they are prone to fatigue fractures under permanent dynamic load.*

As a result of this lesson Sulzer, and soon after several other manufacturers, switched to hight-fatigue strength alloys on cobalt-, iron-, or titanium-basis [68, 70, 71].

Only a few years later, however, when noncemented fixation became increasingly fashionable, cast cobalt-chromium alloys were again used for anchoring stems. The innovation of certain design characteristics such as the "madreporic" surface [47] or the "spongiosa metal" structure [31, 37] required the casting process. As should have been anticipated, the cast metal stems again suffered from fatigue fractures. Thus the same lesson had to be learned a second time, at high costs: *the use of biomaterials must meticulously take their properties into consideration.* It also follows *that in trying to improve some details one should not disregard the lessons already learned.*

Closing Remarks and Open Questions

There are several sources of information on possible improvement and final outcome of artificial joint replacements: laboratory investigations, animal tests, recording of the inital results, long-term follow-up of patients, and retrieval studies. After all of our experiences it has turned out that long-term follow-up of patients and retrieval studies have given the most valuable information about the performance of the endoprostheses over the long run.

Regarding the follow-up of patients only, one must be aware that it takes 7–10 years to realistically assess a given prosthetic device.

Real improvements in artificial joint replacement have been made in small steps, based on sound knowledge and experience. Any innovation carries a risk of failure, but the lessons resulting in improvements we have learned more from failures than from successes.

We all agree that the ultimate goal of total joint replacement is the longest possible undisturbed function of the implants in the patient, without failure. It is quite interesting, that failure has very few causes. These are recurrent luxation, infection, and aseptic loosening. The most important one is aseptic loosening, and the most important reason for aseptic loosening is wear and degradation of the materials.

Nevertheless, many questions remain open and awaiting answers. Some of these open questions are:
- Will the fixation with or without cement win?
- Will polished surfaces of cemented stems dominate the rough finish?
- Will roughshot surfaces of noncemented titanium implants result in a better permanent fixation than porous ingrowth?
- Will hydroxyapatite coating produce better long-terms results than those with other permanent fixing methods?
- Will the CoCrMo metal/metal bearing in hip joints supersede the combination metal or aluminium ceramic/UHMW polyethylene?

References

1. Agins HJ, Alcock NW, Bansal M, Salvati EA, Wilson PD, Pellici PM, Bullough PG (1988) Metallic wear in failed titanium-alloy total hip replacements. J Bone Joint Surg Am 70: 347–356
2. Amstutz HC, Clarke IC (1991) Evolution of hip arthroplasty. In: Amstutz HC (ed) Hip arthroplasty. Churchill Livingstone, New York Edinburgh London Melbourne Tokyo, pp 1–14
3. Amstutz HC, Yao J, Dorey FJ, Gruen TA (1991) Acrylic fixation – Stem and socket replacement: Results, principles, and technique. In: Amstutz HC (ed) Hip arthroplasty. Churchill Livingstone, New York Edinburgh London Melbourne Tokyo, pp 239–260
4. Bergmann G, Graichen F, Rohlmann A (1992) Loading of hip implants by torsional moments. 38 th Annual Meeting, Orthopaedic Research Society, Washington, D.C., February 17–20, p 19
5. Bergmann G, Graichen F, Rohlmann A (1992) Load reduction of hip implants by forearm crutches. VIII Meeting of the European Society of Biomechanics, Rome Italy, June 21–24, p 300
6. Bergmann G, Graichen F, Rohlmann A (1993) Hip joint loading during walking and running, measured in two patients. J Biomech 26/8: 969–990
7. Black J, Sherk H, Bonini J, Rostocker WR, Schajowitz F, Galante J (1990) Metallosis associated with a stable titanium-alloy femoral component in total hip replacement. J Bone Joint Surg [Am] 72: 126–130
8. Bobyn JD, Pilliar RM, Cameron HU, Weatherly GC (1980) The optimum pore size for the fixation of porous-surfaced metal implants by the ingrowth of bone. Clin Orthop 150: 263–270
9. Carlsson AS, Gentz GF, Linder L (1983) Localized bone resorption in the femur in mechanical failure of cemented total hip arhroplasties. Acta Orthop Scand 54: 396–402

10. Charnley J (1960) Anchorage of femoral head prosthesis to the shaft of femur. J Bone Joint Surg [Br] 42: 28
11. Charnley J (1967) Total prosthetic replacement of the hip. Centre for Hip Surgery, Wrightington Hospital, Internal Publication No 4, September 1967
12. Charnley J (1970) Acrylic cement in orthopaedic surgery. Churchill Livingstone, Edinburgh London
13. Charnley J (1975) Fracture of femoral prostheses in total hip replacement: A clinical study. Clin Orthop 111: 105–120
14. Charnley J, Kettlewell J (1965) The elimination of slip between prosthesis and femur. J Bone Joint Surg [Br] 47: 56
15. Engh CA, Bobyn JD, Glassman AH (1987) Porous coated hip replacement. The factors governing bone ingrowth, stress shielding, and clinical results. J Bone Joint Surg [BR] 69: 45
16. Engh CA, Bobyn JD (1988) Results of porous-coated hip replacement using the AML prosthesis. In: Fitzgerald R jr (ed) Non-cemented total hip arthroplasty. Raven, New York, pp 393–406
17. Engh CA, McGovern TF, Engh CA jr, Macalino GE (1993) Clinical experience with the anatomic medullary locking (AML) prosthesis for primary total hip replacement. In: Morrey BF (ed) Biological, material and mechanical considerations of joint replacement. Raven, New York, pp 167–184
18. Fiechter TH, Stanisic M, Frei W (1988) Granulombildung bei nicht gelockerten TEP. Orthop Praxis 6: 397
19. Follaci FM, Charnley J (1969) A comparison of the results of femoral head prostheses with and without cement. Clin Orthop 62: 156–161
20. Galante J (1988) Clinical results with the HGP cementless total hip prosthesis. In: Fitzgerald R jr (ed) Non-cemented total hip arthroplasty. Raven, New York, pp 427–431
21. Galante J, Rostoker W, Lueck R, Ray RD (1971) Sintered fiber metal composites as a basis for attachments of implants to bone. J Bone Joint Surg [Am] 53: 101
22. Geduldig D, Dörre E, Happel M, Lade R, Prüssner P, Willert HG, Zichner L (1975) Welche Aussicht hat die Biokeramik als Implantatmaterial in der Orthopädie? Med Orthop Tech 6: 138–143
23. Gierse H, Maaz B, Pelster C (1988) Probleme der Endler-Pfanne – Diskrepanz zwischen radiologischem und klinischem Befund bei mittelfristigen Ergebnissen. Orthop Praxis 6: 368–369
24. Goldring SR, Jasty M, Roelke M, Petrison KK, Bringhurst FR, Schiller AL, Harris WH (1988) Biological factors that influence the development of a bone-cement membrane. In: Fitzgerald R jr (ed) Non-cemented total hip arthroplasty. Raven, New York, pp 35–39
25. Gluck T (1890) Die Invaginationsmethode der Osteo- und Arthroplastik. Berlin Klin Wochenschr 33: 732–757
26. Gluck T (1891) Referat über die durch das moderne chirurgische Experiment gewonnenen positiven Resultate, betreffend die Naht und den Ersatz von Defekten höherer Gewebe, sowie über die Verwertung resorbierbarer und lebendiger Tampons in der Chirurgie. Arch Klin Chir 41: 187
27. Haboush EJ (1953) A new operation for arthroplasty of the hip based on biomechanics, photoelasticity, fast setting dental acrylic and other considerations. Bull Hosp J Dis 14: 242
28. Harris WH, Schiller AL, Scholler JM, Freiberg RA, Scott R (1976) Extensive localized bone resorption in the femur following total hip replacement. J Bone Joint Surg Am 58: 612
29. Heilmann K, Diezel PB, Rossner JA, Brinkmann KA (1975) Morphological studies in tissues surrounding alloarthroplastic joints. Virchows Arch A Pathol Anat Histol 366: 93–106

30. Henrichsen E, Jansen K, Krogh-Poulsen W (1953) Experimental investigations of the tissue reactions to acrylic plastics. Acta Orthop Scand 22: 141
31. Henssge EJ, Peschel U (1987) Anatomisch angepaßte Hüftendoprothese mit spongiös-metallischer Oberfläche. Chir Praxis 37: 503–512
32. Herren T, Remagen W, Schenk R (1987) Histologie der Implantat-Knochengrenze bei zementierten und nicht-zementierten Endoprothesen. Orthopäde 61: 239–251
33. Hofmann AA, Bloebaum RD, Rubman MH, Bachus KN, Plaster RL (1992) Microscopic analysis of autograft bone applied at the interface of porous-coated devices in human cancellous bone. Int Orthop 16: 349–358
34. Huddlestone HD (1988) Femoral lysis after cemented hip arthroplasty. J Arthroplasty 3: 285–297
35. Jasty MJ, Floyd WE, Schiller AL, Goldring SR, Harris WH (1986) Localized osteolysis in stable, non-septic total hip replacement. J Bone Joint Surg [Am] 68: 912
36. Jones LC, Hungerford DS (1987) Cement disease. Clin Orthop 225: 192–206
37. Judet J, Judet R (1950) Use of an artificial femoral head for arthroplasty of the hip joint. J Bone Joint Surg Br 32: 166
38. Judet R, Siguier M, Brumpt B, Judet T (1978) A noncemented total hip prosthesis. Clin Orthop 137: 76–84
39. Kiaer S (1951) Preliminary report on hip arthroplasty by use of acrylic head. Societé Internationale de Chirurgie orthopédique et de Traumatologie, Stockholm 1951. Lielens, Bruxelles, p 533
40. Kiaer S, Jansen K, Krogh-Poulsen W, Henrichsen E (1951) Experimental investigation of the tissue reaction to acrylic plastics. Societé Internationale de Chirurgie orthopédique et de Traumatologie, Stockholm 1951. Lielens, Bruxelles, p 534
41. Knahr K, Böhler M, Frank P, Plenk H, Salzer M (1987) Fünf-Jahres-Erfahrungen mit der Polyäthylen-Füßchenpfanne Modell Gersthof. Z Orthop 125: 375–381
42. Lennox DW, Schofield BH, McDonald DF, Riley LH jun (1987) A histologic comparison of aseptic loosening of cemented, press-fit, and biologic ingrowth prostheses. Clin Orthop 225: 171
43. Lintner F, Zweymüller K, Brand G (1986) Tissue reaction to titanium endoprostheses – autopsy studies in four cases, J Arthroplasty 1: 183–195
44. Lintner F, Böhm G, Bösch P, Endler M, Zweymüller K (1988) Ist hochdichtes Polyäthylen als Implantatmaterial zur zementfreien Verankerung von Hüftendoprothesen geeignet? Z Orthop 126: 688–692
45. Lombardi AV, Mallory TH, Vaughn BK, Droulliard P (1989) Aseptic loosening in total hip arthroplasty secondary to osteolysis induced by wear debris from titanium-alloy modular femoral heads. J Bone Joint Surg Am 71: 1337–1342
46. Lord G, Bancel P (1983) The madreporique cementless total hip arthroplasty: new experimental data and a seven-year follow-up study. Clin Orthop 176: 67–76
47. Lord G, Hardy JR, Kummer FJ (1979) An uncemented total hip replacement. Clin Orthop 141: 2–16
48. Lorenz M, Semlitsch M, Panic B, Weber H, Willert HG (1978) Dauerschwingfestigkeit von Kobaltbasislegierungen hoher Korrosionsbeständigkeit für künstliche Hüftgelenke. Technische Rundschau Sulzer 1/1978, S. 31–40
49. Maguire JK, Cosci MF, Lynch MH (1987) Foreign body reaction to polymeric debris following total hip arthroplasty. Clin Orthop 216: 213
50. McKee GK (1970) Development of total prosthetic replacement of the hip. Clin Orthop 72: 85
51. McKee GK, Watson-Farrar J (1966) Replacement of arthritic hips by the McKee-Farrar prosthesis. J Bone Joint Surg Br 48: 245–259
52. McLelland SJ, James RL, Simmons N (1986) Atraumatic removal of a well-fixed porous ingrowth hip prosthesis. Orthop Rev 15: 387–392

53. Mirra JM, Marder RA, Amstutz HC (1982) The pathology of failed total joint arthroplasty. Clin Orthop 170: 175–183
54. Moore AT (1952) Metal hip joint. A new self-locking metallic prosthesis. South Med J: 45: 10–15
55. Moore AT (1957) The self-locking metal hip prosthesis. J Bone Joint Surg Am 39: 811
56. Morscher E, Dick W, Kernen V (1982) Cementless fixation of polyethylene acetabular component in total hip arthroplasty. Arch Orthop Trauma Surg 99: 223–230
57. Müller M, Buchhorn GH (1994) Clinical experience with total hip replacements a review of the available literature. In: Buchhorn GH, Willert HG (eds) Technical principles, design and safety of joint implants. Hogrefe & Huberl, Toronto, pp 353–368
58. Patka P, Slingerland ACH, De Groot K, Van Velzen D (1991) Attrition of femoral head and neck prosthesis. In: Willert HG, Buchhorn GH (eds) Ultra-high molecular weight polyethylene as biomaterial in orthopedic surgery. Hogrefe & Huber, Toronto pp 232–235
59. Pazzaglia UE, Ghisellini F, Barbieri D, Ceciliani L (1988) Failure of the stem in total hip replacement a study of aetiology and mechanism of failure in 13 cases. Arch Orthop Trauma Surg 107: 195–202
60. Remagen W, Morscher E (1984) Histological results with cement-free implanted hip sockets of polyethylene. Arch Orthop Trauma Surg 103: 145–151
61. Revell PA, Weightman B, Freeman MAR, Vernon-Roberts B (1978) The production and biology of polyethylene wear debris. Arch Orthop Traum Surg 91: 167
62. Rose RM, Radin EL (1982) Wear of polyethylene in total hip prosthesis. Clin Orthop 170: 107–115
63. Schenk RK, Wehrli U (1989) Zur Reaktion des Knochens auf eine zementfreie SL-Femur-Revisionsprothese histologische Befunde an einem fünfeinhalb Monate post operationem gewonnenen Autopsiepräparat. Orthopäde 18: 454–462
64. Schmalzried TP, Finerman GAM (1988) Osteolysis in aseptic failure. In: Fitzgerald R jr (ed) Non-cemented total hip arthroplasty. Raven, New York, p 303
65. Schmidt M (1992) Spezifische Adsorption organischer Moleküle auf oxidiertem Titan: „Bioaktivität" auf molekularem Niveau. Osteologie 1: 222–235
66. Schmidt M, Steinemann SG (1991) XPS studies of amino acids adsorbed on titanium dioxide surfaces. Fresenius J Anal Chem 341: 412–415
67. Scott WW jr, Riley LH, Dorfman HD (1985) Focal lytic lesions associated with femoral stem loosening in total hip prosthesis. AJR 144: 977–982
68. Semlitsch M (1992) 25 years Sulzer development of implant materials for total hip prostheses. Sulzer Medica Journal Spring 1992
69. Semlitsch M, Panic B (1980) Corrosion fatigue testing of femoral head prostheses made of implant alloys of different fatigue resistance. In: Hastings GW, Williams DF (eds) Mechanical properties of biomaterials. Wiley & Sons, New York pp 323–335
70. Semlitsch M, Panic B (1983) Ten years of experience with test criteria for fracture-proof anchorage stems of artificial hip joints. Engin Med 12: 185–198
71. Semlitsch M, Weber H (1992) Titanlegierungen für zementlose Hüftprothesen. In: Hipp E, Gradinger R, Ascherl R (Hrsg) Die zementlose Hüftprothese. Demeter, Gräfelfingen, S 18–26
72. Semlitsch M, Lorenz M, Wintsch W (1973) Bruchuntersuchungen an gegossenen und geschmiedeten Kobaltbasis-Legierungen mit dem Rasterelektronen-Mikroskop und Verhütungsmaßnahmen gegen Ermüdungsbrüche und Hüftgelenkendoprothesen. Beitr Elektronenmikroskop Direktabb Oberfl 6: 263–286
73. Semlitsch M, Willert HG, Dörre E (1975) Neue Werkstoffpaarung Al$_2$O$_3$ – Keramik/Polyaethylen zur Verminderung des Polyaethylenabriebs bei Gelenkpfannen von Hüfttotalendoprothesen. Med Orthop Tech 6: 143–144

74. Semlitsch M, Lehmann M, Weber H, Dörre E, Willert HG (1977) New prospects for a prolonged functional life-span of artificial hip joints by using the material combination polyethylene/aluminium oxide ceramic/metal. J Biomed Mat Res 11: 536–552
75. Semlitsch M, Streicher RM, Weber H (1989) Verschleißverhalten von Pfannen und Kugeln aus CoCrMo-Gußlegierung bei langzeitig implantierten Ganzmetall-Hüftprothesen. Orthopäde 18: 377–381
76. Semlitsch M, Weber H, Streicher RM, Schön R (1992) Joint replacement components made of hot-forged and surface-treated Ti-6AL-7Nb alloy. Biomaterials 13: 781–788
77. Semlitsch M, Streicher RM, Weber H (1994) Long-term results with metal/metal pairing in artificial hip joints. In: Buchhorn GH, Willert HG (eds) Technical principles, design and safety of joint implants. Hogrefe & Huber, Seattle Toronto Bern Göttingen, pp 62–67
78. Spotorno L, Schenk RK, Dietschi C, Romagnoli S, Mumenthaler A (1987) Unsere Erfahrungen mit nicht-zementierten Prothesen. Orthopäde 16: 225–238
79. Steinemann SG, Mäusli PA (1988) Titanium alloys for surgical implants – biocompatibility from physicochemical principles. In: Lacombe P, Tricot R, Beranger G (eds) Sixth World Conference on Titanium. Les éditions de physique, Les Ulis pp 535–540
80. Streicher RM, Schön R, Semlitsch M (1990) Untersuchung des tribologischen Verhaltens von Metall/Metall-Kombinationen für künstliche Hüftgelenke. Biomed Tech 35: 107–111
81. Streicher RM, Weber H, Schön R, Semlitsch M (1991) New surface modification of Ti-6Al-7Nb alloy: oxygen diffusion hardening. Biomaterials 12: 125–129
82. Thompson FR (1954) Two-and-a-half years' experience with a Vitallium intramedullary hip prosthesis. J Bone Joint Surg Am 36: 489
83. Townley CA (1982) Hemi- and total articular replacement arthroplasty of the hip with the fixed femoral cup. Orthop Clin North Am 13: 869
84. Valls J (1952) A new prosthesis for arthroplasty of the hip. J Bone Joint Surg Br 34: 308
85. Vernon-Roberts B, Freeman MAR (1976) Morphological and analytical studies of the tissues adjacent to joint prostheses: investigations into the causes of loosening of prostheses. In: Schaldach M, Hohmann D (eds) Advances in artificial hip and knee joint technology. Springer, Berlin Heidelberg New York, pp 148–186
86. Waugh W, Charnley J (1990) The man and the hip. Springer, Berlin, Heidelberg, New York
87. Webb PJ, Wright KWJ, Winter GD (1980) The Monk „Soft top" endoprosthesis – clinical, biomechanical and histopathological observations. J Bone Joint Surg Br 62: 174–178
88. Weber BG, Fiechter T (1989) Polyäthylen-Verschleiß und Spätlockerung der Totalprothese des Hüftgelenkes. Orthopäde 18: 370–376
89. Weightman B (1977) Friction, lubrication and wear. In: Swanson SAV, Freeman MAR (eds) The scientific basis of joint replacement. Pitman Medical, Turnbridge Wells, United Kingdom, p 46
90. Wiles P (1957) The Surgery of the osteo-arthritic hip. Br J Surg 45: 488–497
91. Willert HG (1973) Tissue reactions around joint implants and bone cement. In: Chapchal G (ed) Arthroplasty of the hip. Thieme, Stuttgart, pp 11–21
92. Willert HG (1991) Ein neues Hüftgelenkendoprothesensystem für die Implantation mit Knochenzement. In: Neugebauer H (Hrsg) Was gibt es neues in der Medizin? Müller, Vienna, pp 141–148
93. Willert HG (1991) Differences and similarities of osteolyses from particulate polyethylene and PMMA-bone cement. In: Willert HG, Buchhorn GH (eds) Ultra-high molecular weight polyethylene as biomaterial in orthopedic surgery. Hogrefe & Huber, Toronto pp 89–103
94. Willert HG, Puls P (1972) Die Reaktion des Knochens auf Knochenzement bei der Alloarthroplastik der Hüfte. Arch Orthop Unfall-Chir 72: 33–71

95. Willert HG, Semlitsch M (1976) Tissue reactions to plastic and metallic wear products of joint endoprostheses. In: Gschwendt N, Debrunner HU (eds). Huber, Bern Stuttgart Vienna, pp 205–239
96. Willert HG, Semlitsch M (1977) Reactions of the articular capsule to wear products of artificial joint prostheses. J Biomed Mater Res 11: 157–164
97. Willert HG, Lintner F (1987) Morphologie des Implantatlagers bei zementierten und nichtzementierten Gelenkimplantaten. Langenbecks Arch Chir 372: 447–455
98. Willert HG, Buchhorn GH (1992) Biologische Fixation und knöcherne Reaktion auf zementlose Implantate – Heilung, Integration, Irritation. In: Hipp E, Gradinger R, Ascherl R (eds) Die zementlose Hüftprothese. Demeter, pp 49–53
99. Willert HG, Buchhorn GH (1993) Particle disease due to wear of ultrahigh molecular weight polyethylene. Findings from retrieval studies. In: Morrey BF (ed) Biological, material and mechanical considerations of joint replacement. Raven, New York, pp 87–102
100. Willert HG, Ludwig J, Semlitsch M (1974) Reaction of bone to methacrylate after hip arthroplasty. J Bone Joint Surg Am 56: 1368–1382
101. Willert HG, Semlitsch M, Buchhorn GH, Kriete U (1978) Materialverschleiß und Gewebereaktion bei künstlichen Gelenken. Orthopäde 7: 62
102. Willert HG, Buchhorn GH, Hess T (1989) Die Bedeutung von Abrieb und Materialermüdung bei der Prothesenlockerung an der Hüfte. Orthopäde 18: 350–369
103. Willert HG, Bertram H, Buchhorn GH (1990) Osteolysis in alloarthroplasty of the hip, the role of ultra high molecular weight polyethylene wear particels. Clin Orthop 258: 95–107
104. Wiltse LL, Hall RH, Stenehjem JC (1957) Experimental studies regarding the possible use of self-curing acrylic in orthopaedic surgery. J Bone Joint Surg Am 39: 961–972
105. Zichner LP, Willert HG (1992) Comparison of alumina/polyethylene and metal/polyethylene in clinical trials. Clin Orthop 282: 86–94
106. Zweymüller K, Deckner A, Lintner F, Semlitsch M (1988) Die Weiterentwicklung des zementfreien Systems durch das SL-Schaftprogramm. Med Orthop Tech 108: 10–15
107. Zweymüller K, Lintner F, Semlitsch M (1988) Biologic fixation of a press-fit titanium hip joint endoprosthesis. Clin Orthop 235: 165–206

The Importance of Remembering Past Mistakes When Considering Implant Materials for Future Hip Endoprostheses

M. SEMLITSCH, H.-G. WILLERT

Introduction

The clinical performance of various hip prostheses types with revision rates under 20 % and implantation times up to 15 years provides valuable information about the direction in which design, fixation principles, and material concepts should continue to be studied and optimized.

This contribution presents especially our personal experience with various design concepts for the replacement of the hip joint [15, 37] using metallic materials, polymer synthetic materials, ceramic, and coatings.

Fixation Principles for Hip Endoprostheses

The first usable hip prostheses types from Moore, Thompson, McKee, Ring, and Sivash in the 1950s were implanted and anchored directly in the bone without cement. Charnley's cementation technique with self-hardening monomer and polymer methylmethacrylate provided immediate primary fixation for the cup and the stem, and was the real breakthrough in hip endoprosthetics. Optimization of the cementation technique by Ling [6], Weber [31], and Draenert [2] resulted in fixation of over half of all hip endoprostheses today using acrylate cement. Experience has shown that cement thicknesses of 3 mm on average and maximum 5 mm have been successful. Very thin cement layers tend to fracture early, and the resulting cement wear causes foreign-body granulomae, which leads to loosening of the implant. Solid, perfectly anchored cement plugs, hardened according to specifications, exhibit good long-term stability.

In the 1970s and 1980s, many operators began again to consider cementless fixation for hip endoprostheses because unsatisfactory results were occasionally found where hip prostheses had not always been cemented optimally. The various hip prostheses types followed the following fixation principles:
– *macrostructures on cup and stem,* such as cup threads and holes, relief, recesses and steps on the stem, or craterlike, or espacially surfaces with beads or spongiosalike structure;

- *microstructures on cup and stem,* such as sintered-on metallic powder beads or titanium wires or coarse blasting of the metal surfaces;
- *coatings on cup and stem,* using plasma spray methods to apply hydroxylapatite or pure titanium powder.

Particularly successful are those cementless hip cups and stems which provide not only a very good primary fixation by their press-fit design but also achieve secondary fixation, and which are not dependent only upon the ingrowth of osseous tissue into porous surface structures. If connective tissue is allowed to form at any time as a result of too much micromotion between the implant and the osseous bed, this will inevitably lead to loosening of the implant. There have been positive results with regards to bony ongrowth with surfaces which have been roughened by blasting or coating. Hydroxylapatite, as a substance similar to bone, has an additional effect; however, 10-year results are not yet available.

Materials Concepts for Hip Joint Replacement

Hip Ballhead Endoprostheses Without Cups

In certain femoral neck fracture cases a hip ballhead endoprosthesis having a ball diameter as close as possible to that of the acetabulum is implanted. None of the polymer synthetic materials used up to date (Plexiglas, polyethylene, polyacetal, polyester) has performed successfully clinically when articulating against bone/cartilage. In all cases there was massive wear on the synthetic ballheads, with pronounced foreign-body reactions as a result [15].

On the other hand, good long-term performance has been obtained with ballheads made from the cobalt-chromium-molybdenum cast alloy Co-28Cr-6Mo (ISO 5832-4) or from the iron-chromium-nickel-molybdenum forging steel Fe-18Cr-14Ni-3Mo (ISO 5832-1) or aluminium oxide ceramic Al_2O_3 (ISO 6474). Metal ballheads can either be integral with the hip prosthesis stem or attached using a taper spigot. So-called duo-heads are mounted on small ballheads on the stem.

Shell Endoprostheses with Cups

The shell endoprostheses of the 1970s consisted of a cemented CoCrMo metal shell or an Al_2O_3 ceramic shell mounted on the spherically or cylindrically prepared femoral head and a cemented thin-walled polyethylene cup in the acetabulum.

The unsatisfactory long-term results are due, on the one hand, to the thin-walled, easily-deformed polyethylene cups and, on the other, to the biomechanically unsuitable load transfer conditions. The question is still open as to whether new materials concepts such as the CoCrMoC metal/metal combination for cup and shell, and a cementless fixation for future shell endoprostheses will provide a solution.

Low-Friction Head/Cup Combination with Low Wear

The ballhead of total hip endoprostheses must articulate in the artificial cup with minimum friction so that as little force as possible is transferred to the prosthesis anchoring. During their functional life in the patient both components should experience minimum change of shape due to creep and wear in order to avoid jamming of the ballhead in the cup.

Ballheads made from polymer synthetic materials (polyethylene, polyacetal, polyester) have not performed well clinically in combination with CoCrMo metal cups. All ballheads of synthetic materials with convex articulating surfaces suffered massive wear, leading to foreign body reactions [38].

Likewise, cemented hip cups of plytetrafluorethylene (Teflon), Teflon reinforced with mica particles (Fluorosint), and polyacetal combined with metal ballheads have not performed well clinically on account of hight wear rates.

It was only with cups introduced by Charnley in 1963 using ultrahigh molecular polyethylene (ISO 5834-2) with a sufficient wall thickness of 6–8 mm combined with ballheads of FeCrNiMo forged steel (ISO 5832-1) that a satisfactory clinical result was achieved [1]. Yearly wear of the polyethylene cup of 0.1–0.3 mm and increasing scratches on the soft steel ballhead, which causes the wear to be increased still further, must be reckoned with.

In the 1980s Charnley introduced the harder and more corrosion resistant iron-chromium-nickel-manganese-molybdenum-niobium-nitrogen forging steel Fe-20Cr-10Ni-4Mn-3Mo-Nb-N (ISO 5832-9) for the 22 mm ballhead [37]. Long-term cup wear is expected to be lower, as the harder ballheads do not get scratched.

Metall ballheads in the titanium-aluminium-vanadium Ti-6Al-4V forging alloy (ISO 5832-3), used in the United States for many years, have not shown good clinical performance combined with polyethylene cups. There are repeated occurrences of badly scratched titanium ballheads where three-body wear occurs due to cement particles, with strong black discoloration of the surrounding tissue. Coating the titanium ballhead with a 3–5 μm thin titanium nitride layer with very high hardness makes the ballhead surface extremely scratch resistant and thus solves this problem. Titanium nitride has been in clinical use since 1986 [26] for ballheads made from the titanium-aluminium-niobium Ti-6Al-7Nb forging alloy (SN 056 512 and ASTM F-1295, ISO 5832-11). Surface hardening of the polished titanium surface to a depth of only 0,1 μm using nitrogen ion implantation does not appear very promising because the depth of the hardening should be at least 5 μm, better still 30 μm as in the oxygen diffusion hardening process [26]. Such ODH-treated Ti-6Al-7Nb ballheads have been under clinical investigation since 1992.

Most metal ballheads (Figs. 1 and 2) implanted today are made from the CoCrMo cast alloy (ISO 5832-4) or the forging alloy (ASTM F-799). With these

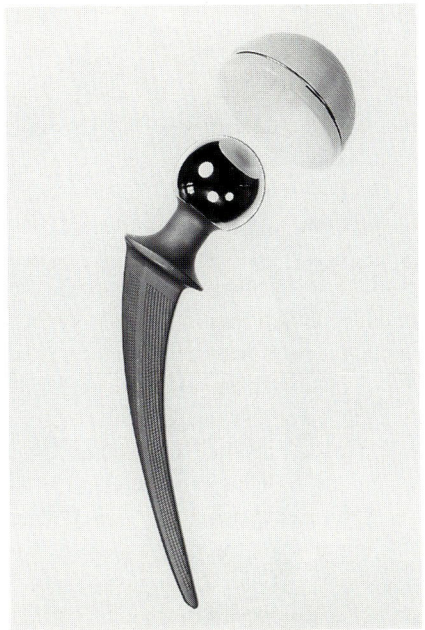

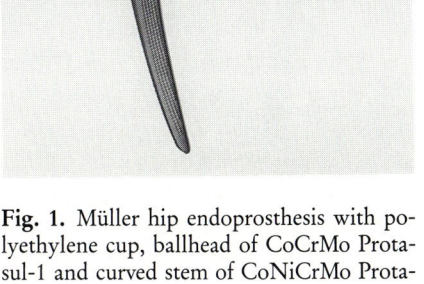

Fig. 1. Müller hip endoprosthesis with polyethylene cup, ballhead of CoCrMo Protasul-1 and curved stem of CoNiCrMo Protasul-10

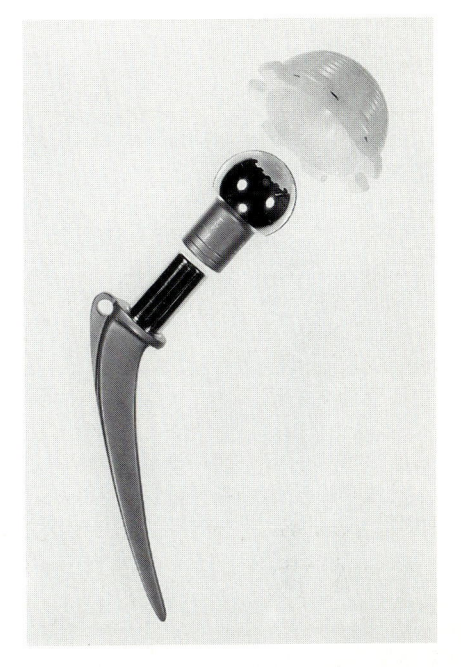

Fig. 2. Weber rotating hip endoprosthesis with polyethylene cup, modular rotating ballhead and cylindrical spigot of CoCrMo Protasul-2 and stem of CoNiCrMo Protasul-10

relatively hard and wear-resistant ballheads, a yearly polyethylene cup wear rate of 0.1–0.3 mm must be rekoned with. To reduce polyethylene cup wear it has been paired since 1975 with Al_2O_3 ceramic ball heads (ISO 6474) with very high hardness and good wettability with body fluid (Figs. 3 and 4). Clinical results show that it is in fact possible to reduce the wear of the polyethylene cup to 0.05–0.15 mm per year [30, 42]. Even lower wear (0–6 μm per year) of cup and ballhead can be achieved with the Al_2O_3 ceramic/ceramic combination of Boutin and Mittelmeier [11]. The ceramic cup must not, however, be implanted at an angle steeper than 45°. Since 1970 there have been repeated clinical cases in which too steep implantation of the ceramic cup has led to massive ceramic wear, not only of the ballhead but also of the cup, due to interference with the ballhead neck and recidivous subluxation.

In the 1960s McKee added a CoCrMo cast cup to the Thompson hip ballhead endoprosthesis to make a total hip endoprosthesis, ensuring adequate clearance between the CoCrMo cast ballhead and cup to permit access of joint liquid to the articulating metal surfaces.

Huggler and Müller selected the same materials concept for cup and ballhead in 1963 and 1965. After 10 to 20-year implantation times these hip prosthesis types exhibit yearly wear rates of maximum 10 μm [18, 25, 32, 36].

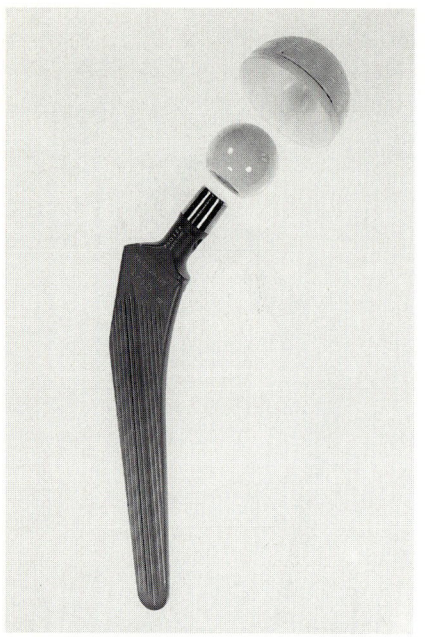

Fig. 3. Müller hip endoprosthesis with polyethylene cup, modular ballhead of Al_2O_3 ceramic Biolox and straigth stem of CoNiCr-Mo Protasul-10

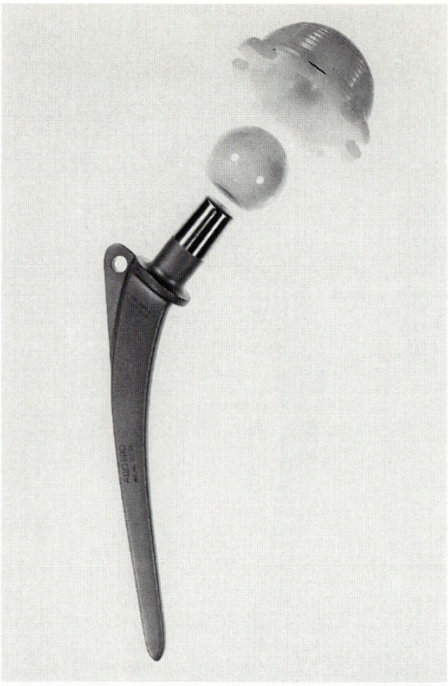

Fig. 4. Weber-Stühmer hip endoprosthesis with polyethylene cup, modular ballhead of Al_2O_3 ceramic Biolox and stem of CoNiCr-Mo Protasul-10

The 28 and 32 mm metal ballheads in the Co-28Cr-6Mo-0,2C forging alloy (Figs. 5–10) introduced in 1988 for Weber [31], Zweymüller, Müller, Wagner, and Stühmer hip endoprostheses gave friction values in the metal/metal combination comparable to the polyethylene/metal combination [28].

Table 1. Clincally verified material combinations for cup and ballhead for total hip endoprostheses

Cup	Ballhead
Ultrahigh molecular weight polyethylene	Fe-18Cr-14Ni-3Mo
	Fe-20Cr-10Ni-4Mn-3Mo-Nb–N
	Co-28Cr-6Mo-0.2C
	Co-28Cr-6Mo-0.08C
	Ti-6Al-7Nb/TiN
	Ti-6Al-7Nb/ODH
	Al_2O_3
Al_2O_3	Al_2O_3
Co-28Cr-6Mo-0.2C	Co-28Cr-6Mo-0.2C

The Importance of Remembering Past Mistakes

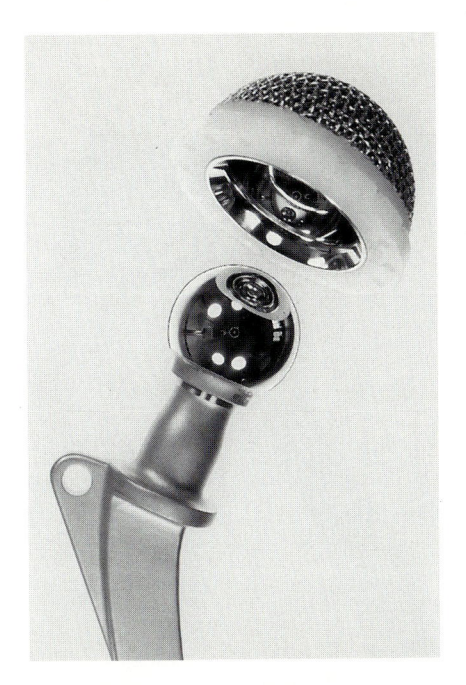

Fig. 5. Weber hip endoprosthesis with Metasul CoCrMo metal/metal articulation

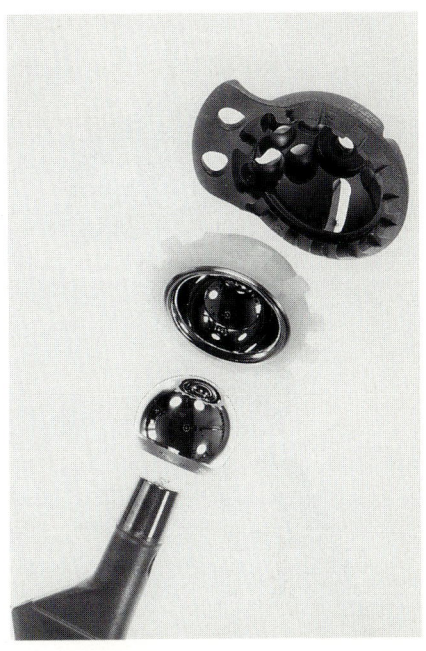

Fig. 6. Müller hip endoprosthesis with Metasul CoCrMo metal/metal articulation

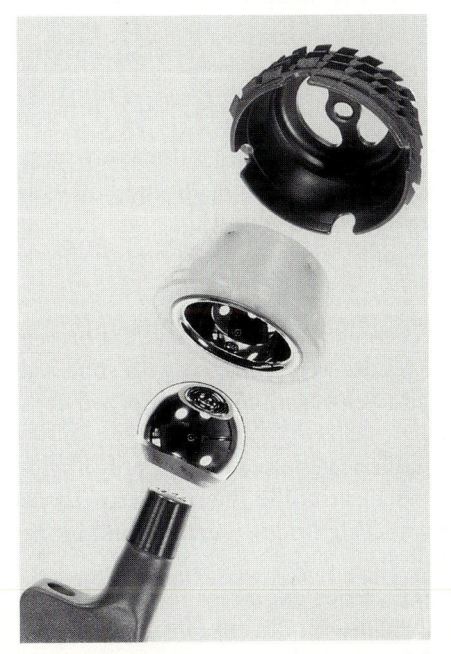

Fig. 7. Zweymüller hip endoprosthesis with Metasul CoCrMo metal/metal articulation

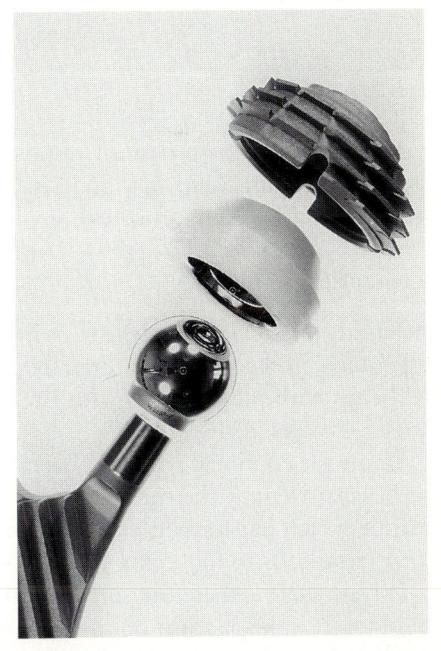

Fig. 8. Stühmer hip endoprosthesis with Metasul CoCrMo metal/metal articulation

Fig. 9. Wagner hip endoprosthesis with Metasul CoCrMo metal/metal articulation

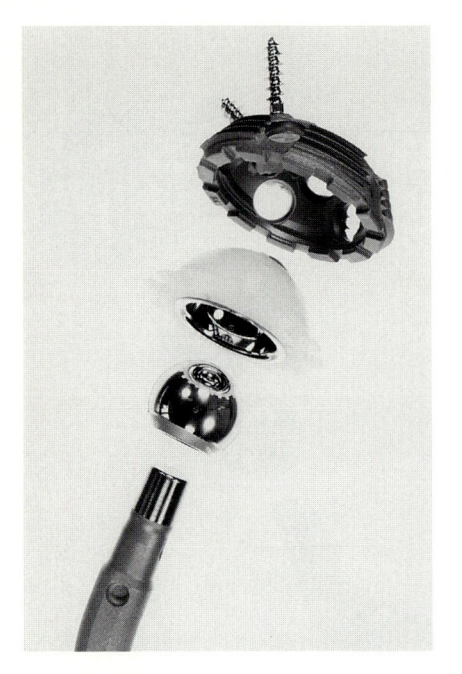

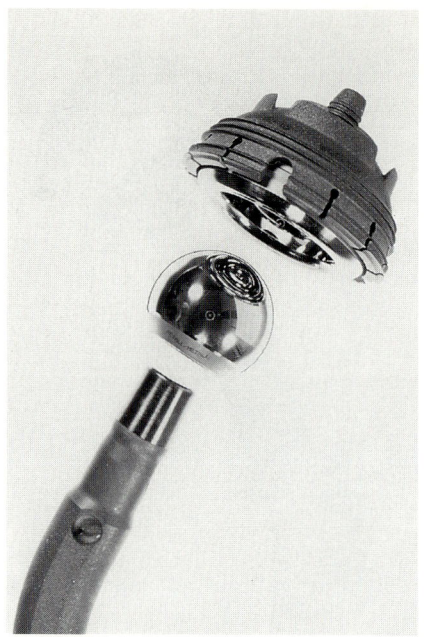

Fig. 10. Wagner hip endoprosthesis with Metasul CoCrMo metal/metal articulation without PE insert

Based on long-term clinical results up to 30 years [21], a sufficiently large assortment of usable to very good material combinations for the cup and ballhead of total hip endoprostheses are availabel today (Table 1).

Cementless Cups

Relatively elastic polyethylene cups in direct contact with bone have not proven themselves in the long term. Equally poor results were obtained with spherical RM cups with plugs [12] as with Endler and Schwägerl conical threaded cups after 6–8 years [4, 10, 40].

Under the continual relative movement in the acetabulum the soft polyethylene is worn away by the cartilaginous and osseous stubs in the connective tissue mantle which has formed [8, 14] and causes foreign-body reactions and in the long term leads to loosening of the polyethylene cup.

Polyethylene is therefore suitable only as an articulation component where it is an insert in a spherical or conical metal shell with direct bone contact.

The spherical or conical shells of quite differing designs can be manufactured in the CoCrMo casting alloy (ISO 5832-4), the TiAlV casting and forging alloy

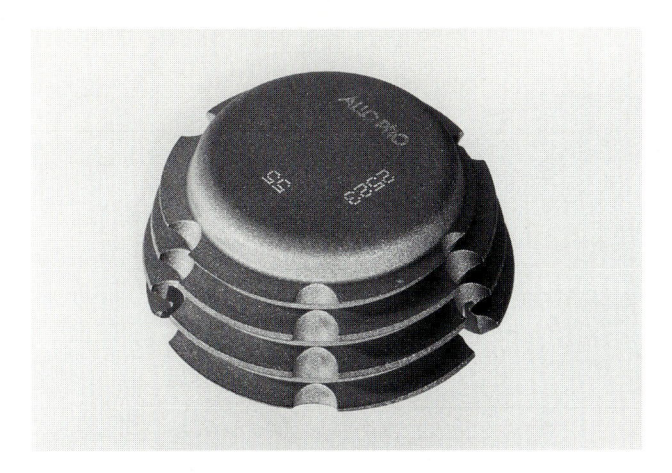

Fig. 11. Willert hip joint cup with conical shell in pure titanium Protasul-Ti and polyethylene insert

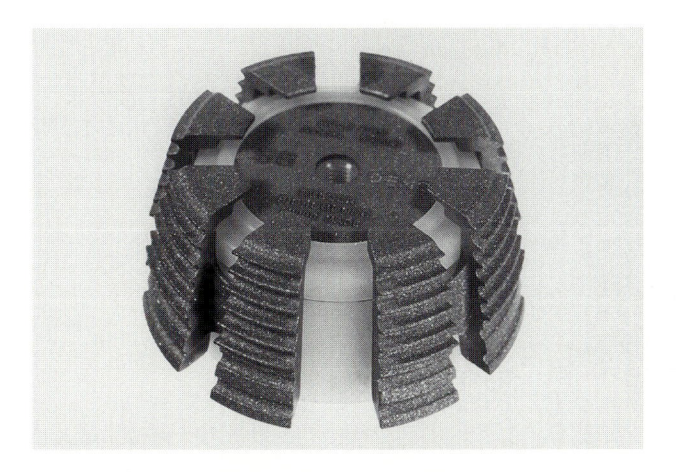

Fig. 12. Balgrist hip joint cup with conical expansion ring and cover-plate of pure titanium Protasul-Ti with polyethylene insert

(ISO 5832-3), forging grade 4 pure titanium (ISO 5832-2), or the TiAlNb forging alloy (SN 056 512, ASTM F-1295, ISO 5832-11).

For better anchoring in the bone, the surface of these metal shells is either coarse-blasted (Figs. 11 and 12) or coated with CoCrMo beads or titanium powder, or with sintered-on titanium wire. Also, titanium powder or hydroxylapatite can be applied to the surface using plasma spray methods.

Polyethylene cups with a sintered multilayer mesh of grade 1 pure titanium (ISO 5832-2) bonded with polyethylene cups as in Morscher and Griss cups

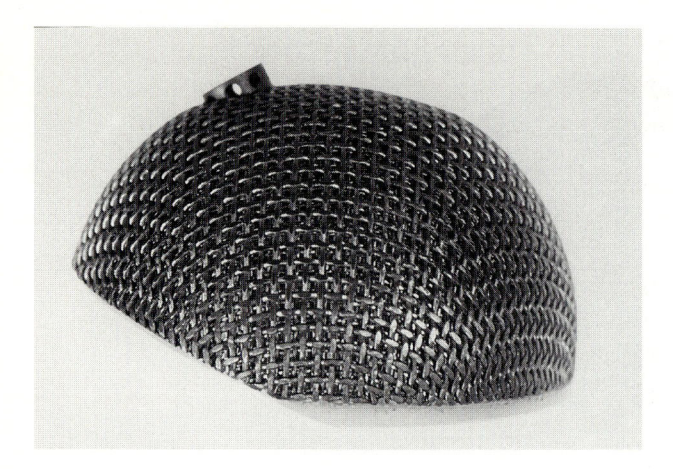

Fig. 13. Morscher hip joint cup of polyethylene with multi-layer Sulmesh shell of pure titanium Protasul-Ti

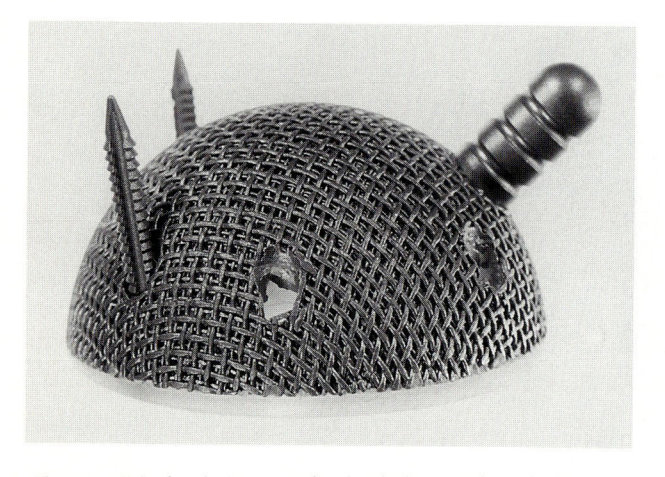

Fig. 14. Griss hip hoint cup of polyethylene with multi-layer Sulmesh shell of pure titanium Protasul-Ti

(Figs. 13 and 14), have controlled porous surface structures to improve the ingrowth of osseous tissue [17].

With optimum implantation orientation in the acetabulum, conical Mittelmeier cups in Al_2O_3 ceramic have good clinical results in contact with bone [11].

For cementless cups a large selection of materials in polyethylene, CoCrMo metals or Al_2O_3 ceramic is thus available for the outer shell and the cup insert.

Fixation Stems for Cemented and Cementless Hip Endoprostheses

The fixation stems of the Moore, Thompson, McKee, Huggler, Weber, and Weber-Huggler hip endoprostheses in the 1950s and 1960s were made from the CoCrMo casting alloy (ISO 5832-4), with high corrosion and wear resistance but limited fatigue strength.

Small cross-sections of loosened stems were severely loaded in bending and torsion, leading to undesirable cases of fatigue fracture.

In 1972, to avoid fracture of loosened stems, Sulzer introduced [16] the high-strength and corrosion-resistant cobalt-nickel-chromium-molybdenum forging alloy Co-35Ni-20Cr-10Mo (ISO 5832-6) for the Müller and Weber hip endoprostheses (Figs. 1–4). Since then stem fracture has been unknown for these prostheses [20].

Fracture-safe prosthesis stems can also be manufactured in the CoCrMo forging alloy (ASTM F-799).

The ballhead and fixation stem of the Charnley hip endoprostheses of the 1960s and 1970s were made from FeCrNiMo forging steel (ISO 5832-1) in the soft-annealed condition. Loosened stems repeatedly suffered permanent distortion and fatigue fractures in the fixation area [41].

Fig. 15. Willert CF-30 hip endoprosthesis with Sulmesh polyethylene cup, modular ballhead and FeCrNiMnMoNbN Protasul-S30 stem with longitudinal bore

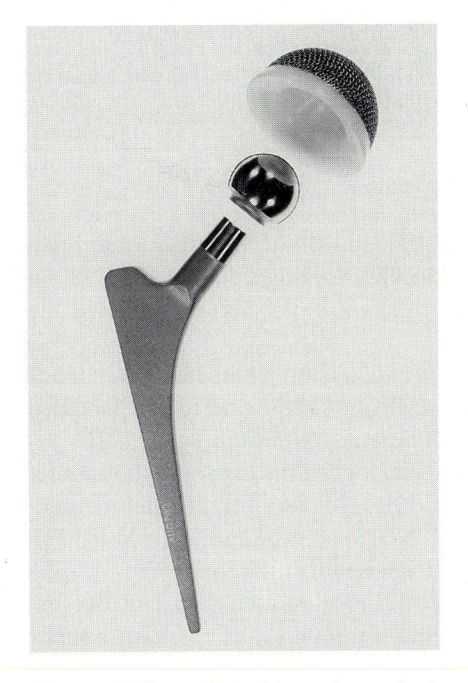

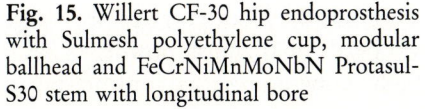

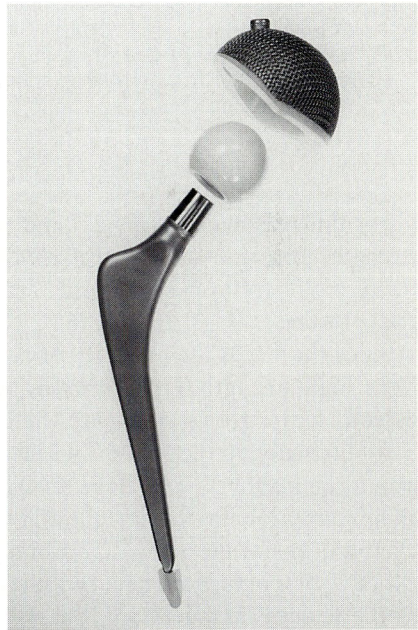

Fig. 16. Morscher-Spotorno MS-30 hip endoprosthesis with Sulmesh polyethylene cup, Biolox modular Al_2O_3 ceramic ballhead and stem of FeCrNiMnMoNbN Protasul-S30

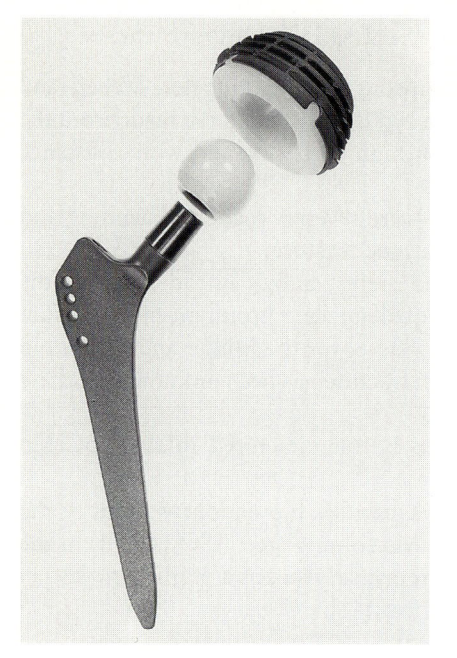

Fig. 17. Zweymüller hip endoprosthesis with pure titanium shell, polyethylene insert, modular ceramic ballhead and SL stem of TiAlNb Protasul-100

Fig. 18. Spotorno hip endoprosthesis with stem and expansion shell of TiAlNb Protasul-100, polyethylene insert, and modular ceramic ballhead

For this reason Thackray[27] and Sulzer [17] in the 1980s introduced high-strength, corrosion-resistant FeCrNiMnMoNbN forging steel (ISO 5832-9) for fracture-safe fixation stems and scratch-resistant ballheads of cemented hip endoprostheses (Figs. 15 and 16).

Since the 1970s the majority of cementless fixation stems have been made from high-strength TiAlV forging alloy (ISO 5832-3) due to the fact that osseous tissue grows well onto the biocompatible titanium [9, 19, 22].

Additionally, in the 1980s, Zwicker [43] introduced the titanium-aluminium-iron forging alloy Ti-5Al-2,5Fe (ISO 5832-10) and Sulzer [24, 26] the titanium-aluminium-niobium forging alloy Ti-6Al-7Nb (SN 056 512 and ASTM F-1295, ISO 5832-11) for the manufacture of highly stressed fixation stems (Figs. 17–20). All three titanium alloys have produced good clinical results up to date. Because of the toxicity of vanadium, the two alloys without vanadium have become preferred in recent years.

For the fixation of cementless stems in bone the stem surfaces are either coarse blasted or are coated with CoCrMo beads or titanium powder or with sintered-on titanium wire. The relatively high temperatures used for sintering of

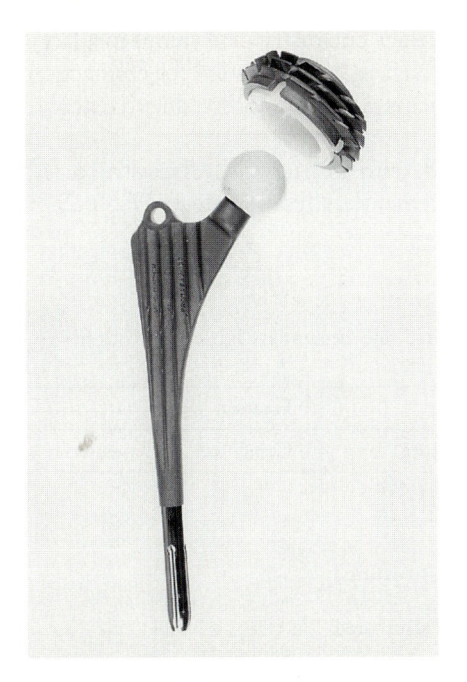

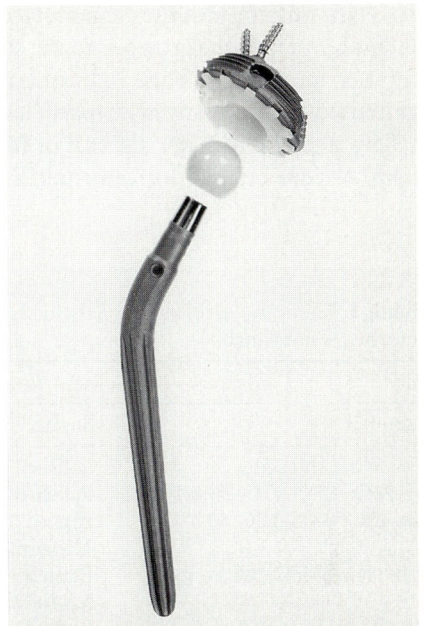

Fig. 19. Stühmer hip endoprosthesis with pure titanium shell, polyethylene insert, modular ceramic ballhead, and stem of TiAlNb Protasul-100

Fig. 20. Wagner hip endoprosthesis with pure titanium shell, polyethylene insert, modular ceramic ballhead, and stem of TiAlNb Protasul-100

the microstructures result in a reduction in the stem fatigue strength, which must be accounted for in the stem dimensioning.

The casting method for the CoCrMo metal in ceramic moulds permits the CoCrMo casting alloy (ISO 5832-4) to be manufactured economically for complicated stem designs with widely varying surface structures. Over the years, however, both Judet hip prostheses with their craterlike surface structure and Lord hip prostheses with their coarse single layer of beads have had repeated cases of fatigue fracture with loosened stems. Revision operations involving fractured, distally well ingrown stems are particularly onerous.

Coarse blasting of forged fixation stems in titanium alloys, as with plasma spray coating with hydroxylapatite, does not result in a reduction in the fatigue strength of the hip prosthesis stem.

The pure titanium coating with a very rough surface and open micropores, applied by Aesculap using vacuum plasma spraying, reduces the fatigue strength of the stem by about 20 %, and this must be accounted for in the dimensioning.

For the assessment of the stem surfaces against bone three factors play a decisive role [19]. The primary stem fixation determines whether osseous tissue can grow onto or into the stem surface. Surface chemistry determines to a large extent how fast bone grows onto the stem surface, and how solid the connection between implant and bone is. Furthermore, implants can loosen due to osteolysis caused by too many wear particles.

Several metallic materials, cast or forged, with a variety of surface structures, can therefore be used for cemented and cementless fixation stems (Table 2).

Table 2. Clinically verified materials for cemented and cementless hip endoprostheses (+, Suitable; -, not suitable)

Stem		Fixation	
Material	Surface structure	Cemented	Cementless
Fe-18Cr-14Ni-3Mo	Polished or blasted	+	-
Fe-20Cr-10Ni-4Mn-3Mo-Nb-N	Polished or blasted	+	-
Co-28Cr-6Mo-0.2C	Blasted	+	
	Micro-macro structured		+
Co-28Cr-6Mo-0.08C	Blasted	+	
	Micro-macro structured		+
Ti-6Al-4V	Blasted	+	+
	Micro-macro structured		+
Ti-6Al-7Nb	Blasted	+	+
	Micro-macro structured		+

Modular Construction of Hip Endoprostheses

A modular construction system for total hip endoprostheses was first achieved by Weber [29] with polymeric ballheads (polyacetal and polyester) with three neck lengths, mounted and capable of rotating on a cylindrical, highly polished neck trunnion. Weber also implanted rotating ballheads with three neck lengths in the very wear resistant CoCrMo cast alloy (ISO 5832-4). The polyacetal and polyester ballheads had to be given up after 6 years of clinical use [34] due to unresolveable wear problems. On the other hand, the metallic rotating ballheads have been successful in more than 20 years of clinical use [30]. In the middle 1970s, based on in-depth laboratory studies [23], the 32 mm Biolox Al_2O_3 ceramic ballhead was introduced for Müller and Weber hip endoprostheses as an alternative to the previous combination of a metal ballhead articulating in a polyethylene cup [35]. The ceramic ballheads with three neck lengths are fixed on the stem using the taper spigot connection with a structured 14/16 or 12/14 taper on the metal stem of iron, cobalt, or titaniumbase alloys. The operator needs to take care to always use ballhead and stem from the same supplier to ensure the fit between the ceramic and metal tapers.

The ceramic taper bore and the metallic stem taper spigot are manufactured to very close tolerances so that stems and ballheads from the same manufacturer can be paired without difficulty. The pairing of components from different sources can lead to wobbling of the ceramic ballhead on the metal spigot. This can lead to fretting corrosion on the metal taper and even to fracture of the ceramic ballhead.

Additionally, before mounting/screwing on and impacting the ceramic ballhead onto the metal taper with a plastic hammer, special care must be taken to ensure the cleanliness of both taper surfaces. There must be no blood, tissue, or bone chips between the two taper surfaces; otherwise the perfect fit of the ceramic ballhead could be compromised. Insufficient taper fit leads to extremely high stress peaks in the ballhead taper, which can ultimately lead to fracture of the ceramic ballhead. Since 1975 only 0.01 % of the over 300 000 implanted Biolox ceramic ballheads have fractured, necessitating replacement with a CoCrMo metallic ballhead [5].

The perfect fit of the tapers is a prerequisite for the absence of fretting corrosion phenomena between metal ballheads of CoCrMo (ISO 5832-4, ASTM F-799) and FeCrNiMnMoNbN (ISO 5832-9), and stem tapers of CoCrMo (ISO 5832-4, ASTM F-799), FeCrNiMnMoNbN (ISO 5832-9), and the titanium alloys TiAlV, TiAlFe, TiAlNb (ISO 5832-3, 5832-10 and ASTM F-1295, ISO 5832-11). Poor taper fit can lead, according to Dujovne and Bobyn [3], to massive corrosion activity due to continual relative movement between the metallic surfaces of the taper.

The Future Development of Implant Materials for Hip Endoprostheses?

Regarding new developments, Neugebauer [13] as editor of the series of books *What's new in medicine?* provides some general answers to the above question:
- Not everything that is "new" is necessarily "good."
- Even if "better is better than good," "even better" is often under discussion before it is even proven to be better than what was originally "good."
- Sooner or later one realizes that the long-forgotten "good" was in fact better than the latest novelty.
- To be able to correctly judge the significance of a method (hip joint replacement) or technology (materials concept) for the human organism, the results over many years (at least 10–20), perhaps even over a whole lifetime, need to be considered.

The history of mistakes over the past 40 years in hip endoprosthetics regarding prosthesis types and materials concepts leads one to hope that one has learned from the mistakes of the past, that the present-day situation is reviewed critically, and that one remains open to future developments, but with extreme caution.

References

1. Charnley J (1979) Low friction arthroplasty of hip. Springer, Berlin Heidelberg New York
2. Draenert K (1986) Beobachtungen zur Zementierung von Implantatkomponenten. Med Orthop Techn 6: 200–205
3. Dujovne AR, Bobyn JD, Krygier JJ, Wilson DR, Brooks CE (1992) Fretting at the head/neck taper of modular hip prostheses. Transactions of 4th World Biomaterials Congress, Berlin (ISBN 90-72101-03-0). Eur Soc Biomater 264
4. Jantsch S, Schwägerl W (1990) Mittelfristige Verlaufskontrollen der zementfreien Schaftverankerung. In: Zweymüller K (Hrsg) 10 Jahre Zweymüller-Hüftendoprothese. Huber, Bern, 117–123, (ISBN 3-456-81903-X)
5. Kempf I, SemlitschM (1990) Massive wear of a steel ball head by ceramic fragments in the polyethylene acetabular cup after revision of a total hip prosthesis with fractured ceramic ball. Orthop Trauma Surg 109: 284–287
6. Ling RSM (1979) Cementing techniques. Revision Arthroplasty, Sheffield, 19–32
7. Lintner F, Böhm G, Bösch P, Endler M, Zweymüller K (1988) Ist hochdichtes Polyethylen als Implantatmaterial zur zementfreien Verankerung von Hüftendoprothesen geeignet? Z Orthop 126: 688–692
8. Lintner F, Böhm G, Zweymüller K, Endler M, Koitz S, Brand G (1988) Die Verträglichkeit von Polyethylen in der direkten Verankerung zum Knochen. Proc. 14. Jahrestagung der Österr. Ges. für Biomed. Technik, 76–79 (ISBN 3-900-60806-7)
9. Lintner F, Böhm G, Brand G (1990) Bone reactions to hip joint replacements made of titanium alloys. Titanium Int. Conf. Österr. Ges. Biomed. Technik 672–688 (ISBN 0-935297)
10. Lintner F, Böhm G, Bösch P, Brand G, Endler M, Zweymüller K (1991) Results of histological and microradiographical examination of cementless implanted polyethylene threaded hip sockets. In: UHMW Polyethylene as Biomaterial in Orthopedic Surgery. Hogrefe & Huber, Göttingen, Publishers, 173–180 (ISBN 3-456-81853-X)
11. Mittelmeier H, Heisel J (1986) 10 Jahre Erfahrungen mit Keramik-Hüftendoprothesen. Med. Lit.Verlagsgesellschaft Uelzen, ISBN 3-88136-117-0)
12. Morscher E, Dick W, Kernen V (1982) Cementless fixation of polyethylene acetabular component in total hip arthroplasty. Arch Orthop Trauma Surg 99: 223–230
13. Neugebauer H (1988) Was gibt es Neues in der Medizin? Müller, Wien, 17
14. Remagen W, Morscher E (1984) Histological results with cement-free implanted hip joint sockets of Polyethylene. Arch Orthop Trauma Surg 103: 145–151
15. Semlitsch M (1974) Technical progress in artificial hip joints. Engin Med 3: 10–19
16. Semlitsch M (1979) Eigenschaften der CoNiCrMo-Schmiedelegierung Protasul-10 für Gelenkendoprothesen mit klinischer Anwendung seit 1971. Swiss Med 1, 9: 15–21
17. Semlitsch M (1992) 25 years Sulzer development of implant materials for total hip prostheses. Medicajournal Spring 92: 4–9
18. Semlitsch M (1993) CoCrMoC metal/metal articulation as a solution to the problem of wear of hip joint replacements. In: IMechE Annual Expert Meeting „Failure of Joint Prostheses", Bournemouth (GB) 40–45
19. Semlitsch M, Lintner F (1991) Metallische Werkstoffe und deren Oberflächen für direkt am Knochen zu verankernde Hüftendoprothesenschäfte. Med Orthop Tech. 111: 60–64
20. Semlitsch M, Panic B (1983) Ten years of experience with test criteria for fracture-proof anchorage stems of artificial hip joints. Engin Med 12: 185–198
21. Semlitsch M, Willert (1988) Metallic materials for artificial hip joints. Encyclopedia of medical devices and instrumentation, Vol. 1 Wiley, New York 137–149
22. Semlitsch M, Weber H (1992) Titanlegierungen für zementlose Hüftendoprothesen. Die zementlose Hüftprothese, Demeter, Gräfelfing 18–26

23. Semlitsch M, Lehmann M, Weber H, Dörre E, Willert HG (1977) New prospects for a prolonged functional life-span of artificial hip joints by using the material combination polyethylene/aluminium oxide ceramic/metal. J Biomed Mater, Res 11: 537–552
24. Semlitsch M, Staub F, Weber H (1985) Titanium-Aluminium-Niobium alloy, development for biocompatible, highstrength surgical implants. Biomed Tech 30: 334–339
25. Semlitsch M, Streicher RM, Weber H (1989) Verschleißverhalten von Pfannen und Kugeln aus CoCrMo-Gußgierung bei langzeitig implantierten Ganzmetall-Hüftprothesen. Orthopäde 18; 377–381
26. Semlitsch M, Weber H, Streicher RM, SCHÖN R (1991) Gelenkprothesen-Komponenten aus warmgeschmiedeter und oberflächenbehandelter Ti-6Al-7Nb Legierung. Biomed Tech 36: 112–119
27. Smethurst E (1981) A new stainless steel alloy for surgical implants compared to 316 12. Biomaterials 2: 1–4
28. Streicher RM, Schön R, Semlitsch M (1990) Untersuchung des tribologischen Verhaltens von Metall/Metall-Kombinationen für künstliche Hüftgelenke. Biomed Tech, 35 5: 107–111
29. Weber BG (1970) Die Rotations-Totalendoprothese des Hüftgelenkes. Z Orthop 107: 304–315
30. Weber BG (1981) Total hip replacement: rotating versus fixed and metal versus ceramic heads. Proc. of 9th Hip Society Meeting. Mosby, St. Louis, 264–275
31. Weber BG (1988) Pressurized cement fixation in total hip arthroplasty. Clin Orthop 232: 87–95
32. Weber BG (1992) Metall-Metall-Totalprothese des Hüftgelenkes: Zurück in die Zukunft Z Orthop Grenzgeb 130: 306–309
33. Weber BG, Fiechter TH (1989) Polyethylen-Verschleiß und Spätlockerungen der Totalprothese des Hüftgelenkes. Neue Perspektiven für die Metall/Metall-Paarung für Pfanne und Kugel. Orthopäde 18: 370–376
34. Weber BG, Stühmer G, Semlitsch M (1974) Erfahrungen mit dem Kunststoff Polyester als Komponente der Rotations-Totalprothese des Hüftgelenks. Z Orthop Grenzgeb 112, 5: 1106–1112
35. Weber BG, Frey O, Semlitsch M, Dörre E (1977) Aluminiumoxid-Keramikkugeln für Hüftendoprothesen nach Baukastenprinzip. Z Orthop 115, 305–309
36. Weber BG, Semlitsch M, Streicher RM (1993) Total hip joint replacement using a CoCrMo metal-metal-sliding pairing. J Jpn Orthop Assoc 67, 391–398
37. Willert HG, Semlitsch M (1981) Biomaterialien und orthopädische Implantate. Thieme, Stuttgart, Orthopädie in Praxis und Klinik, 22.1–22.53
38. Willert HG, Buchhorn GH, Hess TH (1989) Die Bedeutung von Abrieb und Materialermüdung bei der Prothesenlockerung an der Hüfte. Orthopäde 18: 350–369
39. Willert HG, Semlitsch M (1990) Wohin geht die Entwicklung der Hüftendoprothetik? Prakt Orthop 2: 355–374
40. Willert HG, Trautmann M (1990) Verlaufskontrollen bei klinischen Problemfällen. In: Zweymüller K (Hrsg) 10 Jahre Zweymüller-Hüftendoprothese. Huber, Bern, 108–113
41. Wroblewski BM (1990) Revision surgery in total hip arthroplasty. Springer, Berlin Heidelberg New York, 131–138
42. Zichner L, Willert HG (1992) Comparison of Alumina/Polyethylene and Metal/Polyethylene in clinical trials. Clin Orthop Relat. Res 282: 86–94
43. Zwicker U, Bühler K, Müller R (1980) Mechanical properties and tissue reactions of a titanium alloy for implant material. In: Kimura H, Izumi O (eds) Titanium 80, Science and Technology, Proc. 4th Int. Conf. on Titanium, Kyoto 505–514 ISBN 89520-370-7

Tribology of Artificial Joints

R. M. STREICHER

Introduction

More than half a million hip, knee, shoulder, elbow, wrist, finger, and ankle joint prostheses made from engineered materials are implanted world-wide every year to replace diseased natural joints. The breakthrough in artificial joint replacement was achieved with the introduction of approved materials, such as CoCrMo cast alloys with suitable biocompatibility and resistance and with optimized implantation technique using aseptic surgery. Nowadays joint replacement operations are standard, with long-term success rates of more than 10 years [3, 4]. Materials which can be used as biomaterials in endoprosthetics are subjected to complex conditions. For this reason, so-called modular prosthesis systems, which partly resolve the conflicting requirements for components with fixation and tribological requirements, have found wide use in recent years. Using the knowledge from more than 20 years ago, that it is primarily polymer wear particles which significantly affect the long-term results of cemented and cementless prostheses due to osteolysis and subsequent loosening, there is now increased interest in the tribology and material optimization of articulating components of implants [1, 23]. This contribution provides an overview of the tribological validation of new material combinations and designs, together with a brief report on experience.

Tribology

Tribology (DIN 50 323) is a collective term and includes the theories of the processes of friction (DIN 50 281), and of lubrication and wear (DIN 50 320). The beginnings of this science go back to Leonardo da Vinci (1425–1519). A tribological system consists generally of two opposing solid bodies, an intermediate substance, and surrounding medium. The bodies in contact with each other are subjected to normal and tangential forces depending on their geometric dimensions, their mechanical properties, especially those of the surface, and the condition of the marginal surface (surface energy). The actual contact area of the bodies is only a small portion of the nominal surface (1–1000 ppm). It is a function of the dimensional congruence of the components, the modulus of elasticity, and the characteristic mechanical strength parameters. Additionally, the type of loading (e.g., sliding or rolling friction) and the temperature play a role. Wear and friction are thus system dependent and are not specific material properties and therefore require a corresponding analysis as a tribosystem (DIN 50 320).

In principle the wear and lubrication conditions in a technical tribosystem are divided into two conditions. With fluid film lubrication the two solid bodies are completely separated by the intermediate substance, while with dry or boundary lubrication the surfaces of the articulating bodies are in direct contact with each other. The term mixed lubrication covers the area of fluid film lubrication where the intermediate substance can only partially separate the two bodies. While the coefficient of friction μ is a function of the surface energy and of the plastic or elastic deformation, the wear coefficient k depends on fracture initiation and on subcritical or critical fracture propagation. For different material combinations μ is mostly only minimally different, whereas there can be differences of order of magnitude for k. Technically, material removal can occur as abrasive, adhesive, fatigue induced, and tribochemical wear and can be determined by linear (depth and volume of wear), gravimetric (loss of volume or wear particles), or more exotic methods such as ferrography or thin-layer activation.

Human Joints

Considered technically, a human joint consists of two solid bodies (bone), each of which is covered with a porous, elastic layer (cartilage). Between them is a lubricating fluid of viscous structure (synovia), this being a dialysate of blood plasma consisting of water with proteins and salts, and a high-molecular protein (hyaluronic acid) which, depending on cartilage function, more or less completely separates the two solid bodies. This tribosystem is sealed within an impermeable membrane (capsule). The joint is lubricated to achieve minimum friction, and under normal circumstances no wear occurs with several hydrodynamic and elastohydrodynamic mechanisms. These include the squeeze effect, the wedge effect, "weeping," and "boosted lubrication" [21], giving friction coefficients from 0.005 to 0.025 for a healthy joint [13]. In the case of rheumatic disease of the joint, for example, a less favorable tribological situation develops due to the reduced lubricating capability of the synovia. Fluid film lubrication ceases, and extreme wear of the joint surfaces can occur. This leads to increased friction values and pain, and in the long term to the replacement of the affected joint.

Artificial Joints

Joint replacement using artificial materials is used as a last resort to rehabilitate patients with defective joint function. Because of the changed tribological situation due to the use of engineered, non-porous materials under the loading and dynamic conditions existing in the body, a permanent hydrodynamic or elastohydrodynamic lubricating film is not to be expected. Therefore contact of the articulating surfaces is nearly always present in an artificial joint, so that increased friction values and also wear of the materials used is unavoidable. Not only the chemical composition, size, and morphology of the wear particles but also the wear rate is important with respect to possible osteolysis processes [23]. Small amounts of tiny particles can be carried away by the patient's periarticular lymphatic system, and little or no foreign body reaction is to be expected.

After first attempts at implantation with various completely unsatisfactory materials, Plexiglas was used as a ballhead prosthesis in 1946, which – as were the first polymer/metal articulation combinations using polyamide, polyethylene, and Teflon – was also a failure. A selection of material combinations for prosthesis sliding surfaces which have been extensively used clinically to date is shown in Table 1. Since its introduction in 1962 the standard material combination today for artificial joints is ultrahigh molecular weight polyethylene (UHMWPE) with austenitic steel or CoCrMo alloys, with a mean wear rate of about 0. 2 mm/year [17]. Attempts to replace UHMWPE with other polymers (e. g., polyoxymethylene, POM; radiation-hardened polyethylene terephthalate, PET) have all been unsuccessful to date.

Table 1. Material combinations for articulating endoprostheses

Ballhead	Cup					Metal	Ceramic
	Polymer						
	PTFE	UHMWPE	PE-CF	POM	PETP	CoCrMo	Al_2O_3
FeCrNiMo	--	++	--	●	●	-	-
FeCrNiMnMoNbN	●	++	-	●	●	-	-
CoCrMo	●	++	--	--	--	++	-
Ti6Al4V	●	--	--	-	●	-	-
Al_2O_3	●	++	●	●	●	-	++
ZrO_2	●	+	●	●	●	-	-

++, Long-term clinical use; +, clinical investigation; –, technically nonsense; --, clinically failed; ●, not tested yet.

The combination using Al_2O_3 ceramic articulating against itself has shown that it produces, with ideal positioning with the hip prosthesis, very small wear of 8 µm per year [7]. If, however, there is incorrect positioning of the cup (> 50°), the high contact pressure can result in catastrophic wear due to an "avalanche effect" [10]. On the other hand, the clinical results of the combination of UHMWPE cups with Al_2O_3 ceramic ballheads has been good, in that these have about 50 % reduced wear (0.05–0.13 mm per year) compared with metal ballheads [25]. For knee prostheses the combination of UHMWPE tibia parts with CoCrMo alloy femoral condyles is still used, as the brittleness of the ceramic has prevented its application here as an alternative material.

Ball-head and cup combinations of CoCrMo alloys against each other which were introduced before 1960 by one manufacturer [5] showed an increased rate of loosening [14] due to manufacturing imprecision and higher friction moment compared with the "low-friction" material combination of polymer and metal introduced by Charnley. Investigation of metal/metal hip prostheses with up to 20 years implantation time showed wear rates of only a few micrometers per year [14].

Tribological Investigations

Before starting with clinical investigation, the tribological behavior of new materials and designs must be investigated in the laboratory. Apart from the complex tribosystem in patients, there are problems in that there are, as opposed to machines, no generally valid rules regarding joints, because there is always a very wide variation in the input values for individual patient data, so that exact repeatability is scarcely possible. In general, the following applies for the selection of tribological investigation methods: Reduction and simplification of the investigation parameters reduces the specific result, but increases the validity of the general result. To obtain an optimal overview of the tribological behaviour of material combinations it is important not to concentrate on one test but to proceed in a stepwise manner before clinical use, as is shown in Table 2. The preparation of a testing plan for tribological investigations is therefore crucial. A comparison of the various possibilities for testing the tribological characteristics

Table 2. Tribological test phases

Method	Advantages/Disadvantages
Screening test (pin/disc)	Non comparable conditions to in vivo
	Fast (7 days), cheap
	Simple, cheap machines
	Only general information
Model test with implants (pendulum)	Simple comparable conditions to in vivo
	Fast (minutes)
	General information
	Only friction values
Simulator test	Physiological conditions closely accomplished
	Long-term tests (months)
	Expensive, complicated machines
	Complex
	Specific information
Clinical investigation	Physiological conditions
	Complicated and expensive investigation
	Long-term (years)
	Stresses individual
	Scatter of data

Table 3. Comparison of in vivo and in vitro conditions

	in vivo	Simulator	Screening
Ball diameter (mm)	55	22–37	3–6
Force (N)	300–3500	300–2250	25/100
Stress (MPa)	0–5	0–10	3.5
Velocity (m/s)	0–0.055	0–0.013	0.025
Movement (°)	oscillating cyclic	oscillating cyclic	rotating continous
Flexion/extension	20/25	21/21	-
Abduction/adduction	5/8	5/11	-
Internal/external rotation	8/6	8/8	-

of material combinations is shown in Table 3. To ensure that the conditions for tribological investigations are maintained as realistically as possible, and to allow comparison between different laboratories, several guidelines and standards have been prepared or are in the approval process: ISO TR 9325 and 9326, ASTM F 732, etc.

In our laboratory, based on over 15 years of experience with tribological testing, an air-conditioned cleanroom with airlock and class 100 laminar airflow boxes directly over the individual testing units was installed. The possible influence of contamination from the ambient air was thereby significantly reduced. To further avoid artifacts during tribological testing the intermediate medium for all tests is sterilely filtered using a 0.2 μm membrane filter, and the area around each testing chamber is covered or sealed with a polyurethan (PUR) membrane. The intermediate substance for all standard tests is a stabilized mixture of Ringer's solution with 30% calf serum, buffered to pH 7.2 [24]. In this way a medium is achieved which is similar to the biological system, and which additionally prevents material transfer between the sliding surfaces [2, 6]. Compared with natural synovia, however, a polymeric component to increase viscosity is not present, as hyaluronic acid is too expensive, and water-soluble synthetic polymers such as polyvinyl pyrrolidone or polyacrylamide have shown no advantages.

Laboratory Investigations Using Screening Machines

The advantage of this investigation method is its simplicity and the correspondingly low costs. The simple testing unit design allows the production of machines with several testing stations with little effort, which provide many results in a short time. This also provides the basis for calculating the statistical relevance of the results. Screening test set-ups can vary in their designs from interfacing flat surfaces to ball-on-disc, and in their dynamics from continuous rotation to oscillation. The variance in the published results is therefore correspondingly large. The large simplification of the in vivo conditions naturally affects the relevance of such tests, and the results must be applied to clinical use only with caution and correct interpretation. The relevance of the results can be increased using multiparameter tests which specifically address the so-called Pv combination (pressure/speed). In interpreting the results it is important to consider the combination of roughness, wear, and friction behaviour together with observations of changes of the surfaces of the articulating material combinations in the results. Commonly presented results which ignore scratched surfaces not observed clinically, and which describe only polyethylene wear are irrelevant. For the calibration of testing units or test parameters known positive clinical material combinations (CoCrMo and Al_2O_3 against UHMWPE) and negative references (steel against PTFE, CoCrMo against POM) should be used, as for toxicity tests.

In our laboratory, material combinations are tested in pin-on-disc machines with discs of the harder material and pins of UHMWPE. The testing conditions are matched in very simplified form to those occurring naturally, and are shown in Table 3. The volumetric wear $\Delta V = k3*F*s$ ($k3$ in mm^3/Nm) is calculated from the continuously measured linear wear $\Delta l = k4*P*s$ ($k4$ is the wear coefficient in mm/Nm), and vice versa. These two values can also be determined using gravimetric measurements. The friction coefficient is also determined on a continuous basis in our testing machines and provides a complete picture of the varying tribological conditions during the tests.

Figures 1 and 2 show the results of a study of parameters based on CoCrMo alloy and variation of testing speed. The wear of UHMWPE in the serum mixture shows a strong dependence on sliding speed. It decreases with increasing speed, whereas the friction coefficient follows the well-known pattern according to Stribeck with a minimum of 0.01 m/s. With this material combination increased testing speed produces hydrodynamic effects reducing the wear values by one order of magnitude, and friction by 50 %. The selection of the

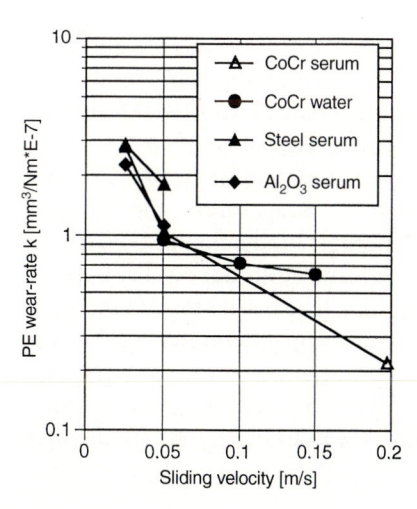

Fig. 1. Relationship between polyethylene wear rate and sliding speed in the screening test

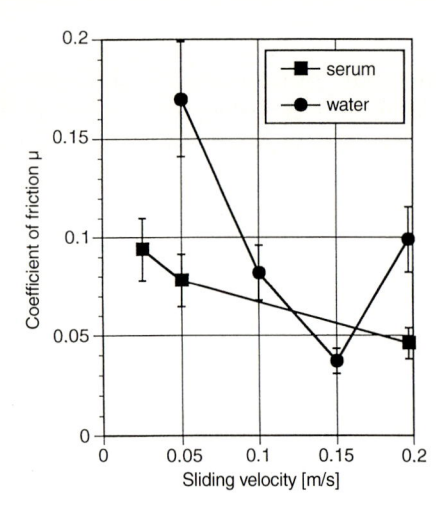

Fig. 2. Relationship between friction and sliding speed for CoCrMo cast alloy combination with UHMWPE in the screening test

liquid intermediate medium shows no significant influence on the wear rate of UHMWPE, although a transfer film of PE onto the other body can be observed when using aqua dest. Friction losses due to the use of serum mixture as an intermediate substance are substantially independent of the sliding speed. On the other hand, the influence of the surface pressure on the main tribological parameters is negligible in the investigated range of 1–3 MPa.

Table 4 summarizes the results (mean values from at least six tests each) of tests using discs of various materials and pins of UHMWPE. The standard deviation of individual results is in the range of 10 %–50 % of the mean values. A linear correlation between roughness and polyethylene wear was found for CoCrMo alloy (correlation = 83 %). This is typical for a combination of two nonpolar materials under mixed lubrication conditions. This correlation between roughness and UHMWPE wear rate for steel alloys has also been mentioned several times in the literature [2].

With a thermomechanical process the carbide size of the CoCrMo alloy was reduced from approximately 20 μm diameter for the cast Protasul-2 to 2–3 μm for Protasul-21WF. The result of the reduced roughness of the CoCrMo alloy is a 20 % lower polyethylene wear and a 15 % lower friction coefficient.

Investigation of the clinically successfully combination of Al_2O_3 [25] with UHMWPE confirmed the known reduction in wear values and friction, although not to the same extent as in vivo. Although a reduction in UHMWPE wear rate of 30 %–75 % in vivo compared with metal ballheads has been reported [22], only 20 % was measured in the laboratory. The reason for this difference is that it is not possible to obtain the same surface quality on flat, hard, oxide ceramic discs as on the ballheads. The alternative ceramics ZrO_2 and Si_3N_4 give higher wear and friction values in all cases. This may well be caused by their lower surface energy values compared with Al_2O_3 and the associated lower adsorption of the intermediate substance.

Table 4. Average values of pin-on-disc tests

Disc	Rz (µm)	Contact angle (°)	HV -	k Value (mm³/Nm×10⁻⁷)	µ
CoCrMo-Guss (Protasul-2)	0.295	93	310	2.693	0.092
CoCrMo-SL (Protasul-21WF)	0.114	78	330	2.265	0.080
FeCrNiMo-SL (316L)	0.153	40	215	3.85	0.086
FeCrNiMnMoNbN-SL[c] (Protasul-S30)	0.092	60	330	2.864	0.078
TiAlNb-SL (Protasul-100)	0.384	43	315	11.67	0.109
TiAlNb-SL+ N+ implanted	0.160	70	700	3.317	0.100
TiAlNb-SL+ PVD-TiN	0.159	66	1800	2.111	0.078
TiAlNb-SL + ODH	0.330	48	1200	1.353	0.051
Al₂O₃ (BIOLOX)	0.064	39	2300	2.131	0.079
ZrO₂	0.155	48	1500	3.216	0.114
Si₃N₄	0.164	-	2500	2.917	0.107

[a] Roughness; [b] Vickers Hardness; [c] Wrought alloey

In none of the single tests using materials based on iron and cobalt were scratches found on the disc surface after the test. On the other hand, when using pure titanium and titanium alloys, there was massive titanium and polyethylene wear, with associated black discolouration of the test medium. To compensate for this disadvantage of titanium and titanium alloys, which are otherwise well accepted clinically for heavily loaded implants, various possibilities for surface modification are available: anodizing, CVD, and PVD coatings as well as N+ ion implantation [15]. Our results from two- to fourfold N+ ion implantation show increasing UHMWPE wear with increasing nitrogen ion concentration and penetration depth. This surface treatment of articulating titanium alloys for implants is therefore inappropriate. On the other hand, a PVD coating with an optimized TiN layer on mirror-finished disc surfaces provides an improvement in the tribological behaviour of UHMWPE compared with cast CoCrMo.

Surface hardening of titanium alloys with oxygen [17] shows particularly positive results, with clearly reduced polyethylene wear similar to clinically verified Al₂O₃ ceramic, and this can represent a fracture-safe alternative with reduced friction and wear. As also found in the testing of other materials, a significant linear relationship is noted between the surface energy of the discs, which is necessary for the adhesion of a corresponding fluid film, and polyethylene wear and friction.

Laboratory Investigations Using Implants

Such testing equipment, generally with only one degree of freedom, produce simplified movements and/or load patterns compared with in vivo. An example of such a test is the simple Charnley pendulum experiment. Pendulum equipment permits rapid evaluation of friction behaviour of various materials and especially of design parameters such as diameter, roundness, and clearance. The principal lubrication mechanism can thus be determined by the variation in the amplitude of the swing.

The friction properties of various material combinations were investigated using an adapted Buchs type pendulum apparatus [11], in which one side of the pendulum is arranged as a ball bearing while the other side is the test prosthesis. Especially CoCrMo alloys articulating against the same material with different ball diameters, and with 32-mm ball diameter against UHMWPE, were tested because excessive friction moment had been blamed for the loosening of earlier metal/metal hip systems [14]. Additionally, the combination of a 32-mm diameter Al_2O_3 ballhead articulating against UHMWPE was tested. The criteria was the number of cycles until standstill.

The results showed linear behaviour of the swing amplitude for all metal/metal combinations using serum mixture as intermediate substance, in other words, only slight dependence of friction upon sliding speed. The 37 mm CoCrMo alloy metal/metal combination had a friction moment 70 %–100 % higher than the 32 mm diameter ball combined with polyethylene, as shown in Fig. 3. The combination of a 32 mm Al_2O_3 ceramic ball with polyethylene showed a further 10 % lower friction loss. The reduction in ball diameter of the metal/

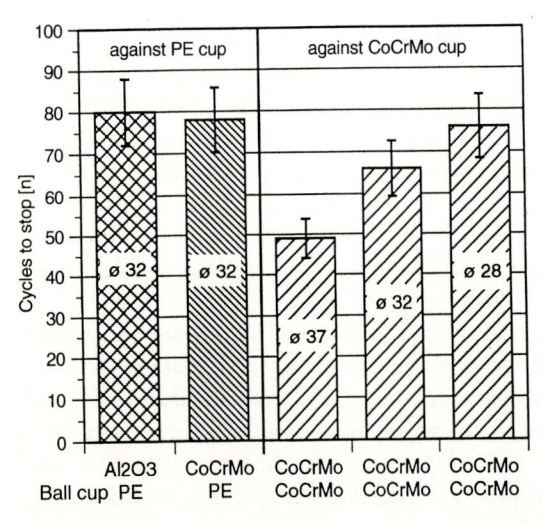

Fig. 3. Results of pendulum tests using various material combinations and diameters

metal combination to 32- and 28-mm, as well as the use of the CoCrMo forging alloy Protasul-21WF instead of the cast alloy Protasul-2, reduced the friction losses in the lubricated condition to the values of the polymer/metal combination. A comparison with prostheses retrieved after clinical use or hip simulator tests done before the pendulum tests showed closed correlation in friction behaviour, although these prostheses achieved a reduced number of cycles because of scratches.

Simulators

For the testing of implants, hip and knee simulators are used which employ similar loading combinations to in vivo by the use of complicated mechanical, pneumatic, or hydraulic systems. Generally in such cases two or more degrees of freedom and kinematics as in vivo are applicable in hip and knee simulators (ISO TR 9325). Many so-called simulators are in fact nothing more than powered model-testing equipment. The anatomical positioning of the implant is important to correctly assess the influence of wear particles on the tribosystem. When the tests are carried out with the prosthesis inverted contamination or wear particles which have a higher density than the intermediate substance can lead to completely erroneous tribological results.

The Stanmore Mk III [24] mechanical hip simulators used in our laboratory are based on values established indirectly by Paul in 1967 [8] and by Rydell in 1966 [12] using telemetry, which were measured under physiological conditions on healthy individuals. The natural loading pattern with double peak is achieved using the appropriate kinematics of these machines via an unloading cam. The operating frequency is set at 0.5 Hz. Because of this, 2–6 months is necessary to evaluate several million load cycles. Because of the long testing period principally CoCrMo combinations with different diameters have been investigated, as the investigation of reoperated prosthesis with this material combination has indicated that an improvement in wear behaviour of orders of magnitude can be expected compared with polymer/metal of ceramic combinations.

In the hip simulator metal/metal combinations show the clear influence of the geometry of the interfacing surfaces. Due to the different moduli of elasticity and a yield point ratio of 1:50 completely different contact surface conditions exist for the metal/metal and metal/UHMWPE combinations. The local contact conditions of the articulating components in the metal/metal combination therefore play a critical role. All combinations tested in the hip simulator have running-in wear in the region of 10–20 μm on each component (Fig. 4). After this surface adjustment period wear on each component in the region of 2–4 μm/million cycles was measured. Where unsatisfactory geometrical conditions were present, the transition from running-in wear to low values did not take place even after several million cycles, and there was heavy wear on both components. The wear measured in the simulator was practically identical for implants with different diameters with optimum manufacturing and was in the

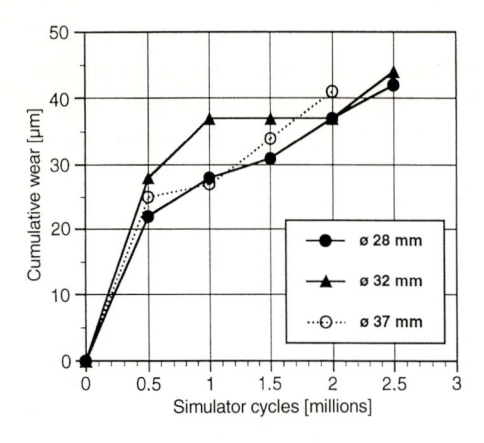

Fig. 4. Comparison of the results of hip simulator tests using metal/metal combinations of different diameters

upper area of that measured on explants retrieved after long-term use [17]. In comparison with retrieved implants, those from the simulators showed a somewhat preferential wear direction (orientation) with increased scratching.

The friction moment measured in the hip simulator for combinations with ball diameter of 37 mm were 5–7 Nm; two to three times higher than for the polymer/metal combinations with 32 mm diameter. With decreasing head diameter and the same nominal clearance the contact surface of the protruding M_3C_7 block carbides is reduced and therefore also the friction resistance. The small, finely distributed carbides of the CoCrMo forging alloy Protasul-21 WF, together with the somewhat increased hardness due to the reduced roughness, and the increased deformation resistance in comparison with the cast alloy are all beneficial. Metal-on-metal combinations using ballheads of the wrought alloy and with a reduced diameter of 32 and 28 mm and optimized clearance yielded friction moment values similar to that of the metal-on-polymer combination measured in the pendulum test. In these cases both the friction moment and the wear were elevated in the running-in period. Where the clearance between the ball and the cup was correctly selected and manufactured, there followed, after 0.5–1 million cycles, a steady wear period with stable, low-value friction and wear conditions.

The knee simulator used in our laboratory is the mechanical model of Stallforth and Ungethüm (1978). The mechanics permit flexion (rolling movement) of 60° maximum with simultaneous implant-specific sliding movement. A body moment of 13 Nm was set for a rotational neutral position. The testing period was 2–3 million cycles for nonstabilized knee prostheses with self-centering UHMWPE tibia parts articulating against CoCrMo cast alloy femoral parts in a blood/serum mixture at 37°C. Tests with nonstabilized knee prostheses showed a good correlation for UHMWPE wear with the results of the screening tests. For example, following running-in of the polyethylene tibia, a steady phase with a constant UHMWPE wear rate of 60 μm per million cycles was measured for femoral parts of cast CoCrMo alloy and with TiN coating. The coated

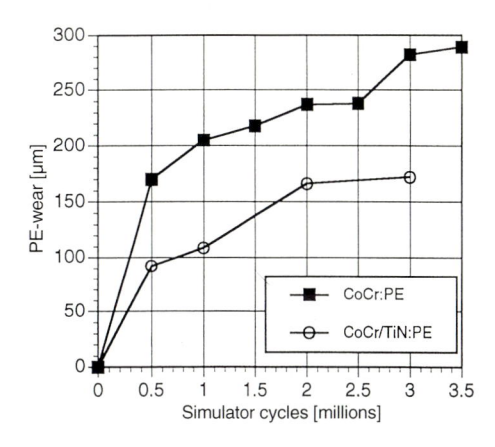

Fig. 5. Comparison of polyethylene wear rates in the knee simulator

articulation surface produced less wear, as shown in Fig. 5. The in vivo wear rate of congruent prostheses is lower and is approx. 25 μm per year [9]. Similarly to many explanted knee prostheses of similar design, the femoral part of CoCrMo cast alloy indicates scratches in the sliding direction of the prosthesis after the test. In some cases these scratches could be traced to exposed catalyst residues in the UHMWPE.

Clinical Investigation

This tribological investigation is the only one with very high relevance, although the results can vary significantly by clinic and assessment method. Measurements from radiographs can, in principle, provide different results, depending on the positioning and assessment methods used. The accuracy using this technique is approx. 0.2 mm, as is its reproducibility. Because of this, realistic assessment is only meaningful with high wear rates. Wear values taken from explants usually give worse values than measurements from radiographs due to the negative selection process. Comparison of the results of various authors is not completely possible here either due to the use of different measurement and assessment procedures.

The measurement of linear wear rates on the 134 hip joint cups in Chirulen available to us, used in combination with 32-mm-diameter CoCrMo alloy ballheads for 10 years in vivo showed a mean of 0.23 mm/year, corresponding to 180 mm^3 polyethylene. Explants from male patients had a 25 % increased wear rate. With increasing implantation time the linear penetration of the ballhead is reduced by the reduction of creep and by the lower surface pressure from the larger contact surface, i.e., the unidirectional wear behaviour of UHMWPE is not linear [18]. The inner surface of used artificial hip joint cups in UHMWPE can be divided into three zones in nearly all cases: a polished bearing zone, a zone of nonbearing, and a transitional zone corresponding to the border between the original cup inside diameter and the newly formed ball support surface formed by wear and creep. In those explanted cups with bone cement particles or traces of same in the tribologically active inner surface of the UHMWPE the wear rate was increased by more than 50 % due to the three-body movement. After about 10 years implantation time, however, the difference from those without cement ingress is no longer significant. The elimination of bone cement particles from the articulating surface by correct cementation procedure, where possible using cement compacting, can reduce this problem significantly and is therefore of primary importance. The use of cementless implant fixation can also eliminate the increase of polyethylene wear due to bone cement. Patient weight, age at operation, and the angle of main loading indicated no significant correlation with the PE wear rate on the investigated implants; only the implantation time. For cups without indication of three-body wear due to cement particles, no negative influence on wear could be detected between chemically disinfected and irradiation sterilized specimens with up to 15 years of use in vivo.

Examinations on 37 explanted all-metal prostheses of Huggler, Müller, McKee-Farrar, and Ring designs with diameters of 35–42 mm and implantation times of up to 25 years showed low wear rates of 2–8 μm per component (ballhead and cup), depending on the prosthesis type. The lowest values of 2 μm/year were measured on 12 Müller prostheses with 37- and 42-mm diameter in the CoCrMo alloy Protasul-2. The optical appearance of the articulating surfaces of the prostheses improves with time. Scratches from the running-in of the ballhead and the cup and from three-body wear from bone cement particles are repolished. The McKee cups in particular indicated partial deformation in the loading direction due to their thin wall thickness without stiffening structures. Additionally, many cups had a recess at the pole from manufacturing which caused increased wear in this design, particularly on the ballhead. In some cases high wear could be traced back to other manufacturing and fit problems in production at that time.

Summary

Beore a new material or design for articulating endoprostheses can be released for clinical investigation, the tribological behaviour of the articulating components must be examined in the laboratory. The complexity of friction, wear, and lubrication as a tribosystem is problematic, so that the tribological behaviour of the interfacing surfaces depends only partly upon material properties, depending on the loading pattern. In addition, there is the individual and unstable patient system which is to provide input values for the tests. For this reason a sound selection of tribological test methods to be used and specialized interpretation of the results, taking account of all observations and measurements, are absolutely essential for a good prognosis of tribological behaviour under clinical conditions. To achieve an optimum overview of the tribological behaviour of material combinations or designs it is important to not only select one test method but also to proceed stepwise with increasing degrees of complexity before proceeding to clinical use. Comparisons with negative and positive reference values and examination of the wear mechanism should always be used to assess the clinical relevance of the results obtained.

Our screening tests indicate that UHMWPE is, as a long molecular chained material, a good partner for various metal and ceramic materials, on account of its high molecular weight with its entanglements, giving good wettability. Its combination with CoCrMo alloys of lower surface roughness and especially with high-grade Al_2O_3 ceramic and ODH-treated titanium alloy provides advantageous tribological behaviour for their use as biomaterials for various articulating endoprostheses. The excellent results of the metal/metal combination with relatively low friction and wear in laboratory tests and in clinical use mean beneficial, reduced loading of the patient's body tissues with detrimental wear particles and should therefore reduce the risk of aseptic late loosening of implants.

References

1. Bobyn JD, Collier JP, Mayor MB, McTighe T, Tanzer M, Vaughn BK (1993) Particulate debris in THA: problems and solutions. Scientific exhibition at the 61st AAOS, pp 1–6
2. Cooper JR, Dowson D, Fisher I (1993) The effect of transfer film and surface roughness on the wear of lubricated UHMWPE. Clin Mater 14: 295–302
3. Joshi AB, Poter ML, Trail IA, Hunt LP, Murphy JCM, Hardinge K (1993) Long-term results of Charnley low-friction arthroplasty in young patients. JBJS 75-B: 616–623
4. Malchau H, Herberts P, Ahnfelt L, Johnell O (1993) Prognosis of THP. Scientific exhibition at the 61st AAOS, San Francisco, pp 1–9
5. McKee GK (1982) Total hip replacement-past, present and future. Biomaterials 3: 130–135
6. McKellop HA, Clarke IC (1984) Evolution and evaluation of materials screening machines and joint simulators in predicting in vivo wear phenomena. In: Ducheyne P, Hasting GW (eds) Functional behavior of orthopedic biomaterials, vol II: Applications. CRC, Boca Raton, pp 51–85
7. Mittelmeier H, Heisel J (1990) Fifteen years of experience with ceramic hip prosthese. In: Aldinger G, Sell S, Beyer A (eds) Noncemented total hip replacement. Thieme, Stuttgart, pp 142–150
8. Paul JP (1967) Forces transmitted by joints in the human body. Proc Inst Mech Eng 181: 8–15
9. Plante-Bordeneuve, P, Freeman MAR (1993) Tibial HDPE wear in conforming tibiofemoral prostheses. J Bone Joint Surg [Br] 75/4: 630–636
10. Plitz W, Hoss HU (1980) Untersuchungen zum Verschleißmechanismus bei revidierten Hüftendoprothesen mit Gleitflächen aus Al_2O_3-Keramik. Biomed Tech 25: 165–168
11. Ruesch R, Thöny C (1981) Reibungsversuche an künstlichen Hüftgelenken. Diplomarbeit, Technikum Buchs
12. Rydell NW (1966) Forces acting on the femoral head prostheses. Acta Orthop Scand Suppl 88

13. Schurz J (1983) Biorheologie. Probleme und Ergebnisse in der Medizin. Naturwissenschaften 70: 602–608
14. Semlitsch MF, Streicher RM, Weber H (1989) Verschleißverhalten von Pfannen und Kugeln aus CoCrMo-Gußlegierung bei langzeitig implantierten Ganzmetall-Hüftprothesen. Orthopädie 18: 36–41
15. Sioshansi, P, Oliver RW, Matthews FD (1985) Wear improvement of surgical alloys by ion implantation. J Vac Sci Tech A3: 2670–2674
16. Stallforth H, Ungethüm M (1978) Die tribologische Testung von Knieendoprothesen. Biomed Tech 23/12: 295–304
17. Streicher RM (1991) Examinations of explanted hip joint cups made of UHMWPE. In: Willert HG, Buchhorn G, Eyerer P (eds) UHMWPE as biomaterial in orthopedic surgery. Hogrefe & Huber, Bern, pp 196–201
18. Streicher RM (1993) UHMW-Polyethylen als Werkstoff für artikulierende Komponenten von Gelenkendoprothesen. Biomed Tech 38/12: 303–313
19. Streicher RM, Schön R, Semlitsch M (1990) Untersuchung des tribologischen Verhaltens von Metall/Metall-Kombinationen für künstliche Hüftgelenke. Biomed Tech 35/5: 107–111
20. Streicher RM, Weber H, Schön R, Semlitsch M (1991) New surface modifiaction for Ti-6Al-7Nb alloy: oxygen diffusion hardening (ODH). Biomaterials 12: 125–129
21. Ungethüm M (1980) Tribologie der Gelenke und Endoprothesen. Osteosyn Endoproth 2: 91-100
22. Weber BG (1981) Total hip replacement: rotating versus fixed and metal against ceramic heads. In: Salvati E (ed) The Hip. Mosby, USA, pp 264–275
23. Willert HG, Semlitsch MF (1977) Reactions of the articular capsule to wear products of artificial joint prostheses. J Biomed Mater Res 11: 157–164
24. Wright KWJ (1982) Friction and wear of materials and joint replacement prostheses. In: Williams DF (ed) Biocompatibility of orhtopedic implants vol I. CRC, Boca Raton, pp 141–195
25. Zichner LP, Willert HG (1992) Comparison of alumina-polyethylene and metal-polyethylene in clinical trials. Clin Orthop 282: 86–94

The Reactivation of the Metal-Metal Pairing for the Total Hip Prosthesis

B. G. Weber

Introduction

The late loosening as a result of polyethylene wear is avoidable by choosing the metal-metal pairing. Certainly, such a prosthesis must be better finished than the earlier McKee prosthesis and its successors. A newly developed metal-metal prosthesis is described which was implanted 110 times between 1988 and 1992. To date absolutely no problems have arisen with this new metal-metal pairing.

The Concepts of Metal-Metal (McKee) and Metal-Polyethylene (Charnley)

Thirty-five years ago in 1960, McKee implanted his first cemented metal-metal total hip prosthesis (THP) which, with developments, remained his standard prosthesis since 1965 [16].

In 1961 Charnley [4] described his own cemented THP (first only the shaft, and later the cup, was cemented). His refined low-friction arthroplasty with 22-mm metal head and polyethylene cup then became very widely used worldwide. There have also been many variations of Charnley's first implant. In contrast, the McKee prostheses are used today in only very few places. These are second-generation McKee prostheses or copies with better frictional properties and thinner necks than the original Thompson prosthesis. The THP surgeon and his patients today confront research and clinical findings which, while successful, have not fulfilled all the previous expectations. As McKee [15] said in 1982: "We always learn more from our failures than our successes."

Metal-Metal 1960–1994

The first generation McKee THP failed within 8 years in almost 50 % of cases [15]. The Norwich School, with McKee, also had to accept failure after an average of 14 years of the shaft in 50 % of cases and loosening of the cup in 51 % with the second-generation McKee prosthesis [1]. Jantsch et al. [12] report 34 %

loosened McKee cups and 26 % loosened shafts. The examination report of three loosened prostheses, which had been implanted 13, 14 and 15.5 years, is worth noting: under the microscope only minimal wear of the prosthetic head and cup (each of 0.001 mm) could be observed.

Täger [27, 29, and personal communication] is still using the McKee THP today. His examination of explanted prostheses suggests an unlimited longevity of the prosthesis. The question of tolerance of metal waste remains open, as the antigenecity of such prostheses is not proven [13].

The explanation for the high rate of loosening of metal-metal THPs has been presented by McKee and his group [15], by Ungethüm et al. [28], and Semlitsch [23, 25, 26] (Fig. 1).

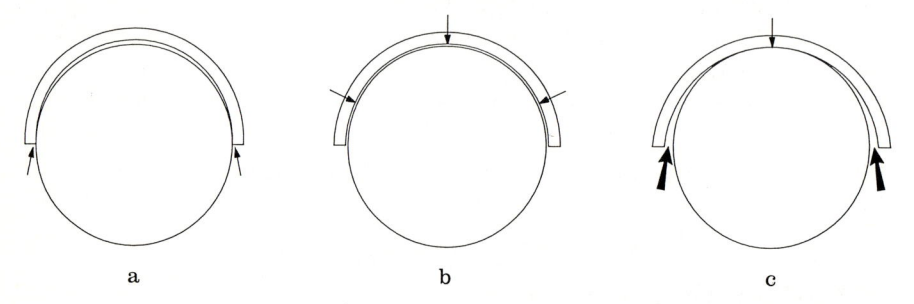

Fig. 1a–c. Different patterns of fit of metal-metal THP. **a** "Equatorial" contact; high friction and sticking. **b** Total contact after lapping process of head and cup; high friction and sticking. **c** "Polar" contact; head smaller than cup, hydrodynamic lubrication possible (*thick arrows*), low friction

The close examination of loosened and explanted prostheses revealed that the manufacturers' quality control of the product was not of a sufficiently high standard, and that the loosening was thus preprogrammed. Although in some cases wear was very small, the required low-friction criteria were not met.

In 1982 McKee [15] stopped using his own metal-metal prosthesis. As far as he was concerned the gliding-pairing material of the future was aluminium oxide ceramic.

In 1983 Ring [22] announced that he has not used metal-metal pairing since 1979 but rather a conical cup made from polyethylene.

Of 60 individual Müller-McKee THPs implanted in the late 1960s the author is aware of five joints that are still functioning perfectly, that is, after a working life of 25–27 years (Fig. 2). This raises an important question: have we, because of the high loosening rate of the metal-metal pairing, given an incorrect explanation of the failures – the unsuitability of the sliding partners? With this explanation the way was open for the other concept, Charnley's. It should be noticed that the cement anchorage of the long-lived metal-metal THPs known to the author is still intact at this time. This experience also raises a question:

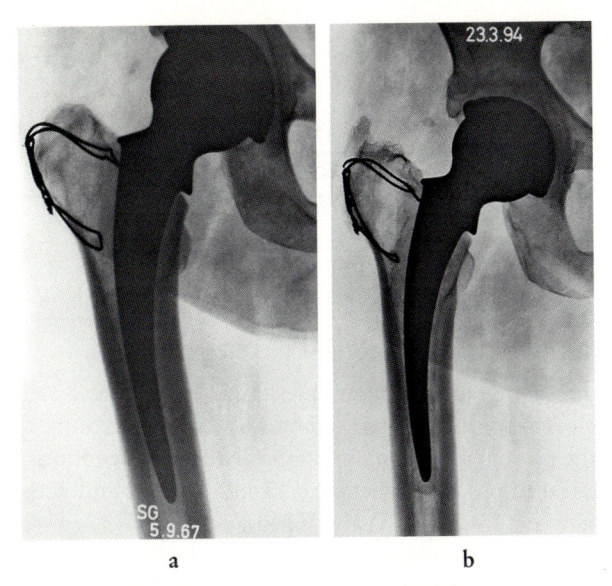

Fig. 2a,b. Example of a metal-metal THP with 27 years' service. **a** At 6 months after surgery for pigmenteous synovitis. Müller-McKee prosthesis, 42 mm. **b** At 27 years after surgery. The cemented prosthesis is stable and is serving as a normal hip joint

there is no sign of aging, rotting, or loosening in any of these joints. In my opinion such deterioration in any system must have another cause than the aging of methylmethacrylate. It is suggested that a prime cause could be a defective cementing technique.

Metal-Polyethylene or Ceramic-Polyethylene Pairing

The common THP with polyethylene cup in use today in all its countless forms has been associated with less loosening than the McKee prosthesis. Because of the smaller head diameter of 22, 28, or 32 mm it behaves as a low-friction prosthesis, in comparison to the insufficiently finished McKee high-friction prostheses with 40 mm diameter head, which had a tendency to stick.

Despite this initial advantage Willert et al. [35] reported loosening of some polyethylene-metal paired prostheses as early as 1978, which could be attributed to what they described as polyethylene debris disease, as we still know it today. The late loosening was caused by particles of polyethylene from the worn cup, which caused a foreign body reaction that gradually spread along the implant-bone interface.

The author's own examination of a comparison group (Table 1) 10 years after operation showed the following: aluminium oxide ceramic heads are less frequently associated with osteolytic phenomena and cause only half as many

Table 1. Radiological findings in THP of different pairing 10 years after surgery

	Metal-polyethylene (n = 139)		Aluminum oxide ceramic-polyethylene (n = 108)	
	n	%	n	%
No radiolucency	92	66.1	86	79.6
Minor radiolucencies without loosening	34	24.4	16	14.8
Loosening	13	9.4	6	5.6

fully developed cases of loosening as analogous prostheses with metal-ball heads. With polyethylene cups and with metal or ceramic heads late loosening is inevitable, provided that the patient lives long enough. With few exceptions, loosening occurs with metal-head prostheses between 10 and 15 years and with ceramic-head prostheses between 15 and 20 years (Fig. 3).

The relationship between polyethylene particle loss and gradual, progressive loosening phenomena along the bone-cement interface, as originally described by Willert [34], has not been sufficiently recognized. The bone cement was held responsible for the loosening, thus encouraging the use of cement-free anchorage. Since then countless suggestions have been made on this subject. We have more than 20 years' more experience, including the experience of failure, with cement anchorage than we have with cement-free anchorage. The optimism associated with cement-free anchorage, which was earlier associated with ce-

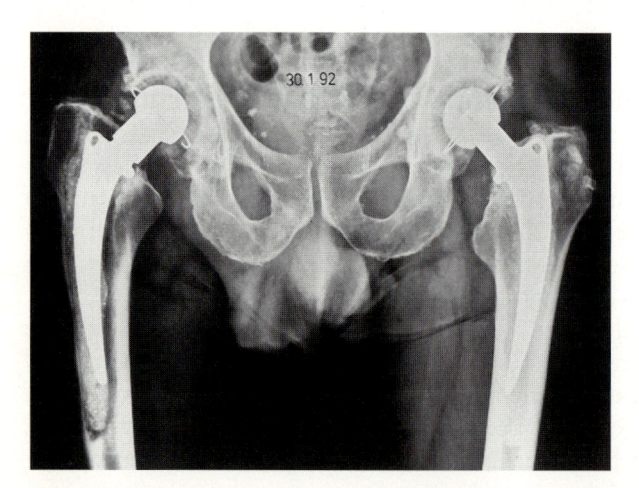

Fig. 3. Degree of wear and loosening. THP on the left side in 1980; THP on the right side in 1982. The follow-up X-ray: *right side*, 10 years after THP with metal head: wear 2 mm, manifest loosening; *left side*, 12 years after THP with aluminum-ceramic head: wear 0.5 mm, stable anchorage

ment anchorage, is now being questioned. The cement-free anchorage suffers from the same defect, tissue reaction to the build-up of foreign body particles produced by polyethylene: late loosening also devlops. If it is granted that, compared to metal-metal prostheses, polyethylene-paired prostheses can be considered low friction, it must also be accepted that polyethylene-paired prostheses suffer from high wear, from polyethylene debris disease.

In Search of Both Low Wear and Low Friction

In view of the problem of late loosening, particularly the problems associated with loosening revision surgery, it is not surprising that new polyethylene-free pairings have been suggested (metal-metal following McKee, ceramic-ceramic following Boutin [2], Mittelmeier [17].

The fundamental difference between the common polyethylene paired and metal-metal functioning prostheses can be seen in the different degrees of wear. The linear wear (Fig. 4), i. e., the penetration or movement of the prosthesis head into the artificial joint, is 0.1–0.2 mm per year for polyethylene and for metal-metal 0.002 mm per year [15, 31, 32], in other words a difference in the ratio of between 50:1 and 100:1 (Fig. 5).

In fact the issue is not really one of millimetres but of the amount of material worn off from the body of the joint. It is of the same order of difference as that of the land mass of Europe and the land mass of Switzerland.

The living tissue is not able to cope with the enormous amount of poisonous worn off material. It produces polyethylene debris disease. On the other hand

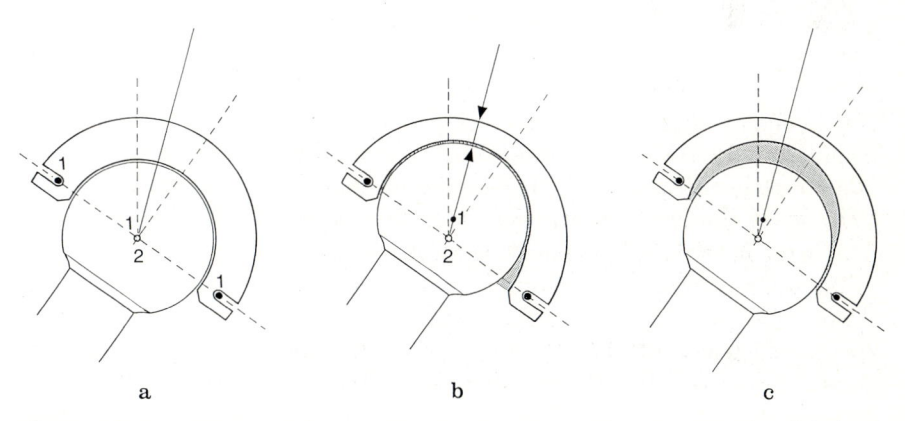

Fig. 4a–c. Linear wear on the X-ray. **a** Perioperative: no wear. The cup centre (*1*) and the head center (*2*) are identical. **b** Years later: the head and its center, has migrated upwards away from the cup center. The distance between 1 and 2 is called linear wear. **c** The amount of wear corresponds to the lost volume of polyethylene (*hatched area*)

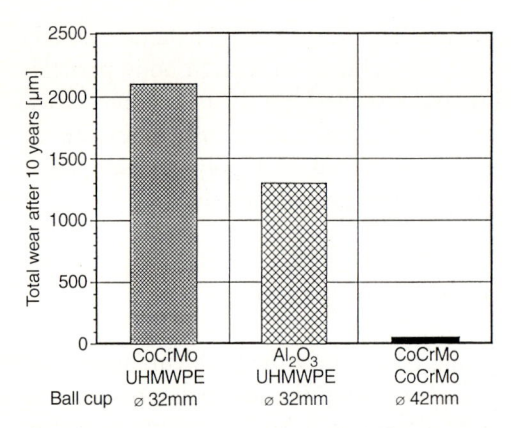

Fig. 5. Linear wear of THPs with different pairing (after Semlitsch)

the minute amount of worn off material from cobalt chromium molybdenum is easily tolerated. Our own five metal-metal THPs of the Müller-McKee type, with a working life of 25 years, were the motive for reactivating the former McKee concept. Low wear and low friction explain the impressive long working life of these prostheses.

Metal-Metal Slide-Pairing Concept: Metasul

Reactivation of the Metal-Metal Concept

At the end of the 1970s the author presented to the engineers Otto Frei and Manfred Semlitsch (Sulzer Inc.) the results of observations made over a 10-year period with Müller-McKee prostheses manufactured by Sulzer. These observations, together with the successful performance of the Weber rotation prosthesis, i. e., the metal-metal trunnion bearing joint, were the motivation to the new, closely quality-controlled, metal-metal paired THP. From 1983 to 1988 Sulzer manufactured the Metasul pairing with a ball head and cup from cobalt chromium molybdenum alloy which had been metallurgically refined. Since 1993/1994 Sulzer has also manufactured Müller, Zweymüller, Wagner, Sportono, Marchetti, and Stühmer prostheses with the Metasul pairing.

The ball heads measure 28 mm or 32 mm diameter, depending on the size of the patient's acetabulum. The metal cup is manufactured as an inlay. The inlays are embedded in a polyethylene cup, which can by choice be manufactured as a normal cup or as an insert into different kinds of metal backing.

The Cemented Weber THP

Between 1988 and 1992 the author implanted 110 of the prostheses shown in Fig. 6a.

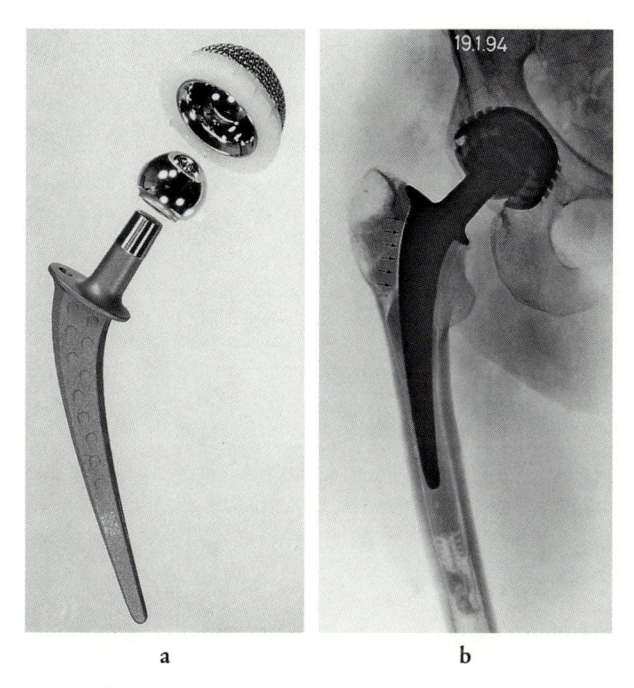

Fig. 6a, b. The new metal-metal THP with titanium shaft. **a** *Titanium shaft*, CoCrMo head. CoCrMo inlay firmly fixed in the polyethylene cup. **b** *Debonding* (arrows)

The titanium shaft has shown a form of loosening previously unknown in three of the author's own cases and more frequently among other users (Fig. 6b). The relatively high elasticity module of titanium (Huiskes [11], Bürgi [personal communication]), is likely to cause vibration in a femur component which is hammered into place, thus causing a cement mantle, which has not completely dried, to widen, and in certain circumstances to split. This causes immediate peroperative debonding so that early loosening is preprogrammed. At any event this is a convincing cause of such cases of loosening.

After 33 years of cement anchorage of total prostheses the following advice can be offered. Whoever cements should not hammer; whoever hammers should not cement. In the viscoelastic cement bed the correct method is to continuously push the wedge-shaped prosthesis shaft into position. Hammering is damaging to the material.

Figure 7 shows the present prosthesis with the CoCrMo shaft, which has remained almost unchanged since 1968, and two new cups. The first cup has a

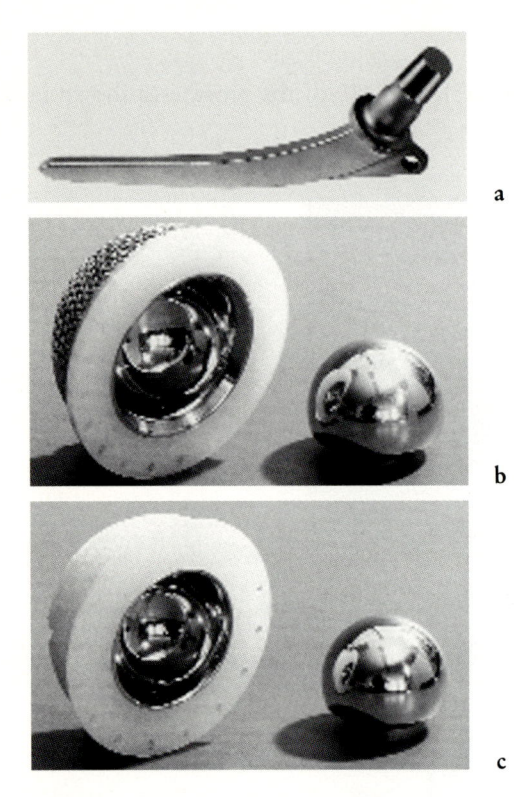

Fig. 7a–c. The new metal-metal THP with the "old" CoCrMo-shaft (Weber). **a** CoCrMo-shaft. **b** Cup with sintered Sulmesh surface. Inlays and heads of 28 or 32 mm diameter (here 32 mm). **c** Cup with special indentations of the surface Inlays and heads of 28 or 32 mm diameter (here 28 mm)

four-layer Selmesh surface, and the second has a special indented polyethylene surface. Both surfaces are designed to enable a very close bonding between the cement and the cup surfaces.

The Weber-Metasul prosthesis system requires a special set of instruments and a sufficiently adapted operation technique. It is not possible to go into further details at this point.

First Experience with the Weber-Metasul System, 1988–1992

It was the wish of both the author and Sulzer that the new system should be tested and controlled in detail before it became generally available.

Patients

From 1988 to 1992, 110 Weber Metasul THPs were implanted.

Five patients have died since operation from causes unrelated to their surgery. Five other patients required further revision surgery which had no relationship to the metal-metal slide pairing.

Three shafts and one cup came loose immediately. This is an example of implant-cement debonding as a result of hammering.

In one further case both components came loose after the second revision operation on the patient who had had his first THP 17 years previously. These five failures were excluded from the study as they had no connection with the metal-metal pairing Metasul. There remained 100 Metasul THPs in 98 patients.

Methods

All 100 THPs were followed up clinically and radiologically in consultation. The oldest implant was 4.5 years old and the youngest 1 year old. The clinical evaluation was made in accordance with the Harris score [10]. The X-rays, both AP and Lauenstein, were evaluated according to the criteria of Gruen et al. [9], and DeLee and Charnley [8].

Results

Preoperatively no patient an excellent Harris score (90–100), 2 had a good score (80–89), 2 a fair score (70–79), and 96 a poor score. The postoperative evaluation showed 88 excellent, 10 good, 2 fair, and none poor. Of the two results rated only as fair one was the result of painful ectopic ossification and one the result of bursitis trochanterica above the circlage wire on the major trochanter.

The X-ray evaluation showed that 90 THPs had no sign of osteolysis or instability in either the cup or the femur. Ten THPs showed minimal radiolucencies without clinical or prognostic significance, i. e., radiolucencies, without progression, which were visible even on the immediate postoperative X-rays. There were "cavities" on the bone-cement interface on the acetabulum, or in zone 1 or 7 of the femur. Such insufficient cement contact always occurs when the finger packing in the Charnley method is not satisfactorily finished or in the area of the cup when the denuding of the bone, the removal of cartilage, is not complete. The subjective estimation of the patients showed almost complete satisfaction, with 89 very satisfied, 10 satisfied, and only one disappointed. Of the five patients who required revision, the results in four cases were good or very good, in the fifth subsequent instability must be expected. Without going further into the necessary, previously obtained, control data (age, etiology, etc.) the current follow-up examinations have shown nothing against the taking up again the, technically improved, metal-metal pairing.

Metal-Metal Wear. In the case of our revision operations, all explants were sent to Sulzer for examination. Their measurements of the wear on the three Metasul ball heads were 0.001, 0.003 and 0.003 mm per year. This confirms earlier observations of other metal-metal explants and the generally accepted laboratory tests on the hip simulator (Semlitsch). Therefore, there is the prospect that the current new Metasul pairing will be able to offer the desired operational life of 25 years or more.

References

1. August AC, Aldam CH, Pynsent PB (1986), The McKee-Farrar hip arthoplasty. J Bone Joint Surg [Br] 68: 520–527
2. Boutin P (1972) Arthroplastie totale de la hanche par prothèse en alumine frittée. Rev Chir Orthop 58: 229
3. Charnley J (1960) Surgery of the hip joint. Present and future developments. Br Med J 1: 821–826
4. Charnley J (1961) Arthroplasty of the hip. A new operation. Lancet 1: 1129
5. Charnley J (1970) Total hip replacement by low friction arthroplasty. Clin Orthop 72: 7
6. Charnley J (1970) Acrylic cement in orthopaedic surgery. Livingstone, Edinburgh
7. Charnley J, Halley DK (1975) Rate of wear in total hip replacement. Clin Orthop 112: 170–179
8. De Lee J, Charnley J (1975) Radiological demarcation of cemented sockets in total hip replacement. Clin Orthop 121: 20–32
9. Gruen TA, McNeice GM, Amstutz HC (1979) „Modes of failure" of cemented stem-type femoral components. A radiographic analysis of loosening. Clin Orthop 141: 17–27
10. Harris WH (1969) Traumatic arthritis of the hip after dislocation and acetabular fractures: treatment by mold arthroplasty. An endresult study using a new method of result evaluation. J Bone Joint Surg [Am] 51: 737–755
11. Huiskes R (1990) The various stress patterns of press-fit ingrown and cemented femoral stems. Clin Orthop 261: 27–37
12. Jantsch S, Schwägerl W, Zenz P, Semlitsch M, Fertschak W (1991) Long-term results after implantation of McKee-Farrar total hip prostheses. Arch Orthop Trauma Surg 110: 230–237
13. Masshoff W, Neuhaus-Vogel, A (1974) Die Gelenkkapsel nach Alloplastik. Arch Orthop Unfallchir 78: 175–198
14. McKee GK (1970) Development of total prosthetic replacement of the hip. Clin Orthop 72: 85–103
15. McKee GK (1982) Total hip replacement. Present and future. Biomaterials 3: 130–135
16. McKee GK, Watson-Farrar J (1966) Replacement of arhritic hips by the McKee-Farrar-Prosthesis. J Bone Joint Surg [Br] 48: 245–259
17. Mittelmeier H (1984) Total hip replacement with the Autophar cement-free ceramic prosthesis. In: Morscher E (ed) The cementless fixation of hip endoprostheses. Springer, Berlin Heidelberg New York Tokyo, p 225
18. Müller ME (1970) Total hip porostheses. Clin Orthop 72: 46
19. Ring PA (1968) Complete replacement arthroplasty of the hip by the ring prosthesis. J Bone Joint Surg [Br] 50: 720–731
20. Ring PA (1978) Five to fourteen year interim results of uncemented total hip arthroplasty. Clin Orthop 137: 87–95

21. Ring PA (1981) Uncemented total hip replacement. J R Soc Med 74: 719–724
22. Ring PA (1983) Ring UPM total hip arthroplasty. Clin Orthop 176: 115–123
23. Semlitsch M (1992) 25 years Sulzer development of implant materials for total hip prostheses. SULZER Med J 1: 1–6
24. Semlitsch M, Vogel A, Willert HG (1971) Kombination moderner Mikroanalysemethoden zur Untersuchung von Gelenkendoprothesenabrieb im Bindegewebe der Gelenkkapsel. Acta Med 19: 38
25. Semlitsch M, Streicher RM, Weber H (1989) Wear behaviour of cast CoCrMo cups and balls in long-term implanted total hip prostheses. Orthopäde 18: 370–376
26. Semlitsch M, Streicher RM, Weber H (1989) Verschleißverhalten von Pfannen und Kugeln aus CoCrMo-Gußlegierung bei langzeitig implantierten Ganzmetall-Hüftprothesen. Orthopäde 18: 1–5
27. Täger KH (1976) Untersuchungen an Oberflächen und Neogelenkkapseln getragener McKee-Farrar-Endoprothesen. Arch. Orthop. Unfall-Chir 86: 101–113
28. Ungetüm M, Jäger M, Witt AN (1972) Sphärizitätsmessungen an Totalendoprothesen nach McKee-Farrar und Weber-Huggler. Arch Orthop Unfallchir 73: 1–6
29. Weber BG (1981) Total hip replacement: rotating versus fixed and metal versus ceramic heads. In: Proc 9th Open Scientific Meeting of the Hip Society. Mosby, St. Louis, pp 264–275
30. Weber BG (1988) Pressurized cement fixation in total hip arthroplasty. Clin Orthop 232: 87–95
31. Weber BG, Fiechter T (1989) Polyethylen-Verschleiß und Spätlockerungen der Totalprothese des Hüftgelenkes. Neue Perspektiven für die Metall-Metall-Paarung für Pfanne und Kugel. Orthopäde 18: 370–376
32. Weber BG, Semlitsch M, Streicher R (1993) Total Hip Joint Replacement using a CoCrMo metal-metal sliding pairing. J Jpn Orthop Ass 67: 391–398
33. Willert HG (1977) Reactions of the articular capsule to wear products of artificial joint prostheses. J Biomed Mat Res 11: 157–164
34. Willert HG, Semlitsch M (1976) Tissue reactions to plastic and metallic wear products of joint endoprostheses. In: Gschwend N, Debrunner HU (eds) Total hip prosthesis. Huber, Bern, pp 205–239
35. Willert HG, Semlitsch M, Buchhorn G, Kriete U (1978) Materialverschleiß und Gewebereaktion bei künstlichen Gelenken. Orthopäde 7: 62–83

Osseointegration of Sulmesh Coatings

R. K. Schenk

Introduction

The term osseointegration has been chosen to characterize the bony incorporation of cementless prostheses. It was originally introduced by Brånemark et al. [2] who defined it histologically as direct bone deposition upon the implant surfaces. The resulting direct bone-implant contact is indeed a decisive prerequisite for a firm and long -lasting anchorage of any prosthetic device [23]. The process of osseointegration, however, continues after this contact is established. The subsequent modeling and remodeling activities along the interface and in the surrounding bone lead to substitution of preexisting and initially formed more primitive woven bone, and in a functional adaptation of the bone structure to load.

The initial stage of osseointegration depends on certain prerequisites, which are linked to material properties and design of the implants as well as to the accuracy of the operation and proper loading prescriptions for the patient. Bioinert materials, surface configurations that favor bone apposition (osteophilic surface), sufficient primary stability, and adequate loading during the healing period are considered essential conditions.

Various procedures are recommended to render an implant surface more attractive for osteoblast attachment and direct bone depositiont or, in other words, to make it more osteophilic. In this respect coating with bioactive materials, such as calcium phosphate ceramics (hydroxyapatite, tricalcium phosphate) provides a specific advantage by forming strong chemical bonds with the mineralizing bone matrix [9, 26]. These coatings, however, pose other problems, related to their mechanical properties and biological instability. Bioinert materials, such as commercially pure titanium or titanium alloys also allow for bony contact, but without chemical binding. A certain degree of adhesion can be obtained by roughening the implant surface. Compared to machined or polished surfaces, a rougher, sand blasted, or plasma-sprayed surface significantly increases the extent of the bone-implant interface [3] as well as the mechanical adhesion [25, 27].

Porous coating of implants goes one step further. Thereby, bone does not only grow upon the implant surface but invades the pores or meshes provided by covering the surface with layers of beads, wires, or lattices [1, 3, 5–7, 10, 11,

13]. Bony ingrowth creates a composite of metal and bone along the interface. This composite transmits compressive, tensile, and shear forces equally well and thus establishes a firm contact, as required for a successful osseointegration.

The first stage of osseointegration, i.e., bony incorporation, can be investigated in experimental animals with unloaded implants. Functional adaptation can be evaluated only in endoprostheses that have been subjected to the manyfold mechanical influences during daily use. This is possible only in autopsy cases, where the specimens can be studied in situ together with the surrounding bone. This paper describes the microscopic findings in three press-fit cups that were retrieved from patients with uneventful postoperative course at various time intervals.

Material and Methods

Individual case histories of the three patients are presented below. All acetabular components were removed, including the surrounding pelvic bone, and fixed in toto in 10 % neutral formalin. The large tissue blocks required long immersion times during further processing. Throughout dehydration in ethanol and infiltration with methylmethacrylate the specimens were kept in continuous motion. Polymerization of the embedding medium was controlled by keeping the jars in a refrigerator at 4°C–7°C to prevent untimely hardening and bubble formation due to overheating during polymerization.

The simultaneous presence of both metal and polyethylene rendered sectioning and grinding of the large blocks rather difficult since the polymer smears and coats the grains of the diamond wafering blades. A heavy duty saw, originally designed for cutting steel bars, finally solved this problem. However, the blade thickness of 1.5 mm caused a greater loss of material.

Sections 1 mm thick were mounted with acrylic glue on opalescent plexiglass slides measuring 7×7 cm and then ground to 100–150 μm. After polishing they were superficially stained with either McNeal's tetrachrome alone or combined with basic fuchsin (for details see Schenk et al. [22]).

Results

Case 1. This material was retrieved at autopsy from an 82-year-old woman. Total hip replacement had been performed because of severe osteoarthritis. The patient died unexpectedly 33 days later from cardiac failure after an uneventful postoperative course. At this time partial weight bearing had been allowed.

The microscopic examination revealed a good fit of the cup in a rather dense pelvic bone. In accordance with the design of the press fit cup [14, 15], primary contact with preexisting bone was achieved along the rim of the cup (Fig. 1a). Compression had caused some local deformation and microcracks of adjacent

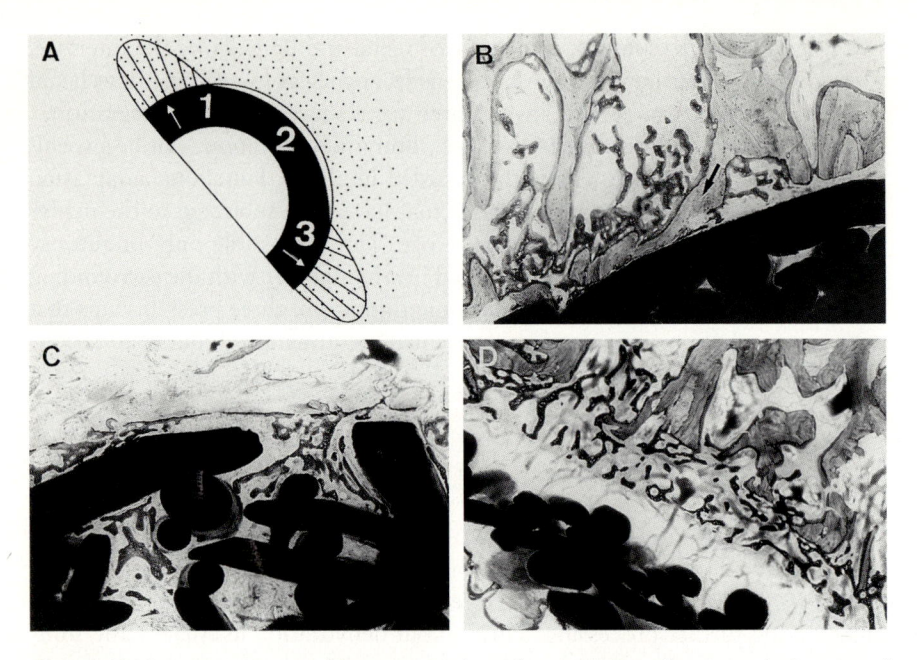

Fig. 1A-D Case 1: an 82-year-old woman, 33 days after total hip replacement. **A** Concept of the press-fit cup. The diameter of the cup is slightly oversized (+ 1.5 mm) and provides, together with the flattened dome, primary stability by a snap-fastener mechanism. **B** In the superior zone 1, compression has deformed some preexisting trabeculae (*arrow*). Newly formed woven bone (*dark staining*) spreads out into the intertrabecular spaces. x 15. **C** Small gap adjacent to the contact area in zone 1. Woven bone formation fills the gap and enters the wire mesh. x 20. **D.** In the area of the dome (zone 2), the gap width of 2 mm exceeds the "osteogenic jumping distance." Newly formed woven bone fills only half of the gap. Fibrovascular granulation tissue has reached the mesh coating. x 18

trabeculae. Together with the destructions caused by the reamer these lesions activated an intensive woven bone formation. This started by bone deposition upon the preexisting bone surfaces and spread out into the intertrabecular spaces and towards the wire mesh (Fig. b). The distance between the implant and the surface of the bony recipient site increased gradually from the margin towards the dome of the cup. The resulting narrow gaps were bridged by woven bone, and secondary contact with the titanium surface had been achieved by bony ongrowth (Fig. 1c). Towards the center of the dome the gap increased further in width and reached a value of almost 2 mm. This distance was too large to be bridged by bone within the given time (Fig. 1d). Along the bony border of the gap the original trabeculae were clearly identified by their weak staining. Their free ends were lined by newly formed woven bone which was growing towards the cup but still remained 300–500 μm away from the implant surface. Woven bone formation was preceeded by blood vessels that had already crossed the gap and started to penetrate the wire mesh.

Osseointegration of Sulmesh Coatings

The soft tissue around the implant and within the intertrabecular spaces is best classified as a granulation tissue. It was well vascularized and occasionally included remnants of the original blood clot and some loose bone debris that were produced during reaming. Some debris were also integrated into newly formed trabeculae. The majority of the newly formed trabeculae consisted exclusively of primitive woven bone.

Case 2. This material was retrieved from a 92-year-old woman who died 21 months after total hip replacement because of cardiac failure. Four months after surgery full weight bearing was allowed; since then she had no pain and good mobility. Radiological controls showed an excellent integration of the press fit cup as was confirmed by the radiographs of the specimen taken after autopsy.

After embedding, the cup with the surrounding bone was first cut in the coronal plane. With this orientation the most central sections usually hit the

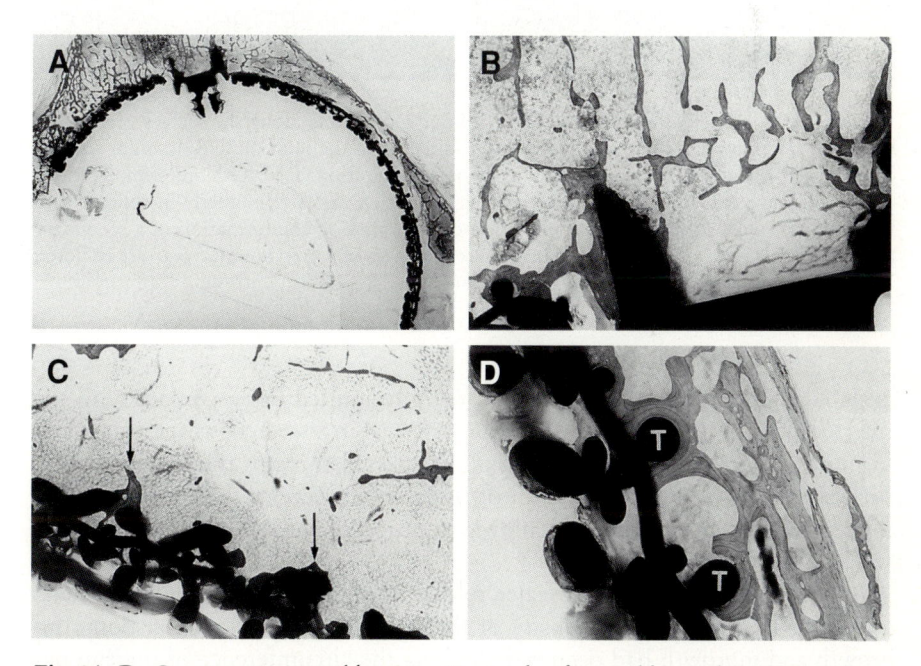

Fig. 2A–D. Case 2: an 92-year-old woman, 21 months after total hip replacement. **A** Coronal section through the center of the dome hits the acetabular notch. The resulting wide gap prevents a bony support in zone 3. x 1. **B** The outer wall of the spigot is covered by a vigorous bone plate which is continuous with radially emerging trabeculae. x 7. **C** Extremely rarefied cancellous bone in zone 2. Some trabeculae have reached the surface of the titanium wires (*arrows*). x 7. **D** A slightly excentric coronal section demonstrates good bony support in zone 3. The superficial, tranversially cut wires (T) are surrounded by concentric layers of lamellar bone, and connected to the internal cortex of the pelvis by continuous bony plates. x 7
Case 2, continued

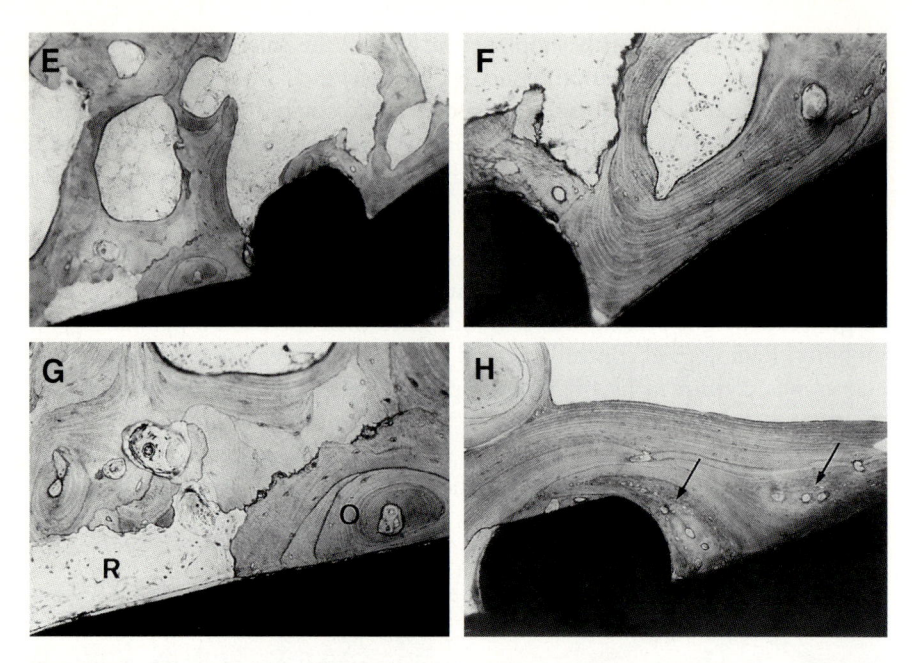

Fig. 2E–H. **E** Lamellar bone deposition and bone remodeling along the surface of the wire mesh. x 32. **F** Lamellar bone was directly deposited upon the sand-blasted titanium surface. This is a characteristic feature of stage 2 of osseointegration. x 80. **G** Bone remodeling is typical for stage 3. Osteoclasts have formed a resorption cavity (*R*) directly in contact with the titantium wire. Filling of such resorption cavities leads to the formation of a secondary osteons (*O*). x 80. **H** One of the rare sites where remnants of woven bone (*arrows*) are enclosed and covered by lamellar bone deposition during stage 2. x 52

acetabular notch where there was no or only limited bony contact with the inferior margin of the cup (Fig. 2a). Bony contact in zone 3, however, was found in more eccentrically located sections that passed through the (former) lunar surface (Fig. 2d). After completion of the coronal sections the remaining segments were cut horizontally to allow inspection of the anterior and posterior walls of the acetabulum.

A survey of these sections revealed relevant progress in bone implant contact as well as in structure and density of the surrounding pelvic bone. Bony ongrowth and ingrowth had occurred all along the circumference of the cup but was especially pronounced in zones 1 and 3, where the rim was found in contact with dense cancellous bone (Fig. 2a). In these areas the spongiosa was clearly anisotropic; the vigorous trabeculae, mostly consisting of plates, ran parallel and emanated in a radial direction from an almost cortical bone layer that extended along the surface of the wire mesh. Some further structural details in zone 1 were noteworthy: One concerns the spigot, a short cylindrical, crownlike protrusion that is supposed to increase rotational stability (Fig. 2b). Its flange was encompassed by a rather thick bone layer that was contiguous with radially emanating trabeculae and supplemented by cross-connecting struts. The second relates to transverse sections through individual wires. These were often completely surrounded by bone that had been concentrically deposited upon their surface. This structural interrelationship is of considerable mechanical importance; it allows not only for transmission of compressive forces but for shear and traction as well.

In zone 2, i. e., in the polar region of the cup, bone had also established contact with the implant surface (Fig. 2c). The density of the cancellous bone was drastically reduced compared to the equator of the cup and the trabeculae represented rather delicate struts that merged with small, discontinuous bony plates upon the implant surface. The intertrabecular space contained normal red bone marrow.

Towards the inferior rim (zone 3), the implant surface approached a part of the medial acetabular wall, which was only 2–3 mm thick. This was connected by vigorous trabeculae and rather thick bony plates with the superficial wires. Again, a large number of wires were almost completely encircled by concentric layers of mature lamellar bone (Fig. 2d).

Sections through the anterior and posterior wall of the acetabulum closely resembled the structure found in the superior and inferior rim. They confirmed a good osseointegration by bony on- and ingrowth as well as by a functional adaptation of the supporting bony scaffold.

Some finer structural details in the bone tissue adjacent or inside of the wire mesh are noteworthy (Fig. 2e). The woven bone formed during the first months had almost completely disappeared. It was replaced by lamellar bone, and only a few scattered remnants could be detected by careful examination (Fig. 2h). The bone-implant interface was considerably increased; especially the most superficial wires were covered or surrounded over remarkable distances by layers of lamellar bone that were 200 μm and more thick. In many contact sites the lamellae ran strictly parallel to the contour of the wires, indicating a continuous bone deposition by osteoblasts that had started directly upon the titanium surface (Fig. 2f). Cement lines of the smooth type, i. e., arresting lines, indicated temporary interruptions of bone formation. In other locations bone remodeling had taken place; activation of osteoclasts resulted in the formation of resorption cavities, which were subsequently refilled by lamellar bone deposition (Fig. 2g).

Case 3. This was a 66-year-old man, who had died 25 months after primary total hip replacement from an apoplectic fit. Fifteen months after surgery he had presented with excellent mobility and no pain. Besides the differences in age and sex, his personality diverged markedly from the preceding patient, especially in terms of physical activity. This was also reflected by the quality of bone stock around the cup, both in view of cancellous bone density and mean trabecular diameter.

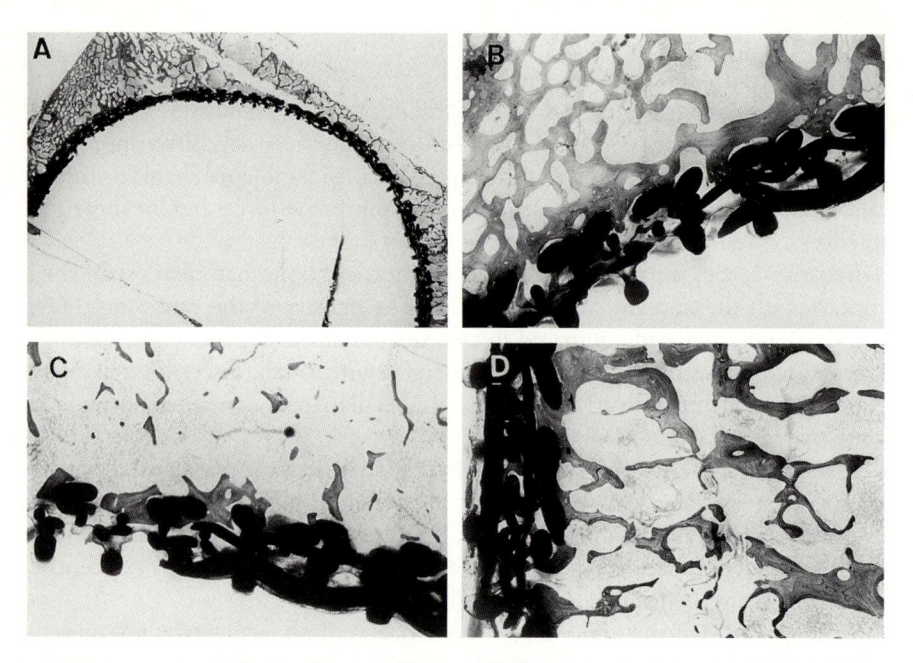

Fig. 3A–D Case 3: a 66-year-old man, 25 months after total hip replacement. **A** Total view of a fully contained coronal section, showing the different bone densities in zones 1, 2 and 3. (An accidental saw cut was produced during dissection). x 1. **B** Ongrowth and ingrowth of lamellar bone in zone 1 results in the formation of an almost continuous secondary subchrondral plate. x 7. **C** Zone 2 features again a very low concellous bone density, although the wires are quite extensively covered by lamellar bone. x 7. **D** Zone 3 shows again good bony on- and ingrowth, and platelike trabeculae emanating in a radial direction. x 7

The overall bone response to the implant, however, showed a striking similarity with case 2 (Fig. 3a). The bony support concentrated, again, upon the rim of the cup. In the respective zones 1 and 3 there was an extensive and intimate bone-implant contact, and mature lamellar bone had penetrated into the pores of the mesh coating (Fig. 3b, d). This resulted in the formation of a composite of titanium wires and bone resembling a subchondral plate. This plate was continuous with cancellous bone, with a rather dense array of platelike trabeculae in zones 1 and 3 and a lower density of discontinuous trabecular profiles (bars or rods) in the polar area (Fig. 3c). The trabeculae again emanated in a radial direction, not only in the coronal sections but also in the anterior and posterior portion of the wall.

The bone remodeling activity was similar to case 2. Besides traces of the younger, woven bone compartment the newly formed and remodeled bone also included some remnants of the original subchondral bone and of preexisting trabeculae. Such avascular, necrotic inclusions become more numerous with increasing distance from the implant, and at about 5 mm they often form the center core of the trabeculae.

Discussion

In its histological appearance osseointegration has much in common with primary or direct fracture healing, which has been characterized mainly by the fact that the fragment ends are united directly by bone without any intermediate connective tissue or cartilage formation [17–19]. The well-known prerequisites for direct fracture healing are precise anatomical reduction and stable fixation. This is achieved by interfragmentary compression. Compression forces the fragment ends into direct contact. Small incongruencies between the fragment ends restrict the contact to localized areas or even pressure points. Contact sites are separated by small gaps which are protected against deformation by the static preload. If these anatomical and mechanical conditions are fulfilled, blood vessels and osteoprogenitor cells invade the gaps and start woven bone formation. Small gaps (1 mm or less) are bridged by woven bone within 1–2 weeks; bridging of larger gaps takes somewhat longer [20].

In fracture repair the pattern of direct gap healing can be subdivided into three stages: (a) bridging of fracture gap by woven bone, (b) reinforcement of this primary scaffold by lamellar bone, and (c) reconstruction of the fracture site and restoration of the original bone structure by bone remodeling. The first stage is completed within 2–4 weeks, and reinforcement within a few months. Bone remodeling requires months or even years since it is limited by the osteoclastic bone resorption rate of approx. 50 μm/day, and the daily rate of lamellar bone deposition of only 1 μm.

The mechanical principles as well as the pattern of direct (or primary) fracture healing can easily be conferred upon the histological features of osseointegration described in the current series of autopsy cases. Case 1, retrieved at only 33 days, closely resembles stage one. In the periphery, the specific design of the press fit cup created primary contact sites that obviously provided sufficient primary stability for direct bone formation to occur. The preparation of the recipient site activated an impressive tissue response, consisting both in a neoangiogenesis and in the recruitment of osteoprogenitor cells. Both the blood vessels and the osteoblast precursors originate from the bone marrow. Woven bone formation results in the formation of primitive trabeculae that bridge the intertrabecular spaces in the adjacent pelvic spongiosa and invade the gap around the implant as well as the wire mesh. Thanks to the incongruency between the spherical recipient site and the flattened dome of the cup the size dependency of the bony bridging becomes obvious: In the polar area, the gap width of 2 mm and more clearly surpasses the threshold value for an instant bridging by woven bone. This confirms observations made in earlier experimental studies of the healing pattern of small cortical defects in rabbits [12, 20]. In the case of implants this distance becomes even more important since bone formation can start from one side of the gap only. The critical gap width around an implant has been experimentally tested in dogs and found to be around 1 mm. Harris et al. [11] have characterized this situation as "osteogenic jumping distance," i. e., the distance that can be bridged by bone formation "by one single jump."

The newly formed bone resembles an early bony fracture callus. It is classified as woven bone and characterized by the numerous, large osteocytes and by the random, feltlike orientation of its collagen fibrils. Woven bone has the outstanding capacity to grow by forming a scaffold of rods and plates and thus is able to spread out into the surrounding tissue at a relatively rapid rate. The construction of the primary scaffold is coupled with the elaboration of the vascular network and results in the formation of a primary spongiosa, which is isotropic, or, in other words, lacks any preferential orientation of its trabeculae. At 33 days woven bone is the only newly formed bone compartment. It has completed the first stage of osseointegration, namely bony incorporation and direct bone ongrowth upon the implant surfaces.

The second stage of direct gap healing consists in a reinforcement of the woven bone and preexisting trabeculae. This process starts after 4–6 weeks and proceeds during the following months. An important and decisive feature of the second stage of osseointegration is the formation of lamellar bone. Lamellar bone can grow only by deposition upon a solid, flat surface. Such surfaces are provided by preexisting trabeculae, the newly elaborated scaffold of woven bone, and by the contour of the titanium wires. Accordingly, lamellar bone deposition not only reinforces the preexisting and newly formed bony scaffold but extends upon the wire mesh as well (Figs. 3b, 4b). This leads to a considerable increase in the bone-implant interface, and a direct contact with mature lamellar bone. Unfortunately, no appropriate specimen of a Sulmesh or similar cup is available in this series to document this stage of osseointegration. Bone reinforcement and its possible dependence on loading conditions, however, have been described in retrieved femoral components at 4.5 and 5.5 months [21, 24]. In addition, the direct lamellar bone deposition upon titanium surfaces is clearly illustrated by cases 2 and 3, where the lamellae often run perfectly parallel to the metal surface or surround the wires in concentric layers. There is no doubt that osteoblasts initially settled upon the metal surface, and that further lamellar bone matrix deposition proceeded in an "implantofugal" manner.

Otherwise, cases 2 and 3 fall clearly into the third stage of osseointegration, which has been characterized, in analogy to the third stage of direct bone healing, by bone remodeling and bone modeling activities. Bone remodeling consists in a replacement or substitution of preexisting, as well as of regenerated bone, by mature lamellar bone. This is accomplished by localized bone remodeling units, which construct secondary osteons in compact, or packets of new lamellar in cancellous bone. Thereby, the shape and internal architecture of the given structural elements are preserved. Modeling designates shape deforming processes, either resorption or formation, along external or internal bone surfaces.

In spite of pronounced differences in the case history, the bone around the two cups reveals striking similarities. In the vicinity of the wire mesh its microscopic structure is uniform. It now consists of lamellar bone; inclusions of woven bone are rare. This proves that the initially formed woven bone, which was almost exclusively present at 35 days, is completely remodeled and substituted after about 2 years. During this remodeling phase most of the preexisting trabeculae and remnants of the original subchondral plate are also replaced by new and vital lamellar bone tissue. The same holds true for incorporated necrotic fragments produced during the operation by the reamer.

Modeling and remodeling are not only involved in bone substitution but are also operative in functional adaptation. Functional adaptation is based on changes in dimension and orientation of the supporting elements. In cancellous bone this becomes apparent in differences in the local cancellous bone density and in the diameter and orientation of the trabeculae. In this respect the results in cases 2 and 3 are remarkably uniform. The whole circumference of the rim is surrounded by dense cancellous bone, consisting mainly of plates and struts aligned in a radial direction to the surface of the cup. Their diameter increases towards the implant surface, where they fuse with an almost complete cortical bone layer that coats the wire mesh. It seems justified to attribute these structural features to the preferential force transmission in the periphery of the cup, as it was indeed intended by its design. A second feature of this concept is the flattened dome, which should prevent a stress concentration in the center of the cup [16, 19]. The initial problem of the gap width is certainly overcome after a few months, and bony contact with the wire mesh is established. But the overall bone density remains low, and only a few trabeculae are connected to the implant. In the dome area the difference between cases 2 and 3 is obvious: the 92-year-old woman is clearly more osteoporotic than the 66-year-old man.

Summary

The success of cementless implants depends on osseointegration, a process that can be compared to fracture healing and converts the primary stability obtained at surgery into a secondary stability, assured by the anchorage of the prosthesis in a vital, healthy bone.

In analogy to direct fracture healing, osseointegration can be subdivided into three considerably overlapping phases. The initial stage consists of a bony incorporation, mainly by bridging the implant-tissue interface or gap by woven bone. In a second stage this bony support is adapted to the increasing load by the mobilization of the patient, mainly by further deposition of lamellar bone upon the preexisting and newly formed scaffold. Reinforcement starts in the second and continues in the following months. The third stage consists in bone remodeling and leads to the substitution of the preexisting and newly formed bone and to changes in orientation of the supporting bony elements. Remodeling starts at 3–4 months and may continue over years.

After about 2 years the cancellous bone structure around the implants corresponds quite well to the force distribution intended by the basic concept of the press-fit cup. It reflects a peripheral introduction of the forces, both by the cancellous bone density and the orientation of the trabeculae.

References

1. Bobyn JD, Engh CA (1984) Human histology of the bone-porous metal implant interface. Orthopaedics 7: 1420–1421
2. Brånemark PI, Hansson BO, Adell R, Breine U, Lindström J, Hallen O, Oemann A (1977) Osseo-integrated implants in the treatment of the edentulous jaw. Experience from a 10-year period. Scand J Plast Reconstr Surg (Suppl) 11
3. Brooker AF, Jr. Collier JP (1984) Evidence of bone ingrowth into a porous-coated prosthesis: a case report J Bone Joint Surg [Am] 66: 619–621
4. Buser D, Schenk RK, Steinemann S, Fiorellini JP, Fox CH, Stich H (1991) Influence of surface characteristics on bone integration of titanium implants. A histomorphometric study in miniature pigs. J Biomed Mater Res 25: 889–902
5. Cook SD, Barrack SL, Thomas KA (1988) Quantitative analysis of tissue growth into human porous total hip components. J Arthroplasty 3: 249–262
6. Cook SD, Barrack RL, Thomas KA, Haddad RJ, Jr (1989) Quantitative histological analysis of tissue growth into porous total knee components. J Arthroplasty 4:33-45
7. Cook SD, Thomas KA, Haddad RJ Jr (1988) Histologic analysis of retrieved human porous-coated total joint components. Clin Orthop 234: 90–101
8. Crowinshield RD, Brand RA, Pederson DR (1983) A stress analysis of acetabular reconstruction in protrusio acetabuli. J Bone Joint Surg [Am] 65: 495–499
9. de Groot K, Geesink R, Klein CPAT, Serekian P (1987) Plasma sprayed coatings of hydroxylapatite. J Biomed Mater Res 21: 1375
10. Galante J, Suner DR, Gächter A (1987) Oberflächenstrukturen und Einwachsen von Knochen bei zementfrei fixierten Prothesen. Orthopäde 16: 197–205
11. Harris, WH, White RE, McCarthy, JC, Walker, PS, Weinberg, EH (1983) Bony ingrowth fixation of the acetabular component in canine hip joint arthroplasty. Clin Orthop 176: 7–11
12. Johner R (1972) Zur Knochenheilung in Abhängigkeit von der Defektgröße. Helv Chir Acta 39: 409–411
13. Morscher EW (1987) Current state of cementless fixation of endoprotheses. Swiss Med 9: Nr. 8
14. Morscher E, Mazar Z (1988) Development and first experience with an uncemented press-fit cup. Clin Orthop 223: 96–103
15. Morscher E, Bereiter H, Lampert Ch (1989) Cementless „press-fit cup" – principles, experimental data and 3-year follow-up. Clin Orthop 249: 12–20
16. Pedersen DR, Crowinshield RD, Brand RA, Johnston RC (1982) An axisymmetric model of acetabular components in total hip arthroplasty. J Biomech 15: 305–315
17. Schenk RK (1992) Biology of fracture repair. In: Skeletal Browner BD, Jupiter JB, Levine AM, Traften PG Skeletal trauma (eds) Skeletal Trauma. Saunders, Philadelphia, PP 31–75
18. Schenk R, Willenegger H (1963) (Zum histologischen Bild der sogenannten Primärheilung der Knochenkompakta nach experimentellen Osteotomien am Hund. Experientia 19: 593–595
19. Schenk R, Willenegger H (1964) Histologie der primären Knochenheilung. Langenbecks Arch klin Chir 308: 440–452

20. Schenk R, Willenegger H (1977) Zur Histologie der primären Knochenheilung. Modifikationen und Grenzen der Spaltheilung in Abhängigkeit von der Defektgröße. Unfallheilkunde 80: 155–160
21. Schenk RK, Wehrli U (1989) Zur Reaktion des Knochens auf eine zementfreie SL-Femur-Revisions-Prothese. Orthopäde 16: 454–462
22. Schenk, RK, Olah, AJ, Herrmann, W (1984) Preparation of calcified tissues for light microscopy. In: Dickson, GR (ed), Methods of calcified tissue preparation. Elsevier, Amsterdam, pp 1–56
23. Schroeder A, Pohler O, Sutter F (1976) Gewebsreaktion auf ein Titan-Hohlzylinderimplantat mit Titan-Spritzschichtoberfläche. Schweiz Monatsschr Zahnheilk 86: 713
24. Spotorno, L, Schenk, RK, Dietschi, C, Romagnoli, S, Mumenthaler A (1987) Unsere Erfahrungen mit nichtzementierten Prothesen. Orthopäde 16: 225–238
25. Steinemann, SG, Eulenberger, J, Maeusli, PA, Schroeder A (1986) Adhesion of bone to titanium. In: Christel, P, Meunier A, Lee AJC (eds) Biological and biomechanical performance of biomaterials. Elsevier, Amsterdam, PP 409–414
26. Thomas KA, Kay JF, Cook SD, Jarcho M (1987) The effect of surface macrotexture and hydroxylapatite coating on the mechanical strengths and histologic profiles of titanium implant materials. J Biomed Mater Res 21: 1395
27. Wilke HJ, Claes L, Steinemann S (1990) The influence of various titanium surfaces on the interface shear strength between implants and bone. In: Heimke G, Soltész U, Lee AJC (eds), Advances in Biomaterials, Amsterdam, Elsevier, pp 309–314

Biomechanics of Osseointegration of a Cementless Hip Joint Cup in Animal Experiments

H. Bereiter

Introduction

The primary movement-free anchorage of the cup implant in the bone must be considered the prerequisite for permanent fixation and osseointegration of an artificial cementless hip joint cup. This requirement is necessary to ensure the physiological conditions around the implant providing osseous reactions which are similar to that during healing of fractures. This means that there must be essentially no movement at the osseous interface to the cup, even where the implant is loaded directly following the operation. The artificial cementless implant should be completely integrated with the surrounding bone to provide firm long-term fixation.

The connection and fixation between implant and bone interface must be of sufficient quality that the physiological forces give rise to no, or only insignificant, relative movement between the implant and the surrounding bone, and that the direct load transfer between implant and bone is ensured. Too much movement between the implant and the bone leads to the formation of connective tissue similar to pseudarthrosis [3, 19, 27, 34, 39, 43, 44, 49].

The mechanical fixation of the implant is present where this condition is met. Strength and stability are terms for material properties in mechanics and cannot be used in the usual sense in this application. Further prerequisites are bio-inert materials in direct contact with bone, and suitably prepared surfaces so that bony ongrowth and ingrowth are possible. In this way direct load transfer between implant and bone is possible and vice versa, and adaptation of the bone by remodelling can be expected [7, 10, 21, 26].

The following conditions for cementless implantation of an artificial hip joint cup must therefore be fulfilled.

Primary Mechanical Fixation

The formation of new bone is possible only where blood vessels are present. Osseointegration therefore requires that such vessels grow onto and into appropriately prepared surface structures beforehand. It has been shown that a pore size of at least 100 μm is necessary. Movements of 50 μm would therefore mechanically damage new vessel branches. Micromovements of 150 μm always lead to the formation of connective tissue without the formation of bone [8, 14, 39, 40]. The necessary primary mechanical fixation in bone is achieved by the use of suitable implant anchoring elements in the bone. Three available techniques for force transfer are available, namely friction hold, Keying hold and material bonding. Several of these possibilities, alone or in combination, are always used for the fixation of implants. Individual anchorage elements can be integrated into the design of the implant or can be additionally applied to the implant [2, 4, 41, 42, 50].

Characteristics of Materials and Surfaces at the Implant Interface with Bone

These are critical with respect to long-term fixation. Titanium and titanium alloys have shown themselves to be the optimal choice among materials tested to date as regards tissue compatibility [1, 9, 12]. The adhesion of bony ongrowth or ingrowth is increased additionally by increasing the surface area, whether by macro-, mini-or micropores. Optimal sizing of pores and porosity has been developed experimentally. These are pore sizes between 100 and 500 μm and porosity of 20 %–60 % [7, 8, 10, 11, 21–23, 32]. The surface relief leads to intermeshing and an improvement in the load transfer between implant and bone [14, 15, 26]. With nonmetallic materials such as calcium phosphate ceramics material bonding can even occur.

Secondary Fixation

Dowels inserted in concrete loose their initial pretensioning and wedging effect due to creep and relaxation in the expansion area. The greatest reduction occurs within a few hours, and the remaining pretensioning can be as low as 60 %–40 % of the original value [2]. Similar conditions occur in bone. On the one hand, there is plastic deformation and, on the other, changes in load transfer direction or deformation initiate bone restructuring according to Wolff's law [3, 16, 33, 38].

To achieve osseointegration the biological activity of the bone must therefore make up this loss of anchorage quality by increased integration of the implant. This implant integration in the bone ensures the long-term fixation.

In the initial appositional bone formation stage, gaps of up to 1 mm can be bridged, the so-called "osteogenetic jumping distance." The same situation applies for the healing of gaps during stable osteosynthesis. However, the situation is less favorable for implants because, in contrast to fractures, the bone formation can proceed only one side [16, 24, 44–46].

Outer Form

The outer form of an artificial cementless hip joint cup takes account of several different factors. On the one hand, there are cup designs with conical or cylin-

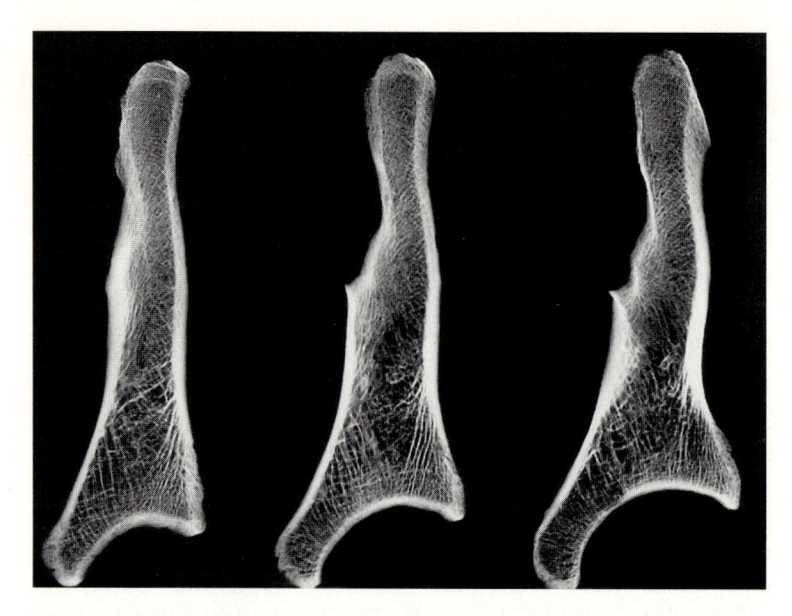

Fig. 1. Bone sections parallel to the linea arcuata show the elegant internal trabecular structure with direct orientation at a right angles to the principal loading zone of the cranial acetabulum and their transition to the corticalis. These bone sections lie mainly parallel to the resulting hip forces in lateral view as calculated by Paul [27]

drical shapes and, on the other, cups with a spherical outer form. A conical outer form necessitates significantly more bone loss during the preparation of the osseous bed, and the previous physiological spherical form of the natural osseous cup for load transfer is lost. Spherical cup forms, however, permit a substantial saving of bone during preparation and preserve the previous physiological load transfer into a spherical shape in the acetabular bone. Load transfer in the pelvis takes place via the corticalis and the associated spongiosa structure [17]. The strongest spongiosa trabeculae are in the peripheral area around the osseous cup, particularly in the main loading area. This morphological situation should be preserved as much as possible (Fig. 1).

Where the anchoring element is an integral part of the implant design, we speak of an intrinsic fixation system. This is the case with threaded or press-fit cups (friction hold) had which are larger than the reamed size. Where the anchoring element is an accessory to the implant, we speak of an extrinsic fixation system. This is the case for cups which are anchored in the bone using additional screws or pins [47].

Value of Animal Experiments

Monitoring the quality of new developments in hip endoprosthetics is not without problems. The clinical and radiographic routine checks require at least an observation period of 5 years or more, and have only limited significance. The most important parameter, namely systematic histological investigations on human specimens, is difficult to obtain. This is why animal experiments are important in this area of work. The reaction of bone to the implant can be investigated systematically. Account must be taken not only of the biomechanical differences of the quadruped but also of the nonequivalence of animal and human bone [5, 6, 13, 18, 20, 33].

The Press-Fit Cup as an Artificial Hip Joint Cup Implant for Humans
The special design and elasticity of this implant achieves a uniform distribution of pressure transfer into the bone, which is concentrated primarily around the rim of the cup. During implantation the acetabulum is reamed to a diameter 1.5 mm less than the nominal diameter of the cup. This "oversize" gives a peripheral interference fit when the cup is impacted into place, providing a solid primary fixation. Anchorage is provided by the friction fit principle. The requirement for good primary fixation is achieved by the so-called "press-fit" mechanism.

The implant surface in direct contact with the bone consists of a mesh shell (Sulmesh; Sulzer, Switzerland). Sulmesh consists of a precisely aligned, resistance-welded four-layer mesh structure with exactly defined pore size and porosity, firmly bonded into the polyethylene. The mesh is manufactured from pure titanium wire. The total mesh thickness is 2.3–2.6 mm. This gives a pore size of 400–600 μm and a porosity of maximum 65 %.

The elasticity of the implant is reduced by the Sulmesh shell. Despite this it is higher than with a solid metal shell. This preserves a relatively high cup elasticity.

The basic spherical form of the press-fit cup permits a minimal amount of removal of bone during surgery. The existing physiological spherical form, and the integrity of the load-transferring trabeculae is maintained. Reaming maintains the subchondral corticalis as far as possible. Reaming is continued to a depth where macroscopic blood spots become visible, permitting direct vital bone contact with the Sulmesh shell [3, 35, 36, 48].

Materials and Methodology

For the animal testing using sheep, appropriately sized press-fit cups were manufactured based on a series of radiographic cadaveric examinations of sheep to determine the average cup size. The outer form of these cups was the same as in the human implants. The cup diameter was 30 mm. The acetabulum was reamed to 29 mm, i. e., only 1 mm smaller than the cup. A good friction fit, or press-fit, is thus achieved with these dimensions.

For the animal test the Sulmesh shell was made from four layers in stainless steel, due to the fact that titanium mesh could not be manufactured with these dimensions. The steel mesh was therefore coated with titanium nitride to improve the biocompatibility. The total mesh thickness was about 2 mm. The pore size was 400 μm and porosity 65 % maximum. The polyethylene on the cup rim protruded a little and was provided with holes for the measuring instruments for rotational and tilting moments.

The mechanical quality of fixation until loosening of the cup was measured using a torque spanner which was directly attached to the artificial hip joint cups. The craniocaudal tilting moment was measured using a calibrated spring scale.

Determination of the Primary Mechanical Fixation

The acetabulum of the sheep cadaver was reamed similarly to human implantation, maintaining as much of the subchondral bony layers as possible. After checking the fit with a trial instrument, the press-fit cup was impacted home into the osseous bed. Immediately following this the torque necessary to rotate out or loosen the cup was measured. Similarly, using the spring scale, the craniocaudal tilting moment (in Newton-meters) was measured.

To compare the quality of various fixation systems a cemented cup and a threaded cup were also manufactured with the reduced dimensions of the sheep acetabulum and were tested using the same measuring methods.

Determination of the Secondary Biological Fixation

The left hip joints of eight mountain sheep were replaced with total endoprostheses. The operation was performed using the standard technique according to the veterinary medicine rules [28]. Following implantation of the press-fit cup, a prosthetic stem with a 16.5 mm diameter ceramic ball head was cemented into the femur using conventional methods. Using a special restrainer for 5 days, the operated animals were permitted controlled loading. Afterwards they were allowed free movement in a larger pen, providing full loading. Three weeks postoperatively all animals were allowed free range in an open meadow with full loading. Adequate movement and loading were spot checked using a load scale under the operated limb. Four animals each were killed at 8 and 52 weeks following implantation of the artificial hip joints. The pelvis was exposed, and the fixation quality of the artificial hip joint cup was determined. Fixation quality was determined using the same methods and measuring instruments as in the in vitro tests.

Histological Preparation

At the end of the implantation period the animals were sacrificed under narcosis, the pelvic region of the cadaver radiographed, and after determination of fixation quality conserved in alcohol. Afterwards the bone with the press-fit cup in situ was embedded in methylmethacrylate. The bone and cup were then prepared in 800 μm sections in craniocaudal direction using a wire saw. The individual 800 μm sections were first radiographed, giving a further assessment of conditions at the bone-implant interface. The most important sections were then ground down to 100 μm thickness. The specimens were colored using light green fuchsine for further histological examination. There were 269 specimens available for radiographic analysis and 52 for histological analysis.

Following this, an assessment was made of the bone penetration into the Sulmesh, its contact area with the Sulmesh, and the direction of the osseous trabeculae away from the Sulmesh surface. This quantitative assessment was carried out on the sections from the largest cup diameter. In each case, three sections were assessed.

Penetration. The depth of contiguous bone surfaces which had penetrated directly into the Sulmesh was measured. Additionally, the maximum depth of individual islands of bone within the Sulmesh was determined. The specimens colored using light green fuchsine were used, with a magnification x20. Determination was done by tracing, using a Nikon profile projector.

Surface contact. Contact between metal implant and bone was also traced out at 20x magnification and the lengths measured. The angle of the trabeculae proceeding from the Sulmesh was measured using the same sections, and compared to the resulting force.

Results

Primary Fixation In Vitro

Figure 2 shows the average measured values of torque and tilting moment needed to loosen the cups from their fixation in the cadaveric acetabulum. The

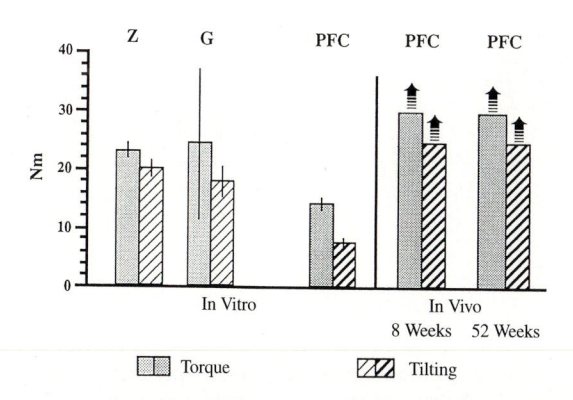

Fig. 2. In vitro and in vivo loosening moment for various cup types. *Columns*, average value (mean ± 1 SD); Z, cemented cup; G, threaded cup; *PFC*, Press-Fit Cup

separation moment values are given in Newton-meters. The accuracy of measurement was 0.5 Nm, corresponding to the accuracy of the instruments as determined at calibration. Six to eight measurements were carried out on each type of cup.

The cemented cups required on average 23 Nm (22–25 Nm) torque and 20 Nm (18–21 Nm) tilting moment to loosen the cup from the osseous bed. In some cases the cement was partly torn from the osseous bed. There were two 4.5 mm anchoring holes in the cranial portion of the cups. The cement thickness was 1–2 mm. We are therefore dealing here, on the one hand, with fixation values between polyethylene and cement and, on the other, between cement and bone. Bone fracture was not observed.

The threaded cups required on average 24 Nm (12–40 Nm) torque and 18 Nm (15–20 Nm) tilting moment to loosen the cup from the bone. The force used to cause bone fracture varied considerably depending upon the fit of the thread and the penetration into the osseous bed, and the variation was large as a result. In this case the relationship of bone strength values to bone thickness was determined.

The press-fit cups required on average 14 Nm (12–15 Nm) torque and 7.5 Nm (7–8 Nm) tilting moment to loosen the cup from the osseous bed. Bone fracture was not detected. The measured values therefore indicate specific cup interference fit values in the osseous bed, i. e., the friction fit or press-fit mechanism immediately following impacting the cup into place.

Secondary Biological Fixation in Vivo

After 8 weeks and after 52 weeks it was found that the previously used measuring methods were not sufficient to rotate or tip the cups from their implanted position. For all eight cups the measuring instrument attached to the polyethylene component was torn out of its anchoring, thereby deforming and destroying the polyethylene. The measured values of 30 Nm torque and 25 Nm

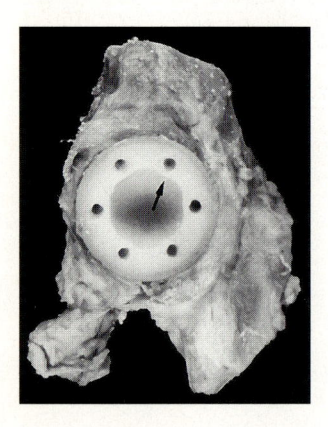

Fig. 3. Loosening test using in vivo specimen. Typical polyethylene deformation caused by torn-out attachment screws for the attachment of the measuring instrument (*arrow*)

tilting moment are therefore in fact those of the quality of the anchoring of the measuring instrument in the polyethylene of the press-fit cup (Figs. 2 and 3).

Microradiography and Histology

The radiographs in the craniocaudal direction of the 800 μm specimen sections of the implanted press-fit Sulmesh shells confirm direct bone contact with Sulmesh in the rim area. This bone contact is visible already after 8 weeks. The bone is not structured. There are not yet any directional trabeculae. On the other hand, 52 weeks after implantation the bone structure near the Sulmesh has clearly changed. The trabeculae are structured and directed into the mesh shell. The subchondral corticalis is integrated into the Sulmesh, and a gap can no longer be distinguished (Fig. 4).

The 100 μm histological sections also confirm intensive osseous ingrowth over one or two mesh layers, with direct bone contact with the titanium nitride coated surface. After 8 weeks there is also an unstructured formation of new bone in the Sulmesh. After 52 weeks a structuring of the bone trabeculae has taken place. These now consist of lamellar bone. Increased magnification shows close and/or direct bone contact with the surface of the Sulmesh. In particular, the mesh has been penetrated by bone, producing three-dimensional interlokking.

The quantitative assessment showed an average penetration depth of two mesh layers (0.5–1 mm). The covered Sulmesh surface was 30 %–40 %.

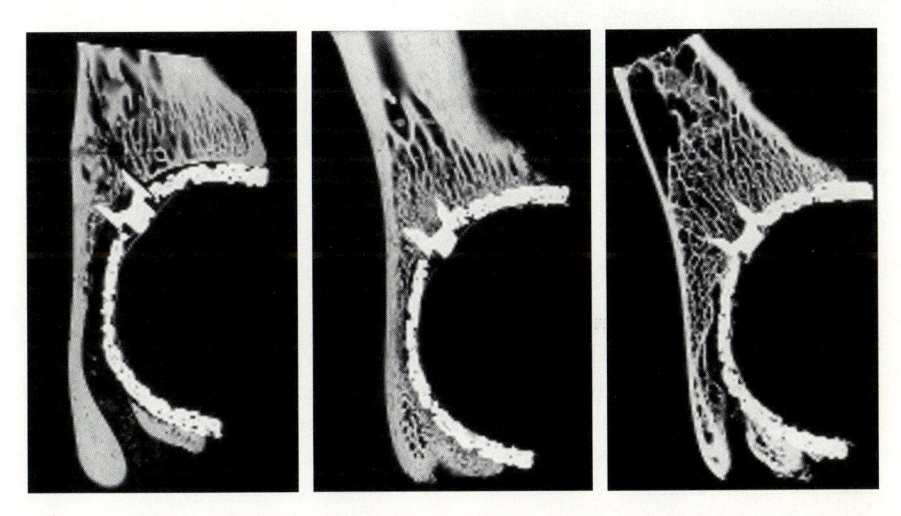

Fig. 4a-c. Radiographs of the 800-μm-thick cup sections. a Situation directly following implantation. Good rim contact with the Sulmesh shell. b Situation 8 weeks following implantation. Visible formation of new bone near the Sulmesh but not structured. c Situation 52 weeks after implantation. Alignment of the trabeculae into the Sulmesh. The gap between the subchondral corticalis is no longer visible

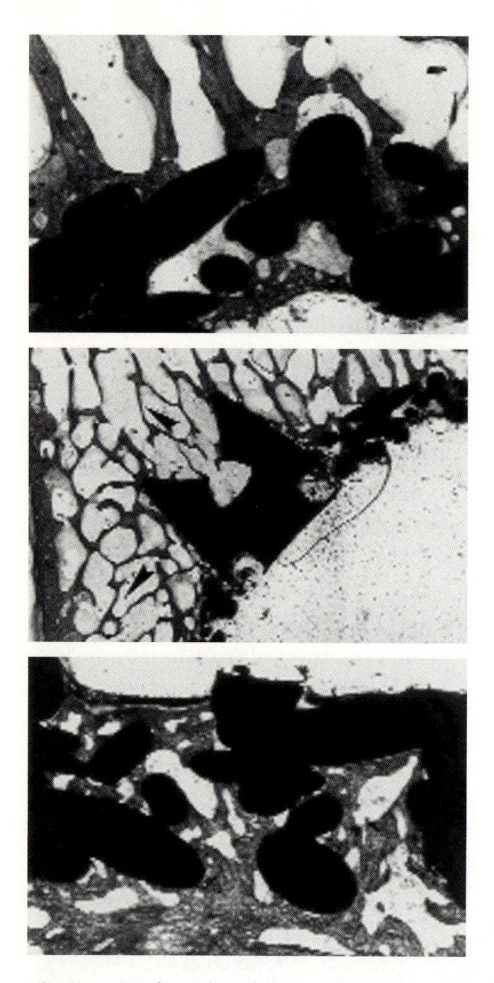

Fig. 5. a "Peduncular" bone contact. Transfer of compression forces in the main cranial loading area. x43. **b** Change in the trabecular alignment. Transfer of shear forces. x14. **c** Integration of the Sulmesh caudal. Transfer of tension forces. x43. *Gray*, bone; *black*, Sulmesh

The alignment of the trabeculae after 52 weeks corresponded precisely to the mechanical loading from the Sulmesh shell, so that the impression is gained that the Sulmesh replaces the subchondral corticalis. Depending on where the mechanical loading occurs, the transfer of compression, tension, and shear forces is provided by the alignment of the newly formed trabeculae (Fig. 5).

Discussion

The investigation of the primary and secondary fixation using animals showed that the fixation quality of the press-fit cup increases at least three times from 8 to 52 weeks in situ. Forces needed to loosen the cup from the osseous bed are higher and could not be determined due to limitations in the instrumentation. The limits of the measurement methodology had been reached. The biological activity of the bone provides an increasing interlocking and connection with the Sulmesh shell. The primary friction hold, which was responsible for the purely mechanical primary fixation, is thus transformed into a so-called keying hold, caused by the bone penetration into the porous Sulmesh surface.

The results of histological and radiological investigations show a restructuring of the loaded spongiosa trabeculae. On the one hand, their alignment corresponds to the forces occurring. On the other hand, newly formed bone grows into the Sulmesh shell with direct contact with the titanium nitride coated mesh wire. This explains the high quality of the fixation. For this reason we can speak of secondary biological fixation.

The newly formed bone proceeds through stages of osteosynthesis. In the first phase apposition causes new fibrous bone to form, improving the mechanical fixation in the first 8 weeks by interlocking. Following this, modeling and remodeling occurs as the bone reacts to the loading and the structure adjusts to the load transfer configuration. Under these circumstances we can speak of optimum osseointegration based on direct bone contact and an osseous structure adapted to the load transfer [9, 43]. Considering this aspect of osseointegration over time, the quantitative assessment of the depth and amount of bony ingrowth is secondary.

Depth of bone penetration and Sulmesh surfaces in contact with bone do not change significantly during the observation period between 8 and 52 weeks. The main difference between 8 and 52 weeks is in the remodeling, which adapts unstructured bone to the loading pattern. The situation after 52 weeks shows spongiosa trabeculae penetrating directly into the Sulmesh. The Sulmesh appears to assume the function of the subchondral corticalis, and the trabecular structure of the spongiosa appears identical to the normal anatomical-morphological structure. The implant scarcely changes the existing morphological conditions. The main force transfer occurs around the periphery, and the gentle spherical operative preparation requires only insignificant new remodeling of the spongiosa because the basic direction of the spongiosa trabeculae is maintained [17, 29].

The results available match well with those from similar animal experiments. Both sintered-on chromium-cobalt beads and pure titanium wire mesh were used to provide porous surfaces. Osseous ingrowth was better using titanium mesh, with very good primary fixation and a good fit of the porous surface with the bone interface. Additional HA sintering brought no significant improvement [15, 24, 25, 30, 31]. The press-fit cup design fulfills all of these requirements.

The in vitro cadaveric tests of fixation quality represent the conditions immediately following the implantation of the artificial hip joint cup. At that time biological reaction of the bone has not yet occurred. The fixation quality of the implant in this situation comes from its mechanical anchorage characteristics alone, provided by its design or attachment elements, in the case of the press-fit cup by friction fit. For this reason we speak of primary mechanical fixation.

Variations in the in vivo results for press-fit cup primary mechanical fixation are explained by differences in the size of the osseous cup. The higher values represent an optimal fit in the bone with deep acetabuli. With the lower values it was noted that the press-fit cup had penetrated less deeply into the bony structure of smaller acetabuli. As only one cup size was available, this inaccuracy had to be accepted. The variance in the measured results is considered minor.

The measurements were made directly following implantation. The effect on primary fixation due to creep and plastic behavior of the bone and the resulting decrease in the quality of primary fixation over time were ignored. The measured moment values reflect the optimal friction fit situation. The reduction in the expansion forces of the friction-fit due to plastic behavior of the bone can, however, be partially compensated for by muscular forces which press the cup into the osseous bed. Afterwards, however, the biological activity of the bone must assume or replace all purely mechanical fixation elements. These must be of sufficient quality that biological activity occurs in the form of osteosynthesis.

In this way adequate osseointegration, in the form of direct bone contact and an osseous structure adapted to the loading pattern, can be expected. Implants which respect the existing morphological conditions of the bone appear to give the bone less "work" to achieve integration.

References

1. Albrektsson T, Branemark Pl, Hansson HA, Lindström J (1981) Osseointegrated titanium implants. Acta Orthop Scand 52: 155-170
2. Amman W (1990) Komponenten des Befestigungssystems. Schweiz Baubl 86: 2–8
3. Bereiter H, Huggler AH, Jacob HAC (1989) Künstliche Hüftgelenke. Probleme und Fortschritte. Swiss Med 4: 7–18
4. Bereiter H, Bürgi M, Rahn B.H. (1992) Das zeitliche Verhalten der Verankerung einer zementfrei implantierten Hüftpfanne im Tierversuch. Orthopäde 21: 63–70
5. Bergmann G, Siraky J, Rohlmann A, Kölbl R (1984) A comparison of hip joint forces in sheep, dog and man. J Biomech 17: 907–921
6. Bergmann G, Graichen F, Rohlmann A (1993) Hip joint loading during walking and running measured in two patients. J Biomech 26/8: 969–990
7. Bobyn JD, Engh CA (1983) Biologic fixation of hip prostheses: review of the clinical status and current concepts. Adv Orthop Surg 7: 137–150
8. Bobyn JD, Pillar RM, Cameron U, Weatherly GC (1980) The optimum pore size for the fixation of porous-surfaced-metal-implants by the ingrowth of bone. Clin Orthop 150: 263–270

9. Brönemark PJ, Hansson BO, Adell R, Breine U, Lindström J, Hallén O, Ohmann A (1977) Osseointegrated implants in the treatment of the edentulous jaw. Experience from a 10year period. Scand J Plast Reconstr Surg Hand Surg 11: 1–32
10. Callaghan JJ (1993) The clinical results and basic science of total hip arthroplasty with porous-coated-prostheses. J Bone Joint Surg [Am] 75: 299–310
11. Cameron HU (1982) The results of early clinical trials with a microporous coated metal hip prosthesis. Clin Orthop 165: 188–190
12. Carlsson L, Röstlund T, Albrektsson B, Albrektsson T, Bränemark Pl (1986) Osseointegration of titanium implants. Acta Orthop Scand 57: 285–289
13. Chen PQ, Turner TM, Rinnigen H, Galante J, Urban R, Rostoker W (1983) A canine cementless total hip prosthesis model. Clin Orthop 176: 24–33
14. Clemow AJT, Weinstein AM, Klawitter JJ, Koeneman J, Anderson J (1981) Interface mechanics of porous titanium implants. J Biomed Mater Res 15: 73–82
15. Cockshutt JR, Schatzker J, Sumner-Smith G, Fornasier VL (1988) Biological fixation of a porous-coated-,metal-blacked-acetabular-component in canine total hip arthroplasty. VCOT 3: 141–145
16. Cowin SC (1990) Structural adaptation of bones. Appl Mech Rev 43/5: 126–133
17. Dalstra M, Huiskes R, Odgaards A, van Erning L (1993) Mechanical and textural properties of pelvic trabecular bone. J Biomech 26, 4/5: 523–535
18. Demeter G, Matyas J (1928) Mikroskopisch vergleichend-anatomische Studien an Röhrenknochen mit besonderer Rücksicht auf die Unterscheidung menschlicher und tierischer Knochen. Acta Anat 87: 45–97
19. Ducheyne P, De Meester P, Aernoudt E, Martens M, Mulier JC (1977) Influence of a functional dynamic loading on bone ingrowth into surface pores of orthopedic implants. J Biomed Mater Res 11: 811–838
20. Eitel F, Seiler H, Schweiberer L (1981) Vergleichende morphologische Untersuchungen zur Übertragbarkeit tierexperimenteller Ergebnisse auf den Regenerationsprozeß des menschlichen Röhrenknochens. Unfallheilkunde 84: 250–254
21. Engh CA, Zeitl-Schaffer KF, Kukita Y, Sweet D (1993) Histological and radiographic assessment of well functioning porous-coated-acetabular-components. J Bone Joint Surg [Am] 75: 814–824
22. Galante J, Rostoker W, Lueck R, Ray RD (1971) Sintered fiber metal composites as a basis for attachment of implants to bone. J Bone Joint Surg [Am]) 53: 101–114
23. Galante J, Sumner DR, Gächter A (1987) Oberflächenstrukturen und Einwachsen von Knochen bei zementfrei fixierten Prothesen. Orthopäde 16: 197–205
24. Harris WH, White RE, McCarthy JC, Walker PS (1983) Bony ingrowth fixation of the acetabular component in canine hip joint arthroplasty. Clin Orthop 176: 7–11
25. Hedley AK, Kabo M, Kim W, Coster I, Amstutz HC (1983) Bony ingrowth fixation of newly designed acetabular components in a canine model. Clin Orthop 176: 12–23
26. Heekin RD, Callaghan JJ, Hopkinson WJ, Savory CG, Xenos JS (1993) The porous-coated-anatomic-total-hip-prosthesis, inserted without cement. J Bone Joint Surg [Am] 75: 77–91
27. Heimke G (1990) Osseo-integrated-implants, vol 1. CRC-Press, Boca Raton FL USA
28. Hohn RB, Olmestead ML, Turner TM, Matis U (1986) Der Hüftgelenksersatz beim Hund. Tierärztl Prax 14: 377–388
29. Huiskes R (1987) Finite element analysis of acetabular reconstruction. Noncemented threaded cups. Acta Orthop Scand 58: 620–625
30. Jasty M, Harris WH (1990) Experience with cementless porous-surfaced-acetabular-components. Orthop Reat Sci 1: 52–61
31. Jasty M, Rubash HE, Paiement GD, Bragdon CB, Parr J Harris WH (1992) Porous-coated-uncemented-components in experimental total hip arthroplasty in dogs. Clin Orthop 280: 300–309

32. Klawitter JJ, Weinstein AM (1974) The status of porous materials to obtain direct skeletal attachment by tissue ingrowth. Acta Orthop Belg 40/5-6: 755–765
33. Kummer B (1992) Knochenstruktur als Ergebnis eines Regelprozesses. Osteologie 1/1: 4–14
34. Morscher E (1992) Current status of acetabular fixation in primary total hip arthroplasty. Clin Orthop 274: 172–193
35. Morscher E, Bereiter H, Lampert Ch (1989) Cementless press-fit-cup. Clin Orthop 249: 12–20
36. Morscher E, Bereiter H, Bürgi M, Koller HJ, Semlitsch M, Weber H, Yurtsever M (1992) Sulmesh – a clinically proven implant surface. Sulzer Med J 92: 13–16
37. Paul JP (1976) Approaches to design: force actions transmitted by joints in the human body. Proc R Soc Lond [Bio] 192: 163–172
38. Perren SM, Huggler AH, Russenberger M et al. (1969) Reaktion der Kortikalis auf Kompression. Acta Orthop Scand Suppl 125: 4–13
39. Pilliar RM, Bratina WJ (1980) Micromechanical bonding at a porous surface structured implant interface – the effect on implant stressing. H Biomed Eng 2: 49–53
40. Pilliar RM, Lee JM, Maniatopoulos DDS (1986) Observations on the effect of movement on bone ingrowth into porous-surfaced implants. Clin Orthop 208: 108–113
41. Rehm G, Eligehausen R, Mallée R (1988) Befestigungstechnik. Betonkalender. Ernst, Berlin, S. 4–15
42. Sass F, Bouché Ch, Leitner A (Hrsg) (1974) Taschenbuch für den Maschinenbau. Springer Berlin Heidelberg New York
43. Schenk RK (1991) Reaktion des Knochens auf Implantate. In: Stuhler T (ed) Hüftkopfnekrose. Springer, Berlin Heidelberg New York Tokyo. S. 533–538
44. Schenk RK, Wehrli U (1989) Zur Reaktion des Knochens auf eine zementfreie SL-Femur-Revisionsprothese. Orthopäde 18: 454–462
45. Schenk RK, Willenegger H (1977) Zur Histologie der primären Knochenheilung. Modifikationen und Grenzen der Spaltheilung in Abhängigkeit von der Defektgröße. Unfallheilkunde 80: 155–160
46. Schwartz JT, Engh CA, Forte MR, Kukita Y, Grandia SK (1993) Evaluation of initial surface apposition in porous-coated-acetabular-components. Clin Orthop 293: 174–187
47. Ungetüm M, Blömer W (1987) Technologie der zementlosen Hüftendoprothetik. Orthopäde 16: 170–184
48. Weber H, Yurtsever M (1992) Sulmesh – a clinically proven implant surface. Sulzer Med J 92: 13–16
49. Weinans H, Huiskes R, Grootenboer HJ (1993) Quantitative analysis of bone reactions to relative motions at implant-bone-interfaces. J Biomech 26/11: 1271–1281
50. Wisniewsky GK (1988) Befestigungstechnik. Systeme und Komponenten stet zur Anwendung im Bauwesen. Moderne Industrie, Bibliothek der Technik 11

Primary Stability of Cemented and Noncemented Implants

E. Schneider

Introduction

The term primary stability refers to the relative motion which occurs at the interface between the prosthesis and bone or between the cement and bone immediately after implantation. This stability is defined as inversely proportional to the amount of movement. A large relative movement therefore reflects a low primary stability and vice versa. Because this relative motion is between 1 and 1 000 μm, it is also called micromotion. The concept of primary stability includes only situations prior to the beginning of tissue reactions. Consequently the relative motion occurring after the onset of ingrowth and remodeling reactions should be defined as secondary stability.

Primary stability is of considerable importance in regard to the loosening of endoprostheses because the amplitude (and perhaps the frequency) of motion at the interface between implant and bone are decisive in whether tissue is formed [72] or resorbed [71] and which properties the tissues produced exhibit. A direct bony attachment of the implant can be achieved only when the relative motion between the implant and the bone remains below a certain level. As the loosening of the implant is the result of all events at the interface, including those at the early stages, it is reasonable to consider primary stability as an important criterion in the development of prostheses [35]. A general request for such measurements as part of all preclinical investigations should therefore be discussed.

The relative motion occurring at the implant of the patient can be influenced in three ways: by prosthesis design, by implantation procedure, and by patient behavior.[a] Prosthesis design includes the application of a particular rationale for prosthesis function and anchorage by selection of the outer geometry, specific material, and surface properties as well as manufacturing and sterilizing conditions. This leads to a multitude of quantities which influence the primary stability. Many of these influence each other. They also depend on the various anatomical, biomechanical, and pathological conditions in the individual musculoskeletal system.[b] The quality of the implantation of a prosthesis, for example, the accuracy of fit achieved or the strength of fixation obtained, influences the relative motion. It depends among other things on the surgical approach, the skill of the operator, the instruments used, the morphology and quality of the bone bed, and the clinical course.[c] The behaviour of the patient, i. e., the extent of his activity, the kind and intensity of his rehabilitation, and chance events such as sudden falls or false steps, are also critical for the relative motion. Given a certain mechanical behavior of the prosthesis, the extent and direction of the load applied by the patient ultimately determines the motion at the interface.

The present work provides a systematic overview and evaluation of the methods to determine the primary stability currently known and discusses the significance of the factors influencing it. The differences between the femoral and acetabular components are considered aswell.

Methods To Determine Primary Stability

Primary stability can be determined mathematically by means of a numerical model, experimentally by in vitro measurements on appropriate specimens, or physiologically by acute measurements on man or animals.

The mathematical procedure has the advantage of allowing determination of the motions at all or at least at specifically selected locations in the interface and in several directions at the same time. It is suitable for parametric investigations in which, for example, the geometry or the material properties of the implant and the bone or the properties of the interface are varied. Numerous load situations considering all muscle forces can be analyzed. The disadvantages of the mathematical procedure are the relatively high effort in the formulation of the models, the simplified modeling of the tissues, and the difficulties in reproducing a realistic anchorage of the implants.

The experimental procedure in the laboratory allows a nearly realistic investigation of the actual implant with its true fixation in the bone. The same methods may be used to analyze implants which have already been implanted in humans or animals. The drawback of this method is the high effort for the measuring technique, the lack of available specimens, the differences between the specimens in regard to their anatomical, mechanical, and interfacial qualities, and the anatomical restrictions present (e. g., the minimal distance between two measurement points, which might reduce the number of transducers applicable). Only the situation immediately after the operation or at the time of extraction can be analyzed; later changes occurring by bone remodeling or ingrowth cannot be assessed.

Acute investigations on human beings or animals are limited today to single situations. The advantage here is that the changes under real conditions and over a period of time can be evaluated. The disadvantage is that the conditions of measuring, such as the magnitude, direction, and frequency of the loads applied, are difficult to control.

Numerical Methods

Finite element analysis (FEM) can be used to determine primary stability. Here the implant and the tissues are reproduced in a mathematical model consisting of numerous elements. The models reported in the literature are quite different in terms of their geometry, the selection of the element types and properties, the load cases, the conditions of the interface, and the criteria selected to estimate the relative motion. The majority of investigations using FEM concern themselves with the femoral component and noncemented implants. Cemented prostheses were investigated among others by Brown and Pedersen [10]. They analyzed the mechanical consequences of decreasing stiffness between the cement and the bone due to formation of a fibrous membrane. They found increasing stresses in the lateral cancellous bone, an increase in the bending moment in the prosthesis, and higher stresses in the cement. Although motions were not monitored explicitly, they must also have increased.

Cheal et al. [16] used an indirect measure, the shear force in the interface between a noncemented prosthesis and bone, as the criterion for assessing relative motion. They modeled a completely ingrown prosthesis by fully connected neighboring points at the interface. They compared its behavior to a prosthesis with identical geometry but consisting of different material and having a different load situation. Although the mathematical model would have allowed a calculation of three-dimensional motions, the authors confined their work to motions tangential to the plane of the prosthesis surface.

Several authors have calculated in their models of the femoral shaft the actual relative motion and worked out the effect of different conditions of friction. For this purpose Kuiper and Huiskes [47] used a planar, Rohlmann et al. [74], and Mandell et al. [55] a tubular simplified model of the femur. They modeled the behavior in the interface either by a special nonlinear element with [47] or without friction [55] or by stepwise elimination of the element connections [74]. Mandell et al. [55] also investigated the influence of the collar and the cone of the prosthesis.

Several authors have used three-dimensional models. Keaveny and Jaloszynskie [43] determined the components and the sum of the relative motion in space for two noncemented prostheses and investigated the influence of partial ingrowth and the effect of a collar. Natarajan et al. [60] worked on the effect of the coefficient of friction and the influence of interface stiffness. Konieczynski and coworkers [44, 45] determined the relative motion of a noncemented shaft in the femur axis (axial, torsional) for four different load situations during walking, and they also varied the quality of bone (normal and osteoporotic). Rubin et al. [75] studied another noncemented prosthesis under the loads occurring during single leg stance and stair climbing. In their model they allowed adhesive friction in the interface with corresponding shear stress or sliding friction with a value between 0.2 and 1.2. Weinans et al. [93] verified with their FEM model and additional mathematical procedures the close connection between the degeneration of interface fixation and the formation of a fibrous membrane in several implants. Davy and Katoozian [20] used the relative motion (and the shear stresses) in the interface as the criterion for calculation of an optimal shaft design.

The relative motion in the pelvis has not yet been examined by means of FEM. While the study of Kurtz et al. [48] concerns relative motion, they examined by means of an axisymmetric model how the gaps between polyethylene and titanium cup behave due to poor conformity between the constituent parts, and how important these motions are for the contact stresses between the femoral ball and the acetabular cup.

Experimental Methods

The experimental investigations are characterized by a wide variety of properties of the specimens, the kinds of loads applied, and the principles of the measuring methods. The bone specimens used are usually human and are preserved in different ways. It would be preferable to use freshly prepared specimens since previous research has shown that the viscoelastic properties of bone change after death [8, 51]. Storage of bones at $-20°C$ and single use after slow thawing is acceptable. The measurement of primary stability, for example, in bones preserved in formalin [24, 34, 57, 84, 85], must still be questioned as the influence of this method of preservation has so far only been examined for the elastic modulus of bone. Its influence in this case, however, has been found to be minor [81].

Various authors have used femora or pelves made of composites to exclude the influence of different geometries or bone properties [1, 9, 18, 23]. Some of these anatomical models of the musculoskeletal system were originally intended to improve the geometric perception or as a material to practice implantation, not as a bone substitute with comparable mechanical properties. Single studies [23] provide hints (but not with further documentation) that artificial and human bone behave similarly. Only one of these studies [7] is explicitly concerned with the primary stability of artificial bones.

Differences are found among many studies in the kind of loading. In most cases the load is quasistatic, i. e., a few (1–15) load cycles at a frequency of approximately 1 Hz are applied, and the relative motion is then taken at a fixed load amplitude. In dynamic load situations (Tab. 1) the number of cycles applied is the main difference:

    300   [27],
  2 000   [18],
  2 400   [77],
  2 500   [34],
  5 000   [23, 58],
 10 000   [63],
 20 000   [9],
 50 000   [26],

60 000 [39],
100 000 [84], and
1 000 000 [21].

Due to the setting process during the initial load cycles, there is practically always a big difference between quasistatic and dynamic measurements [34], so that the validity of the quasistatic measurements must be seriously doubted [84]. The number of cycles to reach an equilibrium depends on the implant, but normally it is less than 10 000. Both total motion and amplitude of motion under dynamic load must be determined.

The direction of the loads applied also differs and complicates a direct comparison between different studies. When examining femoral shafts, pure torsion of 5 Nm [3], 10 Nm [4], or 22 Nm [66] is used around the shaft axis. In other studies torsion is mixed with a transverse force [64], torsion is mixed with an axial force [23, 77], or a bending moment is generated by an oblique force with an angle of 9° [94] or 12° [92] in the frontal plane. Other mixtures of load situations, for example 12° and 5 Nm [15], 10° frontal and 9° sagittal [9] are also offered. Often, single leg stance, for example, at 20° and 8° [5], at 0° and 12° [12], or at 10° and 12° [34] as well as stair climbing [5, 25, 65] are utilized. Rising grom a sitting position at 68° and 8° [5] or 70° [34] is used less often.

Also in the pelvis different force directions are used. One group of studies derives its coordinate system from the orientation of the cup and applies either a pure compression force [56, 87], a torsional moment [17, 19, 90], or a tangential loosening moment [1, 67, 95]. The other group of studies uses a force directed relative to the pelvis, for example, in the direction of the hip reaction force during single leg stance at 21° medial and 12° ventral [50], at 16° and 10° [79], and at 15° and 10° [45]. Dynamic loads as in the femur have not as yet been applied to the pelvis.

Some authors do not measure the relative motion as a criterion of primary stability but the strength of the anchorage. In the femur Jansson et al. [36] determined the extraction resistance of the entire shaft in relation to the applied pressure during curing of the bone cement. Ohl et al. [66] determined the torsional strength of a prosthesis anchored in three different ways. Otani et al. [68] compared the torsional strength of different fixation methods after occurrence of a femoral fracture at prosthesis implantation. In the pelvis Curtis et al. [19] determined the maximum torque transferable from a specific hip cup to the pelvis. Lachiewicz et al. [50] compared the fixation strength of different models in torsion. The failure mechanism in the two studies does not agree with the loosening observed in the patients [67], so that such research cannot clarify the relationship between relative motion and ingrowth.

Relative motion as a criterion for primary stability has been measured in the pelvis by Markolf et al. [56], Giraud et al. [28], Schneider et al. [80], Perona et al. [70], and Kwong et al. [49]. Differences exist in the method of fixing the cup and the pelvis. In only two studies was the whole pelvis fixed physiologically [28,

80]. In all other studies the bone which surrounds the acetabulum was confined, or the pelvis was cast [69] and with that its deformation was reduced.

The measuring sensors have different working principles. Some authors [33, 69, 89] have used eddy current sensors. One or more linear variable differential transformers were used by others [3, 5, 26, 27, 32, 34]. The motion is often not measured at the place of occurrence but is transmitted by pins to the sensors. The accuracy of a good sensor lies in the region of ± 1.4 μm and ± 0,003° [5]. Optical sensors [7] and extensometers [12, 13, 14, 15, 24] were used.

Measuring motion in the pelvis is more difficult than that in the femur because there is less accessible space around the acetabulum, and because most sensors measure not only the relative motion but also the implant and bone deformation. Schneider et al. [79] and Perona et al. [69] measured the relative motion between three landmarks on the pelvis and three reference points on the implant. Markolf et al. [56] and Schneider et al. [79] also measured the relative motion between bone and implant in the highest point (apex) of the cup.

Gilbert et al. [27] postulated that for primary stability measurements the bone and implant may be regardet as rigid body. However, Berzins et al. [5] proved by comparative measurements in the proximal and distal shaft that this presumption is not justified.

Acute Methods

The methods termed acute in this context include radiological and intraoperative procedures on patients, measurements in animals, and determination of stability on retrieved prostheses.

The radiological measurements taken by means of conventional X-rays or by Einbildröntgenanalyse [88] during clinical examinations are not discussed here as these involve migration in the range of millimetres and not micromotions.

A higher resolution can be achieved by roentgen stereophotogrammetric analysis (RSA) developed by Selvik [82] or a similar procedure. This method uses two X-ray cameras to obtain the three-dimensional location of metal balls attached to the prosthesis and implanted into the surrounding bone. Migration can then be determined as the displacement of the prosthesis relative to the bone. This method has been applied, for example, by Kärrholm et al. [41] to determine the migration of noncemented prostheses. Subsidence of one type of implants of up to 2.1 mm, a lateral migration of up to 3.5 mm, and a rotation around the long axis of 3.4° was found. In a further study [40] these cases were classified correctly as being loose after only 6 months. RSA is especially suitable to detect the rotation of an implant. Nistor et al. [61, 62] found by RSA that a polyethylene-coated titanium prosthesis exhibited rotation of up to 7.4° and that a carbon fiber polysulfone prosthesis even turned by 16.2° after 36 months of use. A comparative study [53] of the primary fixation of screws made of polylactic acid and titanium carried out on 39 patients revealed that the use of resorbable screws led to increased migration after 12 months. The RSA method can determine migration earlier than conventional X-rays, but its use in measuring micromotion is further restricted because it is difficult for the patient to generate standardized loads to the prosthesis.

Harris et al. [31] reported on a simple mechanical device to measure the torsional stability of the femoral shaft intraoperatively. In revisions this method can be used to confirm, for example, a stable shaft in the presence of a loose cup. Attempts were also made by Vresilovic et al. [91] intraoperatively to quantify the stability and to correlate it with X-ray pictures, but the applied load was not quantified, and the motion was observed only with the naked eye.

In animal experiments the effects of controlled linear [83] and rotatory movements [11, 13] on the formation of the interface between implant and bone were examined. The use of hydroxyapatite [83] made it possible to replace by bone the motion-induced fibrous layer at movements below 150 μm. The experiment of Burke et al. [11] and its mathematical modeling using FEM [73] confirmed that ingrowth occurred at movements of approximately 40 μm, and that these were greatly dependent on the initial interface preload selected.

Histological investigations have been carried out, for example, to check the effect of fixation elements such as screws made of various materials by means of their ingrowth behavior [2] or to study the bony incorporation of particular implants [76]. Such measurements only show the situation at a single moment in time, i. e., at removal of the specimen. This state is the result not only of the stability created by the fixation elements but of all the processes prior to removal (loading, wear, details of surgery, etc.). The relationship to stability can only be estimated using this technique, not measured.

Measurements of stability on retrieved human femora were performed by O'Connors et al. [65]. In nine clinically stable specimens they found very small motions in the order of 5–25 μm between the implant and the cement and also between the cement and the bone. Tooke et al. [87] determined the micromotion in two kinds of cups from animal experiments and found that the cups with porous coating exhibited lower motion than the cups having a screw geometry. Zalenski et al. [96] compared the relative motion under in vivo conditions to those in the postoperative situation. The stability obtained in this animal test was extraordinarily high, and the motion measured after 6 months was only a few micrometers in the axial direction and approximately double under torsion.

Factors Influencing Primary Stability

A multitude of factors have an influence on the primary stability. These are discussed separately for the shaft and the cup. Many of these factors influence each other. The modification of one of these factors in the design process, for example, the coating of part of the prosthesis with hydroxyapatite, would in all probability influence the entire fixation behavior of the prosthesis.

Primary Stability of the Femoral Shaft

Length of the Prosthesis and Design of the Shaft

Bechtold et al [3] and Gustilo et al. [29] compared a short straight stem with a long curved one and found that the longer implant had a greater stability under torsion. Berzins et al. [5] and Callaghan et al. [15] also confirmed from a literature survey and their own measurements that a curved stem is more stable, but only under larger forces and only in the proximal part. Hua et al. [34] confirmed that only small differences exist between various shaft designs (symmetric, asymmetric, custom made) in the axial direction. On the other hand, the symmetric shaft was the least stable in torsion. The investigation by Walker et al. [92] also showed the smallest relative motion by an "anatomical" or exact fit prosthesis. The increasing misfit increased the motion although no torsional load was used.

Prosthesis Size

A larger prosthesis in the measurements by Gebauer et al. [26] resulted in an increasing stability because with every larger size (in the anatomical range) a better fit was obtained. At the same time, however, the danger of a fissure also increased.

Material Properties of the Shaft

Krushell et al. [46] calculated in a two-dimensional model and Rohlmann et al. [74] in a simplified tubular model that an elastic prosthesis with properties comparable to bone exhibits greater motion than a stiffer shaft made of titanium. Contrary to this, Cheal et al. [16] found in their FEM studies using shear stresses as a measure of relative motion that a prosthesis made of a stiffer material (cobalt-chrome) exhibits a higher degree of motion in the distal region of the shaft than a less stiff composite prosthesis. The result in the proximal part was exactly opposite and coincided with the first two studies. The model of Cheal is three-dimensional and may better represent the physiological reality by including all the active muscle forces in the respective activities. It is furthermore meaningful that in particular for the larger prosthesis sizes, the stiffness of the prosthesis is higher than that of bone. In contrast to this, the stiffness of a smaller prosthesis made of identical material can even be less thant that of the femur [22].

Surface Characteristics

A comparison of three different surfaces [39] showed the smallest motion at the macrotextured surface, follwoed by that of a sandblasted surface and a surface covered by sintered beads. A surface believed to be suitable with respect to ingrowth thus does not necessarily result in lower relative motion. A study of autopsy specimens [24] revealed that porous-coated prostheses in general show small relative motions. An increasing area of ingrowth led to a decrease in the motion. The movement of the distal shaft is especially sensitive to the dimensions of the coating [42], i. e., the more coating the prosthesis has in the long direction, the lower the motion is. The elimination of the coating on the lateral side in comparison to a full coating showed no difference [43], also not with different prostheses or with different coating lengths. A reduced friction in the distal shaft region of a prosthesis, for example, by means of a polished surface leads to increased relative motion [44], which must be compensated by appropriate means in the proximal part of the implant. Tooke et al. [87] showed with measurements in a dog model that a prosthesis with porous coating is stable after 4 months but that it always has more motion than a cemented stem.

Proximal or Distal Fixation

In the study by Gebauer et al. [26] a purely distal fixation led to large amplitudes of motion proximally. The effect of the distal end of the shaft is documented in the animal research of Jasty et al. [38]. A long smooth stem reduced the proximal micromotion. After ingrowth of bone in this area the distal shaft lost its additional stabilizing effect, but it also did not exhibit other negative effects. A temporary distal locking mechanism with screws in a shaft with press fit fixation significantly improved the primary stability in the axial and torsional direction [52]. This technique led to similarly positive results in the study of Blömer et al. [9]. Noble et al. [63] found that a good fit between the implant and the bone decreases the relative motion of noncemented stems, but that it also diminishes contact in the proximal part, which can lead to an increase in motion there. In the research of Ohl et al. [66] the lowest micromotions occurred under rotational loads when the distal and proximal regions were fixed at the same time. Mere proximal fixation was somewhat less stable; only distal fixation showed significant motion due to the flexibility of the shaft.

Collar

The effect of a collar was investigated [25] using an implant with a conical collar. It showed only an effect at loads with a rotatory component (e. g., stair climbing). The study of Keavey [42] showed that with a collar the size of the surface with ingrowth material is less important; the micromotion increased upon removal of the collar. The numerical study of Mandell et al. [55] also confirmed the reduced motion in the axial direction due to the effect of the collar. However, this analysis further showed that a collar has also a strain-reducing effect, and that with it the bone is more protected from stress. This effect can be reduced by a conical shape of the implant but only at the cost of increasing micromotion. Additional screw fixation of the collar in the region of the calcar also leads to reduced relative motion, especially in the axial direction [57].

Whiteside et al. [94] investigated the interplay between the collar and the distal fixation. The collar reduced the subsidence but not the lateral motions. A collar and a good distal fit were necessary to minimize micromotion.

Stabilizing Elements

Cook et al. [18] investigated various stabilizing elements, which through their additional filling of the medullary canal should improve stability. This was not the case. However, in the study by Nunn et al. [64] prostheses with longitudinal ridges of 1 mm height showed better rotational stability than smooth prostheses but remained less stable than the same prostheses with cement. Berzins et al. [6] found that a revision prosthesis implanted by means of allograft pieces in combination with cement was more stable than a noncemented prosthesis but still less stable than a conventional cemented shaft. Blömer et al. [9] also documented in revision prostheses the stabilizing effect of different elements such as double cone and interlocking screws. Heiner et al. [33] maintained that there is no differenc whether the distal part of a shaft inserted into an allograft is secured by press fitting or cement.

Interface Properties

Different investigations, first of all with FEM [60], have shown the importance of appropriate interfacial conditions (stiffness, coefficient of friction). But the effects depend on the directions of motion.

Types of Prostheses

Comparative studies have been carried out by several authors [58, 78]. The more similar the examined prostheses are, the more precise the consequences drawn from these studies can be. As the individual prosthetic models can often be distinguished in several aspects, only very detailed analyses of the motions in specific directions allow relevant conclusions. At the very least it was shown that the motions of single prostheses are as small as those of a cemented prosthesis.

Bone Properties

The primary stability of an implant in soft (cancellous) bone is less than in normal cortical bone [18]. The FEM study of Konieczynski et al. [44] shows that the increased motion of the prosthesis in a bone with reduced quality (osteoporosis) reflects the relation of the corresponding elastic moduli.

Load Conditions

It is not surprising that the direction and magnitude of the loads applied are decisive in the generation of relative motion. Investigations by Konieczynski et al. [43] with four different load situations further showed that the relative motion increases with load but not fully proportional. A change in the load conditions also changes the size of the contact area and the load distribution between the implant and the bone and with it the stiffness proportions. The primary stability should therefore always be determined at several load conditions (in different directions) and also perhaps at more than one load level.

Fissures

Fissures may occur as complications during prosthetic implanation. Unexpectedly, they did not lead to a higher relative motion [26]. On the other hand, in the study of Otani et al. [68] it was shown that after the occurrence of a fissure the torsional stability became particularly inadequate. An improvement was achieved by cerclage wires. The stability became comparable to a control group of unfractured femora when the cerclage was carried out prior to reinsertion of the prosthesis.

Implantation Technique

The study of Sugiyama et al [86] showed that an implantation technique based on press fit causes less micromotion than one based on exact fit.

Cement

Along with other authors, Butler et al. [14] and Burke et al. [12] confirmed the stabilizing effect of cement, especially for nonaxial load directions. This means for the noncemented prosthesis that bone apposition may be hindered because of the motions occurring under bending and torsion types of loads [37]. In a study of 11 retrieved autopsy specimens Maloney et al. [54] demonstrated the small relative motion in prostheses fixed by cement even after 17 years of service. This also means that at this point in time the bone strains had still not recovered the values of the intact femur. Various methods of cement fixation were compared by Sugiyama et al. [85]. Vacuum mixture and pressurized injection of cement were superior to other methods. Nevertheless, the authors found indications of failure for all cementation mehtods even at relatively low levels of torsional loads.

The Primary Stability of the Acetabular Cup

Design of the Cup

Adler et al. [1] found that the addition of screws or spikes was less important for primary stability than a clean surgical preparation and a good geometrical fit of the implant. This was indirectly confirmed by Anderson et al. [2] who examined dogs histologically and found no difference in ingrowth between the cups with press fit and after fixation with screws (titanium or polylactic acid). In the research of Clarke et al. [17] pegs resulted in a remarkably stronger fixation than screws. Lachiewicz et al. [50], however, found that screw fixation is stronger than pegs. Perona et al. [70] found the highest relative motion for a hemispherical cup with press fit, screws diminished the motion, but the cemented cup was the most stable. The ilium showed the least stability; the pubis and the ischium showed better stability. Kwong et al. [49] showed that with an undersized reaming of 1 mm, the use of screws did not improve the relative motion. Identical dimensions for reamer and implant led to more micromotion, which then could be compensated with screws. No difference was found by Lachiewicz et al. [50] in the relative motion at differnt fixation methods. The fixation strength of a surface mesh manufactured from titanium wires was confirmed in animal testing [59].

Fit of the Cup

Adler et al. [1] found that the diameter and depth of the surgically prepared acetabulum is important. They measured the highest moments of loosening torque at an acetabulum reamed 1 mm too small. Poor bone quality increased this value to 2 mm. Curtis et al. [19] found this misfit to be even higher (2–3 mm). The limit to the pelvic fissure was reached at 4 mm. In the study of Kwong et al. [49] the implant could not be completely inserted with a misfit of 2 mm. The optimal value of misfit seemed to be 1 mm. The experimental study of Yerby et al. [95] showed that a hemispherical cup has several advantages over a cup with double radii. It requires a smaller effort for implantation and still provides greater strength against breaking loose. Moreover, the stresses induced in the pelvis are smaller. The FEM study of Hansen et al. [30] showed that the yield stress of bone is reached at a misfit of 1 mm. Bones submitted to a higher misfit undergoes plastic behavior. The study also showed that the stresses induced in the pelvis during walking are an order of magnitude smaller than the stresses induced by misfit. Volz et al. [90] found that a higher torsional strength for a cemented cup is obtained when (a) the acetabulum is reamed sufficiently to completely seat the implant, (b) when all the cartilage is removed, and (c) when the subchondral plate is removed, and holes for additional fixation of the cement are drilled.

Subchondral Bone Plate

Removal of the subchondral bone plate increases the relative motion [56].

Summary

To summarize, in a numerical study the details of the model are of considerable importance, especially interface properties. Reasonable friction coefficients alone can simulate the motion patterns observed experimentally [47, 75]. The loads must be physiological and should include different load cases. The local distribution of the mechanical properties and the dimensional relationship between the implant and bone must be considered. In experimental studies an implantation technique that is near reality is important. The number of specimens used must be sufficiently high and their properties known. The great differences between the results from statically and dynamically loaded prostheses [46, 84] underline the necessity of dynamic loading. Comparative experiments between largely different implants [84] must be interpreted reluctantly. A better possibility is the comparison of geometrically similar prostheses [78] or the specific variation of a single design parameter.

Knowledge of the scale of micromotions and the factors that influence it will be important for future biomechanical studies. Such data can serve to study changes in the properties of bone and the formation of intermediate layers, for example, by ways of mathematical simulations [93] and to predict, if possible, the future behavior of the implants.

In general, primary stability is assumed ideally to be zero, or at least as small as possible to guarantee ingrowth. However, further studies may show that in parallel to current thinking in the field of fracture healing, a certain relative motion is necessary and could lead to better results.

References

1. Adler E, Stuchin SA, Kummer FJ (1992) Stability of press-fit acetabular cups. J Arthroplasty 7: 295–301
2. Anderson G, Greis PE, Klein AH, Rubash HE (1992) Alternative methods of acetabular fixation in a canine total hip replacement model. Trans 38th Annu ORS 17: 318
3. Bechtold JE, Bianco PT, Kyle RF, Gustilo RB (1988) Experimental evaluation of strain and stability for short stem and long curved stem uncemented femoral prostheses in torsion and stance loading. Trans 34th Annu ORS 13: 348
4. Bechtold JE, Bianco PT, Gustilo RB, Kyle RF (1989) Rotational stability of uncemented femoral prostheses – the role of stem curvature and length. Trans 35th Ann ORS 14: 380
5. Berzins A, Sumner DR, Andriacchi TP, Galante JO (1993) Stem curvature and load angle influence the initial relative bone implant motion of cementless femoral stems. J Orthop Res 11: 758–769
6. Berzins A, Wasielewski RC, Sumner DR (1993) Implant stability in revision THA: the role of allograft packing and cementing. Trans 39th Annu ORS 18: 518
7. Bianco PT, Bechtold JE, Kyle RF, Gustilo RB (1989) Synthetic composite femurs for use in evaluation of torsional stability of cementless femoral prostheses. AMD 98: 297–300
8. Black J (1984) Tissue properties: relationship of in vitro studies to in vivo behavior. In: Hastings GW, Ducheyne P (eds) Natural and living biomaterials. CRC Press, Boca Raton, pp 5–26
9. Blömer W, Fink U, Ungethüm M (1994) Biomechanische Aspekte zementfreier Revisionsendoprothesen des Hüftgelenks. Trans Biomech (in press)
10. Brown TD, Pedersen DR (1988) Global mechanical consequences of reduced cement/

bone coupling rigidity in proximal femoral arthroplasty: a three-dimensional finite element analysis. J Biomech 21: 115–129
11. Burke DW, Bragdon CR, O'Connor DO, Jasty M, Haire T, Harris WH (1991) Dynamic measurement of interface mechanics in vivo and the effect of micromotion on bone ingrowth into a porous surface device under controlled loads in vivo. Trans 37th Annu ORS 16: 103
12. Burke DW, O'Connor DO, Zalenski EB, Jasty M, Harris WH (1991) Micromotion of cemented and uncemented femoral components. J Bone Joint Surg [Br] 73: 33–37
13. Burke DW, Bragdon CR, Lowenstein JD (1993) Mechanical aspects of the bone-porous surface interface under known amounts of implant motion: an in vivo canine study. Trans 39th Annu ORS 18: 470
14. Butler CA, Jones LC, Hungerford DS (1988) Initial implant stability of porous coated total hip femoral components; a mechanical study of micromovement. Trans 34th Annu ORS 13: 549
15. Callaghan JJ, Fulghum CS, Glisson RR, Stranne SK (1992) The effect of femoral stem geometry on interface motion in uncemented porous-coated total hip prostheses. Comparison of straight-stem and curved-stem designs. J Bone Joint Surg [Am] 74: 839–848
16. Cheal EJ, Spector M, Hayes WC (1992) Role of loads and prosthesis material properties on the mechanics of the proximal femur after total hip arthroplasty. J Orthop Res 10: 405–422
17. Clarke HJ, Jinnah RH, Warden KE, Cox QG, Curtis MJ (1991) Evaluation of acetabular stability in uncemented prostheses. J Arthroplasty 6: 335–340
18. Cook SD, Averill RG, Manley MT, Cohen RC (1991) Effect of stem fit, shape, bone quality, and proximal modularity on the torsional stability of pressfit hip stems. Trans 37th Annu ORS 16: 530
19. Curtis MJ, Jinnah RH, Wilson VD, Hungerford DS (1992) The initial stability of uncemented acetabular components. J Bone Joint Surg [Br] 74: 372–376
20. Davy DT, Katoozian H (1994) Three-dimensional shape optimization of femoral components of hip prostheses with frictional interfaces. Trans 40th Annu ORS 19: 223
21. Dienel R, Jungnickel I, Holzweissig F, Manitz L, Hellinger J (1984) Mikrobewegungen von zementfixierten Hüftendoprothesenschäften in Leichenfemora. Beitr Orthop Traumatol 31: 151–158
22. Dujovne AR, Bobyn JD, Krygier JJ, Miller JE, Brooks CE (1993) Mechanical compatibility of noncemented hip prostheses with the human femur. J Arthroplasty 8: 7–22
23. Ebramzadeh E, McKellop H, Wilson M, Sarmiento A (1988) Design factors affecting micromotion of porous-coated and low modulus total hip prostheses. Trans 34th Annu ORS 13: 351
24. Engh CA, O'Connor D, Jasty M, McGovern TF, Bobyn JD, Harris WH (1992) Quantification of implant micromotion, strain shielding, and bone resorption with porous-coated anatomic medullary locking femoral prostheses. Clin Orthop 285: 13–29
25. Fischer KJ, Carter DR, Maloney WJ (1992) In vitro study of initial stability of a conical collared femoral component. J Arthroplasty (Suppl) 7: 389–395
26. Gebauer D, Refior HJ, Haake M (1990) Experimentelle Untersuchungen zum Einfluß operationstechnischer Fehler auf die Primärstabilität zementloser Hüftendoprothesenschäfte. Z Orthop 128: 100–107
27. Gilbert JL, Bloomfeld RS, Lautenschlager EP, Wixson RL (1992) A computer-based biomechanical analysis of the three-dimensional motion of cementless hip prostheses. J Biomech 25: 329–340
28. Giraud P, Schneider E, Kempf I (1991) A study of primary motion and deformation of the peri-acetabular area under static load. Chirurgie 117: 732–736
29. Gustilo RB, Bechtold JE, Giacchetto J, Kyle RF (1989) Rationale, experience, and results of long-stem femoral prosthesis. Clin Orthop 249: 159–168

30. Hansen TM, Koeneman JB, Hedley AK (1992) 3-D FEM analysis of interference fixation of acetabular implants. Trans 38th Annu ORS 17: 400
31. Harris WH, Mulroy RD,Jr., Maloney WJ, Burke DW, Chandler HP, Zalenski EB (1991) Intraoperative measurement of rotational stability of femoral components of total hip arthroplasty. Clin Orthop 266: 119–126
32. Hayes DEE Jr, Bargar WL, Paul HA, Taylor JK (1992) Three dimensional micromotion of femoral prostheses. Trans 38th Annu ORS 17: 380
33. Heiner JP, Manley PA, Kohles SS, Vanderby R Jr., Markel MO (1993) Canine hip replacement with proximal femoral grafts: a comparison of cemented versus press-fit distal fixation. Trans 39th Annu ORS 18: 523
34. Hua J, Walker PS (1994) Relative motion of hip stems under load. An in vitro study of symmetrical, asymmetrical, and custom asymmetrical designs. J Bone Joint Surg [Am] 76: 95–103
35. Huiskes R (1993) Failed innovation in total hip replacement. Diagnosis and proposals for a cure. Acta Orthop Scand 64: 699–716
36. Jansson V, Zimmer M, Kuhne JH, Sailer FP (1993) [Initial stability of an implanted cement-canal prosthesis. Results in experimental studies on human cadaver femurs]. Z Orthop 131: 377–381
37. Jasty M, Burke D, Harris WH (1992) Biomechanics of cemented and cementless prostheses. Chir Organi Mov 77: 349–358
38. Jasty M, Krushell R, Zalenski E, O'Connor D, Sedlacek R, Harris W (1993) The contribution of the nonporous distal stem to the stability of proximally porous-coated canine femoral components. J Arthroplasty 8: 33–41
39. Kamaric E, Noble PC, Alexander JW (1989) The effect of proximal surface texture on the acute stability of cementless fixation. Trans 35th Annu ORS 14: 382
40. Kärrholm J, Borssen B, Löwenhielm G, Snorrason F (1994) Early micromotion in cemented femoral stems subsequently revised due to pain or osteolysis. Trans 40th Annu ORS 19: 246
41. Kärrholm J, Snorrason F (1993) Subsidence, tip, and hump micromovements of noncoated ribbed femoral prostheses. Clin Orthop 287: 50-60
42. Keaveny TM (1992) Relative motion for a Moore-type cementless hip prosthesis in the early post-operative situation. Trans 38th Annu ORS 17: 379
43. Keaveny TM, Jaloszynski RL (1994) Effects of circumferential vs. medial-only porous coating for THA cementless fixation. Trans 40th Annu ORS 19: 220
44. Konieczynski DD, Bartel DL (1993) The effects of bone quality and interface friction on early post-operative performance of an anatomic noncemented implant. Trans 39th Annu ORS 18: 447
45. Konieczynski DD, Bartel DL (1994) The role of loading on the immediate post-operative stability of a noncemented hip implant. Trans 40th Annu ORS 19: 222
46. Krushell RJ, Burke DW, Harris WH (1991) Elevated-rim acetabular components. Effect on range of motion and stability in total hip arthroplasty. J Arthroplasty (Suppl) 6: 53–58
47. Kuiper JH, Huiskes R (1993) Finite element simulation of dynamic micro-motion at the interface of bone and prosthesis. Trans 39th Annu ORS 18: 440
48. Kurtz SM, Bartel DL, Edidin AA (1994) The effect of gaps on contact stress and relative motion in a metal-backed acetabular component for THR. Trans 40th Annu ORS 19: 243
49. Kwong LM, O'Connor DO, Sedlacek RC, Krushell RJ, Maloney WJ, Harris WH (1994) A quantitative in vitro assessment of fit and screw fixation on the stability of a cementless hemispherical acetabular component. J Arthroplasty 9: 163–170
50. Lachiewicz PF, Suh PB, Gilbert JA (1989) In vitro initial fixation of porous-coated acetabular total hip components. A biomechanical comparative study. J Arthroplasty 4: 201–205

51. Linde F, Sorensen HCF (1993) The effect of different storage methods on the mechanical properties of trabecular bone. J Biomech 26: 1249–1252
52. Mahomed N, Schatzker J, Hearn T (1993) Biomechanical analysis of a distally interlocked press-fit femoral total hip prosthesis. J Arthroplasty 8: 129–132
53. Malchau H, Kärrholm J, Thanner J, Wallinder L, Geijer M, Herberts P (1994) Bioresorbable vs. titanium screws in acetabular cup fixation: a prospective randomised evaluation using stereoradiography. Trans 40th Annu ORS 19: 287
54. Maloney WJ, Jasty M, Burke DW, O'Connor DO, Zalenski EB, Bragdon C, Harris WH (1989) Biomechanical and histologic investigation of cemented total hip arthroplasties. A study of autopsy-retrieved femurs after in vivo cycling. Clin Orthop 249: 129–140
55. Mandell JA, Beaupré GS, Goodman SB, Carter DR (1994) The influence of femoral component collar or taper on stress transfer and micromotion. Trans 40th Annu ORS 19: 224
56. Markolf KL, Amstutz HC (1983) Compressive deformations of the acetabulum during in vitro loading. Clin Orthop 173: 284–292
57. Martin JW, Sugiyama H, Kaiser AD, Van Hoech J, Whiteside LA (1990) An analysis of screw fixation of the femoral component in cementless hip arthroplasty. J Arthroplasty (Suppl) 5: 15–20
58. McKellop H, Ebramzadeh E, Niederer PG, Sarmiento A (1991) Comparison of the stability of press-fit hip prosthesis femoral stems using a synthetic model femur (erratum, J Orthop Res (1991) Nov; 9 (6): 933.) J Orthop Res 9: 297–305
59. Morscher E, Bereiter H, Lampert C (1989) Cementless pressfit cup. Principles, experimental data, and three-year follow-up study. Clin Orthop 249: 12–20
60. Natarajan RN, Andriacchi TP, Sumner DR (1994) Micromotion in curved uncemented femoral stem depends on both the interface friction and stiffness. Trans 40th Annu ORS 19: 221
61. Nistor L, Blaha JD, Kjellstrom U, Selvik G (1991) In vivo measurements of relative motion between an uncemented femoral total hip component and the femur by roentgen stereophotogrammetric analysis. Clin Orthop 287: 220–227
62. Nistor L, Lundberg A, Ackerholm P (1994) Rotation and subsidence of a composite femoral component analysed by roentgen stereophotogrammetry. Trans 40th Annu ORS 19: 245
63. Noble PC, Kamaric E, Alexander JW (1989) Distal stem centralization critically affects the acute fixation of cementless femoral stems. Trans 35th Annu ORS 14: 381
64. Nunn D, Freeman MA, Tanner KE, Bonfield W (1989) Torsional stability of the femoral component of hip arthroplasty. Response to an anteriorly applied load. J Bone Joint Surg [Br] 71: 452–455
65. O'Connor DO, Burke DW, Sedlacek RC, Lozynsky AJ (1993) Cement bone vs. implant bone micromotion on autopsy retrieved cemented femoral components. Trans 39th Annu ORS 18: 248
66. Ohl MD, Whiteside LA, McCarthy DS, White SE (1993) Torsional fixation of a modular femoral hip component. Clin Orthop 287: 135–141
67. Ohlin A, Balkfors B (1992) Stability of cemented sockets after 3–14 years. J Arthroplasty 7:87–92
68. Otani T, Lux PS, Capello WN (1993) Wiring technique to improve torsional stability of the cementless femoral component in THA associated with a surgically induced femoral fracture. Trans 39th Annu ORS 18: 451
69. Perona PG, Lawrence J, Paprosky WG (1992) Initial acetabular component stability: an in vitro comparison of cemented and cementless acetabular components. Trans 38th Annual ORS 17: 398
70. Perona PG, Lawrence J, Paprosky WG, Patwardhan AG, Sartori M (1992) Acetabular micromotion as a measure of initial implant stability in primary hip arthroplasty. An in

vitro comparison of different methods of initial acetabular component fixation. J Arthroplasty 7: 537–547
71. Perren SM, Boitzy A (1978) La différenciation cellulaire et la biomechanique de l'os au cours de la consolidation d'une fracture. Anat Clin 1: 12
72. Pilliar RM, Lee JM, Maniatopoulos C (1986) Observations of the effect of movement on bone ingrowth into porous-surfaced implants. Clin Orthop 208: 108–113
73. Ramamurti BS, Orr TE, DiGioia (III) AM, Bragdon CR, Jasty M, Harris WH (1994) An investigation of the implant bone interface of an in vivo micromotion canine experiment using finite element analysis. Trans 40th Annu ORS 19: 244
74. Rohlmann A, Cheal EJ, Hayes WC, Bergmann G (1988) A nonlinear finite element analysis of interface conditions in porous coated hip endoprostheses. J Biomech 21: 605–611
75. Rubin PJ, Rakotomanana RL, Leyvraz PF, Zysset PK, Curnier A, Heegaard JH (1993) Frictional interface micromotions and anisotropic stress distribution in a femoral total hip component. J Biomech 26:725–739
76. Schenk RK, Wehrli U (1989) Reaction of the bone to a cement free SL femur revision prosthesis. Histologic findings in an autopsy specimen 5 1/2 months after surgery Orthopäde 18:454–462
77. Schneider E, Eulenberger J, Steiner W, Wyder D, Friedman RJ, Perren SM (1989) Experimental method for the in vitro testing of the initial stability of cementless hip prostheses. J Biomech 22: 735–744
78. Schneider E, Kinast C, Eulenberger J, Wyder D, Eskilsson G, Perren SM (1989) A comparative study of the initial stability of cementless hip prostheses. Clin Orthop 248: 200–209
79. Schneider E, Giraud P, Schönenberger U, Eulenberger J, Wyder D, Seelig W, Schläpfer F, Frick W (1991) Primärstabilität zementierter und zementfreier Hüftprothesen. In: Stuhler T (ed) Hüftkopfnekrose. Springer, Berlin Heidelberg New York Tokyo, pp 565–574
80. Schneider E, Schönenberger U, Giraud P, Bürgi M (1992) Primärstabilität und Beckendeformation bei zementierten und nichtzementierten Hüftpfannen. Orthopäde 21: 57–62
81. Sedlin ED, Hirsch C (1966) Factors affecting the determination of the physical properties of femoral cortical bone. Acta Orthop Scand 37: 29
82. Selvik G (1989) Roentgen stereophotogrammetry. A method for the study of the kinematics of the skeletal system. Acta Orthop Scand (Suppl 60) 232: 1–51
83. Soballe K, Hansen ES, Rasmussen HB, Bünger C (1992) Hydroxyapatite coating converts fibrous anchorage to bony fixation during continuous implant loading. Trans 38th Annu ORS 17: 292
84. Stiehl JB, MacMillan E, Skrade DA (1991) Mechanical stability of porous-coated acetabular components in total hip arthroplasty. J Arthroplasty 6: 295–300
85. Sugiyama H, Whiteside LA, Kaiser AD (1989) Examination of rotational fixation of the femoral component in total hip arthroplasty. A mechanical study of micromovement and acoustic emission. Clin Orthop 249: 122–128
86. Sugiyama H, Whiteside LA, Engh CA (1992) Torsional fixation of the femoral component in total hip arthroplasty. The effect of surgical press-fit technique. Clin Orthop 249: 187–193
87. Tooke SM, Nugent PJ, Chotivichit A, Goodman W, Kabo JM (1988) Comparison of in vivo cementless acetabular fixation. Clin Orthop 235: 253–260
88. Tschupik JP (1988) Grundlagen und Strategien des problemspezifischen Röntgenbildmessverfahrens EBRA (Einbildröntgenanalyse). In: Russe W (ed) Röntgenphotogrammetrie der künstlichen Hüftgelenkspfanne. Huber, Bern, pp 16–41
89. Vanderby R Jr., Manley PA, Kohles SS, McBeath AA (1992) Fixation stability of femoral components in a canine hip replacement model. J Orthop Res 10: 300–309
90. Volz RG, Wilson RJ (1977) Factors affecting the mechanical stability of the cemented acetabular component in total hip replacement. J Bone Joint Surg [Am] 59: 501–504

91. Vresilovic EJ, Hozack W, Rothman RH (1994) Radiographic assessment of cementless femoral components. J Arthroplasty 9: 137–141
92. Walker PS, Schneeweis D, Murphy S, Nelson P (1987) Strains and micromotions of press-fit femoral stem prostheses. J Biomech 20: 693–702
93. Weinans H, Huiskes R, Grootenboer HJ (1993) Quantitative analysis of bone reactions to relative motions at implant-bone interfaces. J Biomech 26: 1271–1281
94. Whiteside LA, Easley JC (1989) The effect of collar and distal stem fixation on micromotion of the femoral stem in uncemented total hip arthroplasty. Clin Orthop 239: 145–153
95. Yerby SA, Taylor JK, Murzic W (1992) Acetabular component interface: press-fit fixation. Trans 38th Annu ORS 17: 384
96. Zalenski E, Jasty M, O'Connor DO, Page A, Krushell R, Bragdon C, Russotti G, Harris WH (1989) Micromotion of porous-surfaced, cementless prostheses following 6 months of in vivo bone ingrowth in a canine model. Trans 35th Annu ORS 14: 377

Gait Analysis: A Biomechanical Tool in the Development of Artificial Joints

U. P. Wyss, P. A. Costigan

Introduction

The geometry and alignment of bones, ligaments, muscles, and other soft tissues are a finely tuned mechanism controlling joint motion. Gait changes if this interplay is altered, especially in joints of the lower extremity. This interplay can be changed by arthritic joint disease (Messier et al. 1992; Harrington 1983), trauma, or corrective surgery, including osteotomies (Prodromos et als. 1985) and joint replacements (Andriacchi et al. 1977). Therefore the analysis of gait is a useful tool in developing artificial joints for the lower extremity. It provides motion, force, and moment data for different individuals or subject groups and for different activities. Results as they relate to the development of joint replacements are discussed, but no new designs are presented.

Development of Artificial Joints

The development of artificial joints involves experts from many different disciplines. The orthopedic surgeon diagnoses a clinical problem and decides together with the patient how it should be treated, including the insertion of artificial joints. Radiologists, anatomists, pathologists, material specialists, mechanical engineers, and biomechanicians must do their part to produce an optimal implant that will not fail prematurely. Therapists play a major role in the successful integration of an artificial joint after the operation (Knüsel et al. 1984), while epidemiologists are responsible for monitoring outcome and follow-up studies properly. All areas of expertise contribute to further improvements of artificial joints, but only the usefulness of gait analysis is discussed here.

Gait Analysis

Human locomotion has been analyzed for over a century. Weber and Weber (1836) were among the first to study human gait. Braune and Fischer (1895) used locomotion studies to optimize equipment for the German infantry. Earlier this century Bernstein (1935) and Bresler and Frankel (1950) studied gait extensively. Morrison (1968) and Winter (1979) pioneered the more recent gait analysis work, which was made possible with the availability of computers that allow collection and processing of data in a reasonable time. They looked at joint angles, joint forces, joint moments, energy, and power during locomotion. Their efforts focused mainly on the mechanism of how we walk, and how walking is controlled. The findings of gait research have been used to some degree in the process of joint replacement (Andriacchi et al. 1982), but the potential for a much wider use of gait research still exists. A remark by Otto Frey from Sulzer Brothers in Switzerland, a pioneer in joint replacement design and manufacturing, illustrates this point. He said that he began to understand much better how joints are loaded, why they work or lead to problems, by looking at joint force and joint moment data in three dimensions, rather than only two-dimensional diagrams as are found in abundance in the literature (personal communication, 1983). These observations by Frey and others led to a recognition in the orthopedic community that gait analysis can be helpful in the understanding of joint problems, understanding changes after surgical treatment, and in artificial joint development.

The most widely used systems for gait analysis are either special videocameras with passive markers and no cables connected to the subject (Winter 1979; Kadaba et al. 1990), or systems using infrared light-emitting diodes as active markers connected with wires to the subject and recorded by special cameras. Some of the analysis techniques combine the alignment and geometry of bones from X-rays with kinematic data (Weinstein et al. 1986; Costigan et al. 1992). This is crucial to obtain accurate data on an individual basis, especially in diseased and deformed joints. Gait analysis can provide three-dimensional information about joint rotations, bone-on-bone forces and moments during walking and stair climbing, which are the most important activities of daily living for the lower extremity. This information is needed to determine the required strength of an implant and how it should be fixed to the underlying bone. Walking speed has been found a good general indicator of the quality of gait (Andriacchi et al. 1977) when looking at the outcome after joint replacements, but it is not useful in the process of designing artificial joints on its own. It is important to be aware of the accuracy of gait analysis data so that they can be used appropriately. Validation of systems, such as described by Deluzio et al. (1993), or direct comparisons with pins inserted in bones (Lafortune et al. 1992), have shown that it is possible to generate data with errors of less than 10 %. Only the very short period of initial foot contact can have larger errors, unless accelerometers are included in the data collection. Implanting transducers in artificial joints produces direct, accurate force measurements (Bergmann et al. 1989) and can be used to validate conventional noninvasive data collection systems.

Gait Data for Designing Artificial Joints

All the data presented in this chapter are based on Questor gait analysis in three dimensions (QGAIT), which includes Questor precision radiography. The data acquisition methods and processing procedures are discussed in detail in previously published work (Siu et al. 1981; Costigan et al. 1992; Li et al. 1993). The three-dimensional motion data were collected with infrared light-emitting diodes as markers. X-rays were taken from all the subjects with radiopaque markers at the location of the kinematic markers for an accurate individual superposition of the kinematic data with the geometry and alignment of the bones. All results presented are from the knee joint, but a similar approach and procedures would

Table 1. Subject data ($n = 35$)

	Height (cm)	Mass (kg)	Velocity (m/s)	Age (years)
Min.	152.0	46.0	0.9	19.7
Max.	191.5	98.5	1.5	29.0
Mean	171.8	64.1	1.2	24.4
SD	10.1	12.8	0.2	3.2
OA Subjects				
B02	172.0	84.5	0.7	62.3
I11	165.1	96.0	0.4	79.5

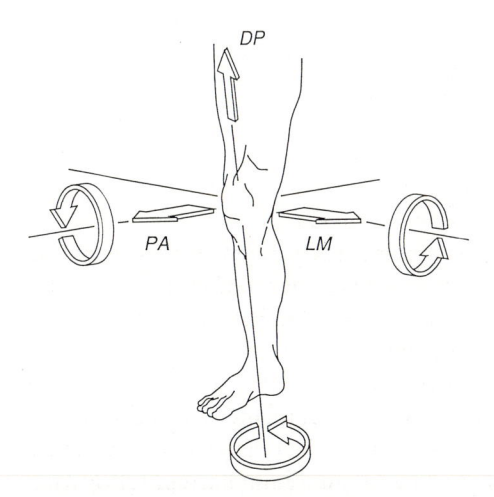

Fig. 1. Sign convention for the rotations, forces, and moments. Distal-proximal *(DP)*, posterior-anterior *(PA)*, and lateral-medial *(LM)* indicates the positive force directions. *Curved arrows (arround DP, PA, LM axes)*, direction of positive rotations and positive moments

provide relevant data for designing other joints. The results of a young healthy population are presented, and the subject-specific information is summarized in table 1. The data from 12 normal asymptomatic elderly subjects were also analyzed, but no significant differences to the young normal group were found. Kinematic and kinetic data are discussed for one subject 1 week before a total knee replacement was implanted (B02), and for one subject 1 week before a hemiarthroplasty was implanted (I11). The subject-specific data for both B02 and I11 are in Table 1. All data are normalized to one walking cycle or stride, and one stair climbing cycle. Time is eliminated by expressing the data as a percentage of a gait cycle from 0 % to 100 %. Figure 1 shows the conventions used to give directions of joint angles, forces, and moments.

Knee Rotations

Knowledge of flexion-extension, adduction-abduction, and internal-external rotation during walking and stair climbing is necessary to determine the range of motion that a joint replacement must accomodate. Other activities such as kneeling or praying must also be assessed in cultures in which these activities are important during daily living. Figure 2a shows mean values for the three rotations from initial foot contact to initial foot contact with a band of ± 1 standard deviation. Figure 2b presents data during stair climbing from toe-off to toe-off. The curves show that the range for adduction-abduction and internal-external rotation is between 5° and 10°, but with considerable variation among subjects as indicated by the standard deviation bands. It also shows that for stair climbing almost 90° of flexion is required, while for walking about 60° flexion is sufficient. The results compare very well with data from Lafortune et al. (1992), whose results are based on measurements with pins inserted in bones, thereby eliminating problems with skin over bone movements. Data for the two osteoarthritic (OA) subjects indicate rotational limitations during walking due to joint degeneration. It was also observed that the knee moves very little during the stance phase for both subjects.

Net Knee Joint Bone-on-Bone Forces

Substantial data have been published on net joint reaction forces, which are not useful for designing artificial joints. Net forces do not account for the torque or moment generated at a joint, thereby neglecting the muscles forces required to produce the moments. Only bone-on-bone forces can be used to determine the strength of an implant and the type of fixation required. It is important to point out, however, that even net bone-on-bone forces do not include cocontraction of muscles that can lead to even higher bone-on-bone forces during parts of the gait cycle. Net bone-on-bone forces at the tibiofemoral joint during walking are shown in Fig. 3a, while Fig. 3b shows the same forces during stair climbing. The curves show the forces normalized to body mass in posterior-anterior, lateral-medial, and distal-proximal directions at the knee joint. The figure shows that

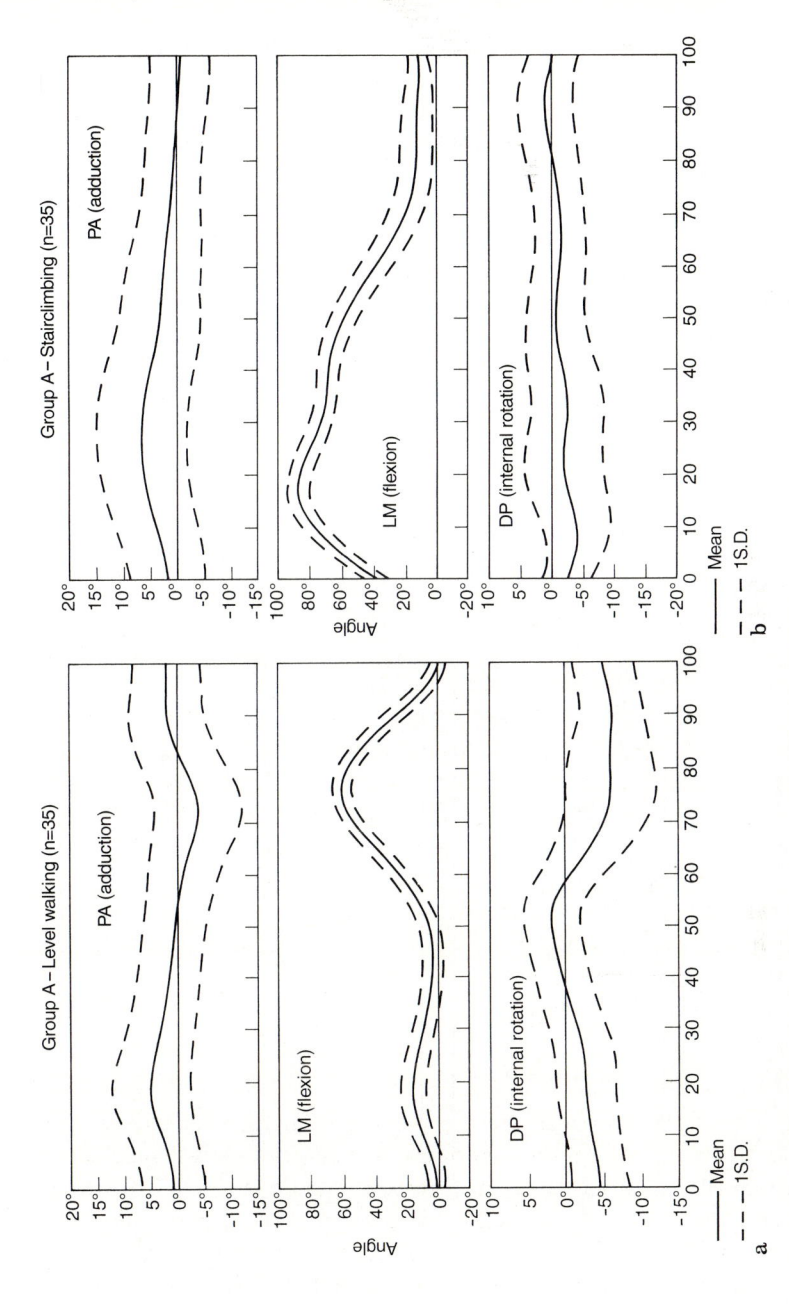

Fig. 2a, b. Three knee rotations during level walking from initial foot contact to initial foot contact (a), and during stair climbing from toe-off to toe-off (b)

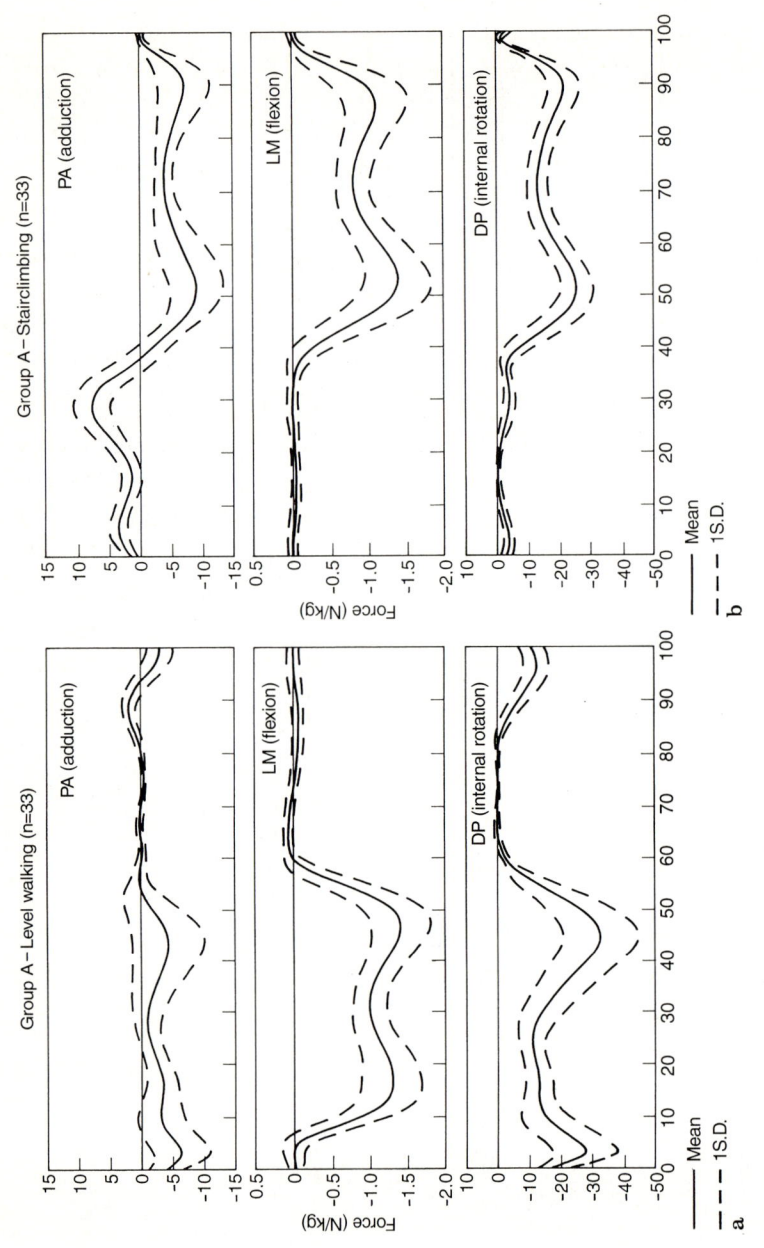

Fig. 3a, b. Net bone-on-bone forces at the tibiofemoral joint normalized to body mass during level walking (**a**), and during stair climbing (**b**)

there are large differences from subject to subject, indicated by large standard deviation bands, which result in forces of up to four times the body weight. The maximum forces during level walking occur during the push-off phase (at about 45 %), where the knee is almost fully extended. There are two peaks during stair climbing that have almost the same magnitude as the one during the push-off phase of level walking. One peak is just after initial foot contact (about 50 %), and another accours during the push-off phase. The flexion angle after the initial foot contact has a mean of 55° for stair climbing. This high load at a larger flexion angle during stair climbing is important and must be considered when designing artificial knee joints. The forces in the posterior-anterior direction are smaller with values of up to the body weight. These forces are also crucial when designing a joint replacement as they represent shear loads which must be absorbed at the implant/bone interface.

It is also very important to include the patellofemoral joint when collecting and analyzing gait data, as it will also be a component of an artificial knee joint. Figure 4 shows the patellofemoral forces for level walking and stair climbing. These forces are zero for gait and stair climbing where the net moment

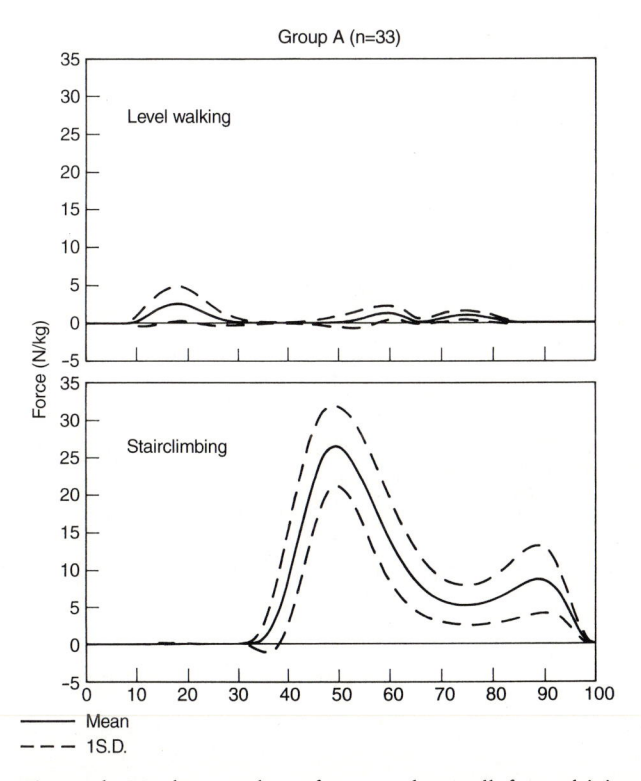

Fig. 4a, b. Net bone-on-bone forces at the patellofemoral joint normalized to body mass during level walking (**a**) and during stair climbing (**b**)

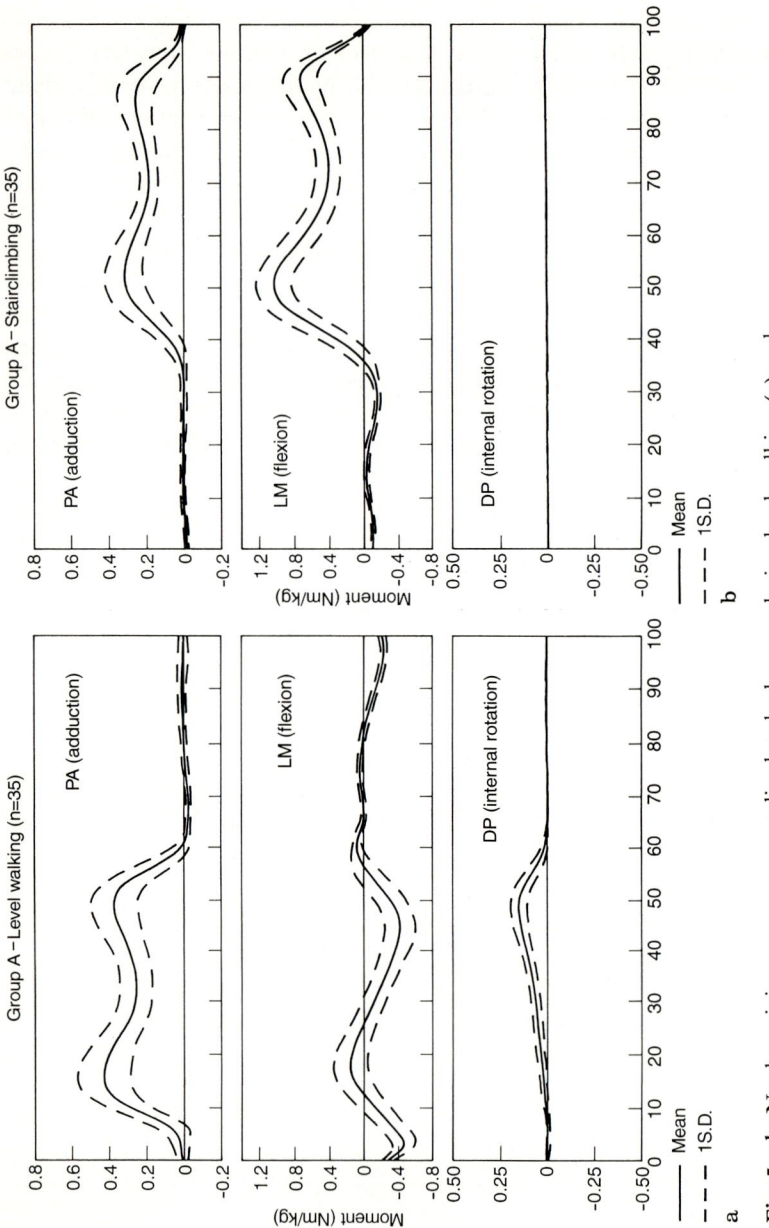

Fig. 5a, b. Net knee joint moments normalized to body mass during level walking (a) and during stair climbing (b)

indicates knee flexor activity. These forces would not be zero if cocontraction of the extensors were considered. It is obvious that stair climbing results in much larger patellofemoral bone-on-bone forces of up to two times body weight. These data are clearly essential when designing artificial knees, but also during follow-up studies. Data for the two OA subjects show that the tibiofemoral forces can be as high or even higher than normal subjects (B02), but also much lower (I11). The pattern is quite different from normal subjects, but also between the two OA subjects. No stair climbing data were gathered for the OA subjects because most preoperative subjects were unable to climb stairs unaided. The bone-on-bone force data for normals compares well in overall shape and magnitude, with data collected on a few subjects by Morrison (1970). His results from various activities showed that stair climbing results in the highest bone-on-bone forces at the knee (1969). Studies by Morrison (1970), Harrington (1976), and Johnson et al. (1980) also show that most of the load is carried through the medial condyles during the stance phase. Johnson et al. (1980) found that despite varus or valgus deformities the load is carried mainly through the medial condyles. They point out that a static analysis does not even give an approximate estimate of the distribution of the load, and that only dynamic gait analysis can show how the loads are distributed.

Net Knee Joint Moments

The net knee joint moments are also a useful indicator for the design of artificial joints since the moments must be balanced with muscle action. Normalized net knee moments are shown in Fig. 5a for level walking and in Fig. 5b for stair climbing. It is interesting to note that the flexor moment (extensor muscle activity) is several times larger during stair climbing, while the adductor moment (abductor muscle activity) is slightly smaller during stair climbing, and the internal-external moment is negligible during stair climbing. The moments for the two OA subjects show the same differences from normal subjects as do the forces. Prodromos et al. (1985) were the first to use adduction moment in the assessment of high tibial osteotomies, but their findings were not conclusive. They indicated that changes in gait pattern could mask the alignment correction achieved during surgery. Weidenhielm et al. (1992), however, concluded that the adduction moments were reduced when total knee replacements were correctly aligned during implantation. This underlines the necessity to pay special attention to correct sizing and optimal surgical techniques.

Gait Analysis to Study Outcome of Total Knee Joint Replacement

One of a few early papers looking at gait after joint replacement was by Andersson et al. (1981). Their conclusion was that the information gathered in a well-equipped gait laboratory is of limited value to the surgeon. They looked only at ground reaction forces and temporal gait parameters, but they indicated that studying forces and moments acting at joints would be more useful for purposes of the design of artificial joints. Andriacchi et al. (1982) studied the gait of five patient groups, where each group received a different knee joint replacement. They found that all subjects still walked differently from normal subjects after joint replacements, but had good clinical outcome. They did find, however, that the flexion angles and flexion moments for the less constrained cruciate-retaining implants were closer to normal during stair climbing. Weinstein et al. (1986) studied factors influencing walking following unicompartmental knee arthroplasty. Their major findings were that anterior malpositioning limited stair climbing ability, and varus-valgus malalignment correlated well with the abduction-adduction moment. These findings confirm earlier conclusions that studying kinematics and kinetics during gait on an individual basis are clinically useful. Whittle and Jefferson (1989) also studied biomechanical gait parameters after knee joint replacement. They found that alignment was generally corrected, but the adductor moment was often still outside the normal range, confirming that clinical results are often better than biomechanical results. Mattsson et al. (1990) also studied gait after hemiarthroplasties and total knee arthroplasties. They found that the clinical outcome was generally better for those patients treated with hemiarthroplasties. They did not, however, measure forces and moments to study the biomechanical factors influencing outcome. Wyss et al. (1994) studied bone-on-bone forces and moments of subjects with hemiarthroplasties before and at least 1 year after surgery. The moment and force data are closer to normal, but still with a much wider variation than for a normal population. This does not mean that the findings are not clinically meaningful, but that the alignment and placement, as well as particular characteristics of the artificial joints must be considered as well. All these studies show that to be clinically useful gait must be studied accurately on an individual basis. Furthermore, the findings will help in determining positive characteristics in artificial knees, their geometry, size, and placement.

Discussion

Data on knee rotation, bone-on-bone forces, and joint moments for various activities over a wide range of subjects will help designing implants with sufficient strength where needed, without making them bulky in areas where the stresses are smaller. Gait analysis also provides data to optimize fixation of implants to host bone. Furthermore, it provides load data (magnitude and direction) for finite element models which analyze implant-bone systems. It even helps in the development of more accurate test procedures for implants. Radin et al. (1991) studied vertical ground reaction forces just after initial foot contact. They found that patients with mild pain had up to 37° higher ground reaction forces than a normal population, indicating that the loads measured for normal populations are smaller than for those whose joint articular surfaces are just beginning to degrade. The data presented here make clear that the bone-on-bone forces at the knee joint are up to five times body weight during parts of level walking and stair climbing. The effect of cocontraction required to keep the leg stable was not included in these results, but results from modeling studies (Seireg and Arvikar 1975), and our own work (Li 1992) have shown that the bone-on-bone force pattern is different, and that the force levels are higher when it is included. The results of cocontraction models are, however, not reliable enough yet due to problems with electromyogram calibration techniques. The bone-on-bone forces can be even higher if a person makes slight jumps or stumbles. Earlier guidelines about forces of levels of up to three times body weight in the development of joint replacement are clearly too low. Levels of five to seven times body weight combined with the additional kinematic information as presented must be adopted to design implants with sufficient strength and adequate bone-implant interfaces.

Conclusions

Gait analysis provides useful information for the development of artificial joints of the lower extremity. The combination of gait data and standardized X-ray, such as QGAIT, also provides a clinically useful tool to follow individual outcome after joint replacement. Motion analysis of other joints provides similarly important motion and load data for the development of artificial joints.

Acknowledgements.
The authors gratefully acknowledge the contributions of Dr. Derek Cooke, Kevin Deluzio, Jian Li, Lynne Kamibayashi, and Dr. Sandra Olney during the development of QGAIT.

References

1. Andersson GBJ, Andriacchi TP, Galante JO (1981) Correlations between changes in gait and in clinical status after knee arthroplasty. Acta Orthop Scand 52:569–573
2. Andriacchi TP, Ogle JA, Galante JO (1977) Walking speed as a basis for normal and abnormal gait measurements. J Biomech 10:261–268
3. Andriacchi TP, Galante J0, Fermier RW (1982) The influence of total knee-replacement design on walking and stair-climbing. J Bone Joint Surg Am 64:1328–1335
4. Bergmann G, Rohlmann A, Graichen F (1989) In-vivo-Messung der Hüftgelenkbelastung. I.: Krankengymnastik. Z Orthop 127:672–679
5. Bernstein N (1935) Untersuchungen über die Biodynamik der Lokomotion, vol 1: Biodynamik des Ganges des normalen erwachsenen Mannes. WIEM, Sovjet Union, Moscow Leningrad

6. Braune W, Fischer O (1895) Der Gang des Menschen. I., Versuche am unbelasteten und belasteten Menschen. Abhandl. d. Math-Phys. Kl. K. Sächs. Gesellsch. Wissensch.
7. Bresler B, Frankel JP (1950) The forces and movements in the leg during level walking. Trans ASME 72:27–35
8. Costigan PA, Wyss UP, Deluzio KJ, Li J (1992) Semiautomatic three-dimensional knee motion assessment system. Med Biol Eng Comput 30:343–350
9. Deluzio KJ, Wyss UP, Li J, Costigan PA (1993) A procedure to validate three-dimensional motion assessment systems. J Biomech 26:753–759
10. Harrington HJ (1976) A bioengineering analysis of force actions at the knee in normal and pathological gait. Biomed Eng 11:167–172
11. Harrington IJ (1983) Static and dynamic loading patterns in knee joints with deformities. J Bone Joint Surg Am 65:247–259
12. Johnson F, Leitl S, Waugh W (1980) The distribution of load across the knee. J Bone Joint Surg Br 62:346–349
13. Kadaba MP, Ramakrishnan HK, Wootten ME (1990) Measurement of lower extremity kinematics during level walking. J Orthop Res 8:383–392
14. Knüsel O, Wyss UP, Frey O (1984) Was bringt die Ganganalyse im Rahmen der orthopädischen Rehabilitation? Swiss Med 6/5a:30–34
15. Lafortune MA, Cavanagh PR, Sommer HJ, Kalenak A (1992) Three-dimensional kinematics of the human knee during walking. J Biomech 25:347–357
16. Li J (1992) An integrated gait analysis system (QGAIT) for evaluation of individual loading patterns at knee joint during gait. Thesis, Queen's University, Kingston, Canada
17. Li J, Wyss UP, Costigan PA, Deluzio KJ (1993) An integrated procedure to assess knee-joint kinematics during gait using an optoelectric system and standardized X-rays. J Biomed Eng 15:392–400
18. Mattsson E, Broström LA, Linnarsson D (1990) Changes in walking ability after knee replacement. Int Orthop (SICOT) 14:277–280
19. Messier SP, Loeser RF, Hoover JL, Semble EL, Wise CM (1992) Osteoarthritis of the knee: effect on gait, strength, and flexibility. Arch Phys Med Rehabil 73:29–36
20. Morrison JB (1968) Bioengineering analysis of force actions transmitted by the knee joint. Bio Med Eng 3:164–170
21. Morrison JB (1969) Function of the knee joint in various activities. Bio Med Eng 4:573–580
22. Morrison JB (1970) The mechanics of the knee joint in relation to normal walking. J Biomech 3:51–61
23. Prodromos CC, Andriacchi TP, Galante JO (1985) A relationship between gait and clinical changes following high tibial osteotomy. J Bone Joint Surg Am 67:1188–1193
24. Radin EL, Yang KH, Riegger C, Kish VL, O'Connor JJ (1991) Relationship between lower limb dynamics and knee joint pain. J Orthop Res 9:398–405
25. Seireg A, Arvikar RJ (1975) The prediction of muscular load sharing and joint forces in lower extremities during walking. J Biomech 8:89–102
26. Siu D, Cooke TDV, Broekhoven LD, Lam M, Fisher B, Saunders G, Challis TW (1991) A standardized technique for lower limb radiography. Invest Radiol 26:71–77
27. Weber W, Weber E (1836) Mechanik der menschlichen Gehwerkzeuge. Dieterichsche Buchhandlung, Göttingen
28. Weidenhielm L, Svensson OK, Broström LA (1992) Change in adduction moment about the knee after high tibial osteotomy and prosthetic replacement in osteoarthritis of the knee. Clin Biomech 7:91–96
29. Weinstein JN, Andriacchi TP, Galante JO (1986) Factors influencing walking and stair-climbing following unicompartmental knee arthroplasty. J Arthroplasty 1:109–115
30. Whittle MW, Jefferson RJ (1989) Functional biomechanical assessment of the Oxford meniscal knee. J Arthroplasty 4:231–243

31. Winter DA (1979) Biomechanics of human movement. Wiley, New York
32. Wyss UP, McBride I, Murphy L, Olney SJ, Cooke TDV (1990) Joint reaction forces at the metatarsal-phalangeal joint in a normal elderly population. J Biomech 23:977–984
33. Wyss UP, Costigan PA, Okuno M, Sorbie C (1994) Net bone-on-bone forces at the knee joint. CORS 94, Winnipeg,

Gait Analysis of Normal Persons and Patients with Coxarthrosis Before and After Conservative Therapy and After the Implantation of a Total Hip Endoprosthesis

O. Knüsel, L. Wiedmer

Introduction

For thousands of years our predecessors concerned themselves with the graphic representation of man, as well as of animals, when walking and jumping. Well known are the prehistoric cliff paintings in France and South Africa which display the elements of movement in an outstanding manner. It is, however, only in the past three centuries that scientists and researchers have paid special attention to upright walking and the sequence of movements involved. In 1852 Gassendi [8] described his observation that forward motion is possible only due to "opposite pressure from the ground" against the forces of the legs pushing downwards and backwards. He also analyzed the rolling action of the sole of the foot, which he compared with the motion of a rolling ball. His compatriot Borelli [3] (1608 - 1679) discovered that the driving force in walking is due to the center of gravity being transferred ahead of its support, where the fall induced by this is prevented by the forward movement of the foot. The actual pioneers of modern gait analysis were the brothers Weber and Weber [25] who, among other things, discovered that the body rotates during the walking process.

Over 15 years in the second half of the nineteenth century Muybridge [19] studied intensively the gait of man and various animals by using up to 24 fixed cameras, but on a purely descriptive basis, without giving any thought to scientific explanation. Based on the high rate of photography, he can be considered the father of kinematographic gait analysis. Marey [17] published his observations in 1894, using a modern gait laboratory; for his studies outside the laboratory he used a "photographic gun" (*fusil photographique*).

Between 1895 and 1905 Braune and Fischer [4] published analyses of human gait which are in part still valid today. These studies formed part of treatises of the mathematical-physical section of the Royal Scientific Society of Saxony and were in response to a military contract from the sovereign, who wanted scientifically to justify the planned new equipment of the German infantry. Braune and Fischer used four synchronized cameras and, with "galvanic" light tubes on the clothing of the test person, reproduced the human form as a line figure, similar to the modern three-dimensional representation of leg kinematics. The experiments and results from this period rendered obsolete all earlier work on gait analysis and still find application today in space technology.

The first experiments on gait analysis in Switzerland were carried out by Scherb [22]. In 1952 he published his analysis of gait disturbances carried out at the Balgrist Orthopedic Department of the University in Zurich using manual palpation of the muscles during walking on a moving walkway. In this way he was able to record an individual activity curve for each group of muscles, the so-called myokinesigram or "musical score" for the muscles.

Over the past 30 years gait analyses have been carried out predominantly in the English-speaking countries. Many gait laboratories were set up in the United Kingdom, Canada, and the United States. The California group of Inman and Saunders [11] determined the walking motion parameters which permit the most economical ambulatory motion. Other well-known experimenters in gait analysis were Chao et al. [5], Murray [18], and Perry [20], and their data and analyses are still referred to today.

Researchers in German-speaking countries were Feldkamp [7] in Münster, Debrunner [6] in Berne, and Baumann [1] in Basle, who's special interest was the gait of patients with cerebral paresis. In recent years technical gait investigation has been carried out on a regular basis at three locations in Switzerland in Basle, Zurich, and Zurzach. The gait laboratory in Basle is attached to the University and that in Zurich is in the Biomechanics Laboratory of the Federal Technical University, now in Zurich-Schlieren. Thanks to H. C. Otto Frey-Zünd, a further clinical gait laboratory has been set up at the Rheumatism and Rehabilitation unit at Zurzach. His former assistant, Wyss, developed the technical basis for this projekt to perform calculations both for basic biomechanical research and for purposes of rehabilitation. This gait laboratory was therefore located at a rheumatism and rehabilitation unit where a sufficient number of patients were always available for research in both areas. Following initial contacts in 1982 much time was taken up in the evaluation of the system. The gait laboratory was opened at the end of 1984. Inaccuracies were soon discovered, however, in both the hardware and the software, and much time was required to correct calibration and programs. Thanks to the fundamental work of Hegi [9] and Wiedmer et al. [25], together with the engineers Bürgi and Barth of Sulzer Medical Technology, an installation was finally available which met all requirements for flexibility and handling.

The Gait Laboratory

Several years ago Baumann and Hänggi [2] defined four requirements which a modern gait laboratory must fulfill:
1. A recording unit with automatic registering of three-dimensional spatial coordinates und angular measurements;
2. At least one force measurement plate for registering floor reaction forces;

3. The ability to calculate dynamic parameters such as speed and acceleration of angular and segmental movements.
4. The determination of muscular activity using electro-myograms on the skin.

The recording systems used today can be divided broadly into three categories:
1. Film or video cameras and passive markers for registering points on the body.
2. Optic-electronic cameras which register impulses principally of infrared light from active diodes.
3. Goniometers.

The following seven conditions should be met to optimize recordings for gait analysis:
1. The measuring system must not prevent normal patient walking motion.
2. The wiring for the active markers must not get in the way.
3. The picture frequency must be at least 50 per second.
4. The system measurement error should not be more than 2 %.
5. Each installation must allow calibration at regular intervals.
6. The evaluation must be carried out immediately following the recording.
7. The patient examination time must be kept short.

Although force measurement plates for determining floor reaction forces and torque in the three planes are part of the standard equipment, the registering of muscle activity still involves considerable investment in equipment and personnel. Most gait laboratories thus perform kinematic and kinetic measurements, but while measurement of muscular activity is desirable, it is not available everywhere.

The Zurzach Gait Laboratory

By the end of 1993 over 600 recordings had been made at the Zurzach Gait Laboraty (Fig. 1), from healthy probands and from patients.

A Selspot-II system is used for the recording unit. At one side of the walkway and at a distance of 4 m from it, two optic-electronic cameras are mounted such that their optical axes intersect at an angle of 60°. These cameras pick up the infrared light emitted by diodes. The three-dimensional spatial position of the diodes is determined at a frequency of 50 times per second using a coordination system built into the cameras, with a maximum capacity of 200 times per second. The infrared light emitting diodes are directed to precisely defined body locations or to ancillary devices. It is important that the diodes are applied to locations with as little soft tissue as possible between the skin and the bone, such as trochanter major, caput fibulae, and malleolus in order to avoid movement

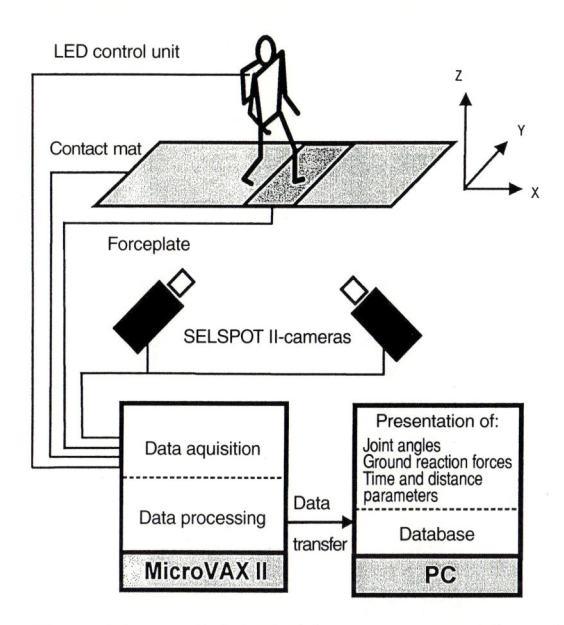

Fig. 1. Scheme of the gait laboratory in Zurzach (Switzerland) with two optic-electronic infrared cameras, a force plate, applications of detecting a floor contact, and computer-assisted evaluation

due to this while walking. Pressure switches operated by foot pressure upon floor contact also activate diodes, giving data for the determination of stride length, stationary and moving phases, walking speeds, and step frequency.

Table 1. Applications for gait analyses include the following

Manufacture of endoprostheses
- Biomechanic reaction of the locomotor system with different endoprostheses
- Development and correction of endoprostheses
- Influence of rehabilitation on the functional result

Orthopedic surgery
- Diagnostic aid for indications for orthopedic operations
- Biomechanic reaction of the locomotor system after orthopedic operations
- Support for new surgery techniques or for implantation of new types of endoprostheses
- Control of postoperative loading

Rehabilitation
- Knowledge about the gait in normal persons and its application in rehabilitation
- Quantitative registration of biomechanical data to supplement clinical examination and personal details of patient, physician, or physiotherapist
- Comparison of different rehabilitation techniques
- Biomechanical notes in the development of new rehabilitation concepts

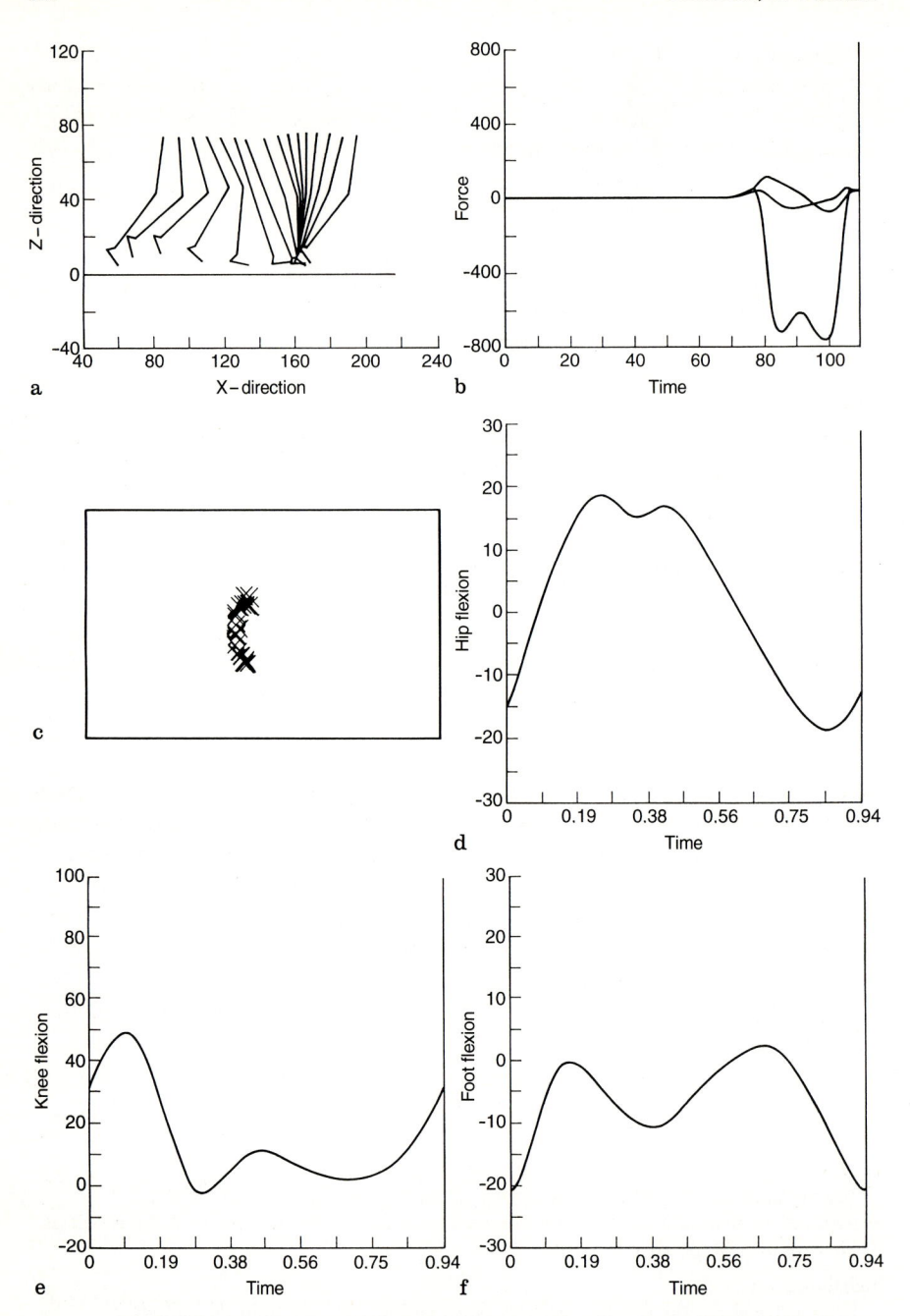

Fig. 2 a–f. Gait analysis records. **a** Line drawing of the leg in standing and during movement. **b** Curves of the floor reaction forces at three levels. **c** Contact area of the foot on the force measuring plate. **d–f** Curves during a double-step. **d** the hips, **e** the knee, **f** the foot

The triaxial forces between foot and floor are measured by a Kistler measuring platform fitted into the walkway and synchronized with the cameras. During recording the patient carries two control boxes on the back which are connected by wiring with the cameras, diodes, and computer. Following digitalization, definitive evaluation is carried out using a Microvax computer consisting of a PC, terminal, monitor, and printer.

Table 1 gives a summary of the various applications, such as angular progression, movements, speed, acceleration and force measurement, as well as energy calculations. A gait analysis sheet is printed out for each patient (Fig. 2)

Following a check of diode visibility the patient walks at usual speed along the walkway accompanied by an assistant. No recording is made the first time, while the patient becomes accustomed to the equipment. When walking at usual speed, five to eight walk cycles are recorded, depending on the fatigue of the patient. Afterwards, the other side is investigated in the same manner. Finally, various anthropometric parameters such as height, weight, leg length, circumference of thigh and calf, etc. are measured and entered on the patient record sheet. If necessary, a repeat analysis is made just before discharge from the hospital to check the success of therapy.

Normal Gait

Walking, the most important form of human motion, is an extremely complex activity. Individual gait pictures give us information on the actual and potential functioning of the human gait apparatus and its control systems. Behavior which deviates from the norm indicates a reaction by the gait apparatus to a disturbance. The considerable compensation ability of the body must, however, be taken into account. Due to the complexity and the rapid movement, the clinical, "visual" description of the gait permits only a rough differentiation of the pathological from the normal.

Technical kinematic and kinetic gait analysis, with its objective data registering and higher resolution, now provides advantages (Table 2):
- The measured and calculated values permit a precise description of the gait pattern, and thus add objective data to the clinical diagnosis of the gait disturbance.
- The complexity and rapid succession of events during walking cannot be visually comprehended in many cases. Gait analysis allows the interplay of segmental and angular processes or isolated aspects of the gait to be studied.
- The combination of kinematics and kinetics gives precise data on the loading of the joints. This makes it possible to examine the vicious circle of protection – a pathological gait pattern with abnormal loading of the diseased joint and compensatory loading of the other side, with progressive arthrosis and damage on the other side.

Table 2. Gait analysis parameters
Measured values

Time and distance parameters
- Gait cadence (steps/min)
- Double support distance (m)
- Gait speed (m/s)
- Stance and swing phase (percentage of double support)

Kinematic parameters
- Movement of the center of gravity of the whole body or of single limbs
- Angle between different limbs
- Movement of anatomic reference markers
- Space orientation of the body or a single limb

Kinetic parameters
- Force plate reactions between foot or shoe and floor

Calculated values
- Speed and acceleration of the body, of single limbs, or of anatomic reference markers
- Approximate rotation axis in the articulations
- Description of the force plate reaction during floor contact
- Torque in the articulations

- Gait analysis can be used to measure the success of various therapies and in the development of prostheses.

Even today, gait analysis requires extensive use of equipment and personnel. It will therefore remain associated with larger orthopedic, rheumatism and/or rehabilitation units. The development of simpler, affordable laboratory set-ups with short investigation times would therefore be welcome.

Gait allows the upright human being to move body weight (and thus the body's center of gravity, which is in front of the second sacral vertebra) as desired and economically, while taking account of ceomplicates balance conditions. To keep the movements as economical as possible the progression should be a smooth as possible, both spatially and temporally. Two-legged locomotion, however, prevents movement in a straight line and constant speed of the body's center of gravity. Inman et al. [11] compared human walking with a wheel with its axis in the hip joint, slightly oval, so that it wobbles as it rolls. Lateral and vertical progression of the center of gravity occurs, with about 5 cm rise and fall, and about 2–3 cm movement over the standing leg (Fig. 3). A complex interaction of the leg segments and the hip gives rise to this track of the body's center mof gravity and the apparently simple mechanical walking process. The determinants of gait defined by Saunders et al. in 1953 [21] are valid today:
1. rotation of the pelvis in the horizontal plane,
2. lateral tilting of the pelvis in the frontal plane,
3. bending of the knee during the standing phase,
4/5. knee and foot interaction in the sagittal plane,
6. lateral swings of the pelvis in the frontal plane.

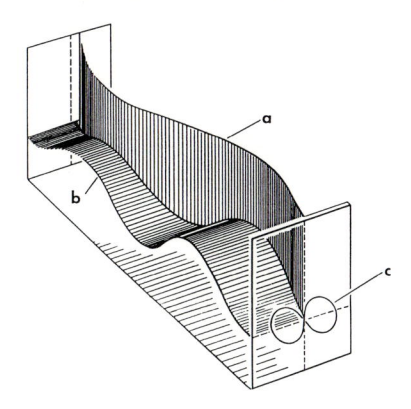

Fig. 3 a–c. The human gait depicted as a wheel that is not perfectly round and wobbles slightly. Its axis is in the hip joint (after [11]). **a** Lateral displacement on the horizontal axis, **b** vertical displacement, **c** projected combined displacement of **a** and **b**

The first three of these determinants reduce the vertical movement of the center of gravity during the advance of the body over the standing leg. The rotation of the pelvis lets the center of gravity sink less during the phase when both feet are on the ground. The tilting of the pelvis in the frontal plane and the bending of the knee of the standing leg allow the center of gravity to move downwards over the standing leg. Loss of potential energy is thus limited. The bending of the knee cushions leg loading upon heel impact on the ground ("loading response"). Rolling the foot allows the knee, analogous to a wheel, to maintain a relatively stable horizontal position during the standing phase and thus supports the smoothing effect of the knee bending on the track of the hips and the center of gravity.

In complex interaction these mechanisms thus lead to the typical gait pattern of sinusoidal smoothed progression of the center of gravity in the direction of motion (Fig. 3). In the frontal plane the body moves over the standing leg with every step. Accordingly, the center of gravity also moves sideways in a sinusoidal path.

The typical human gait pattern repeats itself after every second step with the period between two heel contacts on the same side (Fig. 4). Each step consists of a standing and swinging phase for each leg. Each standing phase consists of the period of time when both feet are in contact with the ground, and the body weight is transferred to the other side. Normal gait is therefore characterized by the symmetry of the step length and step duration, and also of the standing and swinging phases on the right and left sides. Deviations from this symmetry lead to limping.

Given the various recording systems, it is very important to obtain normal data. Hegi [9] investigated 57 healthy probands in terms of gender-specific differences, variations from one side to the other and potential changes in the gait pattern in the very old, with particular regard to patients with hip arthrosis. He observed no gender- or age-related quality differences in the sagittal plane up to the 70th year of age. On the other hand, the variance in values was very high. For the individual patient it is therefore difficult to demarcate a pathologi-

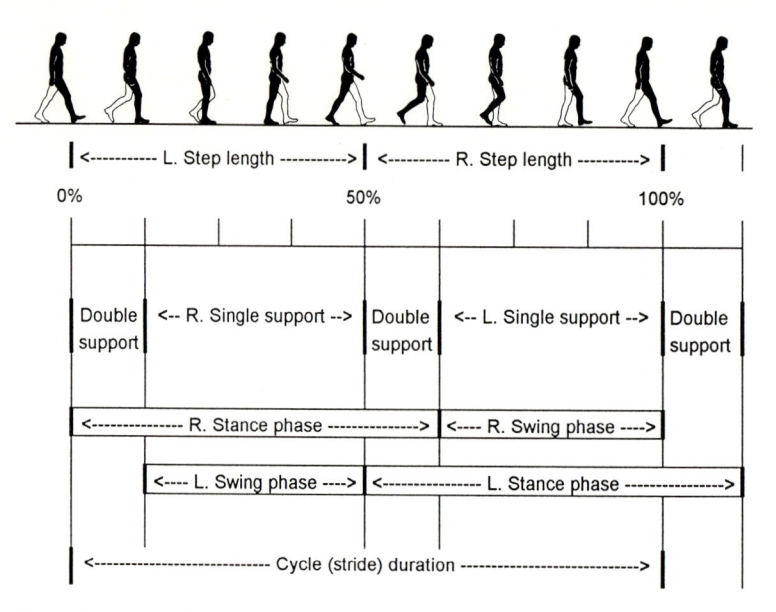

Fig. 4. Time and distance parameters. (From [11])

cal gait pattern, particularly in the very aged. It was, however, important to establish normal values for the different age groups and for the two sexes. These show a clear correlation with the comprehensive investigations by Chao et al. [5].

A study carried out in collaboration with a clinic obtained information from gait analysis of 32 patients with single- or double-sided coxarthrosis to find new aspects for physical or operative therapy [14]. The findings were compared with the norms established by Hegi [9]. Lequesne's [16] functional index for hip disease (FIH) was used for anamnestic data. In addition, subjective pain assessment using the Huskisson [10] visual analogue scale (VAS) was carried out. The subjective opinions of the patient and physician were both significant. The patients received standardized physiotherapy. The clinical assessment included muscular strength and clinical gait phenotype in addition to various functional parameters such as mobility. Radiological classification used the proposal of Lequesne [15]. Correlations of functional diagnosis and gait analysis showed the following: With a high FIH score there was a greater reduction in gait speed and relative length of the double stride and a reduction in the total sagittal hip and knee movement and in the maximum hip extension (Fig. 5). Following the standardized 3-week physical therapy, the subjective clinical and gait analysis parameters were investigated again. In addition to a significant improvement in the subjective and objective parameters of the clinical data, there were also changes in the gait analysis results. There were significant changes in the time and distance factors, in the floor reaction forces, and in the knee angle parame-

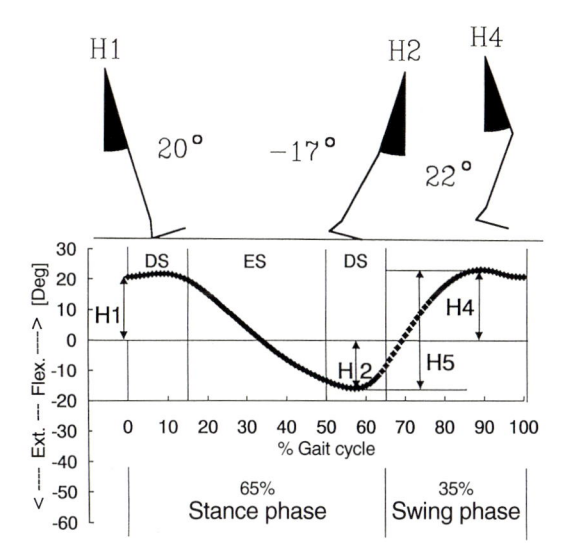

Fig. 5. Flexion and extension of the hip during a gait cycle (stance phase and swing phase). *H1*, Flexion of the hip on heel contact; *H2*, maximum of the hip extension in the late stance phase; *H4*, maximum of the hip flexion in the swing phase; *H5*, movement of the hip during walking; *DS*, double support; *ES*, single support

ters. All these changes were towards norm values. It was noticeable that there were no significant changes in the angular movement patterns of diseased hip joints and those given therapy, even in cases of subjectively very successful therapy. It is probable that the duration was too short to obtain a significant change. The results for hip and knee angles in the sagittal plane (Fig. 5) differ for the various stages of disease. In the early stage the effect on time and distance factors is predominant while at more severe stages there is an easily measurable reduction in total sagittal hip movement, with a secondary reduction in knee extension in the middle of the standing phase. In the severe stage of bilateral coxarthrosis, the hip movement changes to more hip flexion upon heel impact. In this case the total sagittal hip movement is only slightly reduced, but there is greatly increased hip flexion.

We detected two different types of loading behavior (Fig. 6). One group (Fig. 6a) compensates the deficit in hip extension with more hip flexion upon heel impact. The range of motion is thereby reduced to a lesser degree. The increased hip flexion leads, however, to a further "falling forwards" of the body and the center of gravity, and thus to increased acceleration. The center of gravity falls further, from the highest point in the middle of the standing phase down to heel impact. The impact at the extremity is higher, resulting in greater loading. The benefit for the patient is that only slightly shorter steps are made, permitting maintenance of a gait speed which frequently approximates the

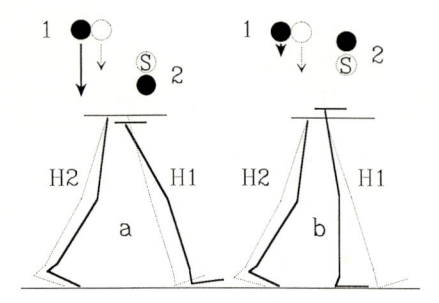

Fig. 6. Lateral view of the position of the legs during maximum of the hip extension H2 and during heel contact H1. *Dotted line,* healthy control; *S,* center of gravity; *a,* osteoarthritis of the hip with additional compression of the affected side; *b,* osteoarthritis of the hip with decompression of the affected side

norm. This gait pattern is typical for patients suffering from bilateral moderately severe osteoarthritis of the hip. Apparently these patients can force the flexibility of their hips so that the range of motion can be maintained at least partly. The increased knee angle at toe lift-off on the less affected side was the only measurable parameter which at least partly explained step length increase after physiotherapy. It is probable that compensatory movements of the pelvis as a whole can explain this. Murray [18] and Steindler [23] have shown greater sagittal and transverse pelvic movement as compensation for restricted hip extension.

The other group (Fig. 6b) does not compensate the deficit in hip extension. As a result there is a severe restriction in the range of motion, also due to the reduced hip flexion upon heel impact. The body does not fall forward as far, and the center of gravity does not sink as much. Impact, and thus loading, is less. Patients with this unloading pattern frequently have a moderately severe to severe one-sided coxarthrosis. This results in major gait asymmetry. Most patients compensate partly for this asymmetry with a restriction in movement in the healthy or less affected side. Walking ability is then reduced, and a relatively low walking speed results. Langer [14] found increased floor reaction forces in all directions as a result of the increased step frequency.

A prospective long-term study [12] investigated most of the patients in the Langer study again for clinical and gait analysis factors. Four of the 28 prospective patients had to be operated on, of whom three received total hip replacement (THR). The assessment of this subgroup provided special data which were significantly different from those in the ohter 24 patients. The THR patients rated pain according to the VAS as 72 % ±10 % at the first examination, compared with 48 % ± 23 % for the 24 others, and an intermalleolar distance of 52 ±19 cm, compared with 72 ±15 cm, and a more significantly reduced passive hip inner rotation.

According to Lequesne [16] scores on the FIH among the later THR patients increased from 8.8 ±0.5 at the first examination to 15.2 ±1.3 preoperatively but decreased to 4.3 ±3.2 at the end of the first postoperative year. This was compared to patients with conservative therapy who had 7.23 ±2.88 at the first examination and 9.15 ±3.62 points after 1 year. The VAS of the THR patients sank from 86 preoperatively to 12 after 1 year.

Itin [12] found worsening of the coxarthrosis symptoms in nonoperated patients ($n = 24$) to be correlated significantly with body size, especially with leg length, and the extent of asymmetry of the coxarthrosis. Subjectively these patients reported clearly more pain and a progressive restriction of the distance walked and in everyday activities. These patients also reported shorter and reduced improvement due to therapy. Clinically, there was a reduction in passive hip inner rotation. The worsening was also more noticeable where there was a greater radiological difference between the worse and better sides. In terms of gait analysis there was a strong correlation between worsening and a reduction in the total sagittal hip and knee movement and strong gait asymmetry (Fig. 6). Worsening was also correlated with increased knee angle after the 3-week therapy. In this case the patients also showed the same tendency, with reduced vertical floor reaction force, and load increase rates. The data suggest that patients with severely reduced hip extension in the late standing phase may in fact fare better. This reduction in forces on the joint spares the joint structures and can be seen as a protection mechanism. On the other hand, those who do not make use of this protection mechanism but respond with increased hip flexion and secondarily with increased knee angle suffer a more rapid deterioration in their coxarthrosis. These patients respond with restricted hip extension in a way such that there is increased loading of the lower extremities. It is probable that this accelerates the process of arthrosis where this was not previously halted to a large extent by light knee flexion. This leads, however, to nonphysiological loading of the knee.

Tall patients, especially those with proportionally long legs, progress less well, possibly due to increased torsional moment in the hip area. This was not measured in the Zurzach installation.

There was a large number of farmers in the patient population (15 %). These showed a worsening on the less affected side over time, very probably due to overloading of the better side to spare the pathological side.

Based on the above, various therapeutic measures are conceivable, for example, partial reduction in the increased loading using appropriate shoes or correction of the gait pattern so that compensation of the hip extension deficit by increased hip flexion is not necessary. Concerning endoprosthetics, this gait behavior raises the possibility of patients with endoprostheses compensating possible deficits in extension in this way, such that an overloading situation occurs, of this overloading leading to a change in prosthesis lifetime. Do individual prosthesis types or the surgical technique affect the resulting gait pattern? It is certain that differentiation of biomechanical disturbances, especially of gait disturbances of coxarthrosis patients, can provide new ideas both for rehabilitation and for orthopedic surgery.

References

1. Baumann JU (1984) Clinical experience of gait analysis in the management of cerebral palsy. Prosthet Orthot Int 8:29
2. Baumann JU, Hänggi A (1977) A method of gait analysis for daily orthopaedic practice. J Med Eng Technol 1:2
3. Borelli A (1682) De mota animalium. Lugduni Batavorum, Roma
4. Braune W, Fischer O (1895–1905). Der Gang des Menschen. Abhandlungen der königlich-sächsischen Gesellschaft der Wissenschaft Mathematisch-physicalischer Classe, Leipzig
5. Chao EY, Laughman RK, Schneider E, Stauffer RN (1983) Normative data of the knee joint motion and ground reaction forces in adult level walking. J Biomech 16:3–219
6. Debrunner HU (1975) Ganganalyse mit der Mehrkomponenten-Meßplattform. Aktuel Probl Angiol 30:34–38
7. Feldkamp M (1979) Ganganalyse bei Kindern mit zerebraler Bewegungsstörung. Pflaum, München
8. Gassendi D (1682) De motu animalium secundems totum, ac primum de gressu. Opera tom. II Liv. XI Cap. V Florenz
9. Hegi T (1991) Der gesunde Gang: Kinematische und kinetische Ganganalyse von 57 gesunden Probanden mit dem Selspot-II-System und einer Kraftmeßplatte. Inauguraldissertation, Universität Basel
10. Huskisson EC (1974) Measurement of pain. Lancet 4:1127–1131
11. Inman VT, Ralston HJ, Todd F (1981) Human walking. Williams & Wilkins, Baltimore
12. Itin C (1992) Verlaufsbeobachtungen über ein Jahr von 28 Koxarthrose-Patienten mittels klinischer und ganganalytischer Parameter. Med. Dissertation, Universität Basel
13. Knüsel O, Wiedmer L (1990) Die Ganganalyse-Geschichte, Methoden und Grundlagen. Z Phys Med Baln Med Klim 19:110–123
14. Langer TH (1991) Quantitative Ganganalyse bei 32 Koxarthrose-Patienten vor und nach physikalischer Therapie. Inauguraldissertation Universität Basel
15. Leguesne M (1982) Diagnostic criterial, functional assessments and radiological classification of osteoarthritis (Excluding the spine). In: Huskisson EC, Katona G (eds) Rheumatology. Karger, Basel, p1
16. Leguesne M Samson M (1981) A functional index for hip disease. Reproducibility. Value for discriminating drugs efficacy (abstract). 5th Int. Cong. Rheum. Paris, p778
17. Marey EJ (1894) Le mouvement. Flammarion, Paris
18. Murray MP (1967) Gait as a total pattern of movement. J Phys Med [Am]1:290–332
19. Muybridge E (1955) The human figure in motion. Dover, New York
20. Perry J (1992) Gait analysis, normal and pathological function. Monterey, Slack
21. Saunders JB, Inman VT, Eberhart HD (1953) The major determinants in normal and pathological gait. J Bone Joint Surg 35:543–588
22. Scherb R (1952) Kinetisch-diagnostische Analyse von Gangstörungen. Technik und Resultate der Myokinesigraphie. Enke, Stuttgart (Beiheft 82 oder Orthop)
23. Steindler A (1955) Kinesiology of the human body under normal and pathological conditions. Thomas, Springfield
24. Weber W, Weber E (1836) Mechanik der menschlichen Gehwerkzeuge, eine anatomisch-physiologische Untersuchung. Dietrich, Göttingen
25. Wiedmer L, Langer T, Knüsel O (1992) Das Gangmuster von Patienten mit Hüftarthrose. Orthopäde 21:35–40

Part II

Cemented Acetabular Fixation

The Cemented Hip Cup: The Weber Polyethylene-Ceramic and Metasul Cups and the High-Pressure Cementing Technique

B. G. Weber

Introduction

The total hip prosthesis (THP) can be said to fail as soon as it comes loose. With cemented anchorage [1, 2] there are two possible results: either immediate loosening, occurring as a consequence of faulty cementing technique, or immediate stability, as a result of good cementing technique. The subsequent fate of the prosthesis after immediate stability depends on possible factors of interference: (a) premature loosening resulting from infection, (b) late loosening following reaction of the tissues to polyethylene debris on the implant-bone interface as described by Willert [5], and (c) long-term stability lasting 30 years or more in the event of the absence of any significant wear, i. e., when the metal-metal pairing funcitons ideally [4].

Cup-Cementing Philosophy

Whether the cup "sits" well is determined during the operation (Fig. 1):

a) With many cups the cement runs out freely between the inserted cup and the acetabulum. In practice the cement undergoes no pressure. The bonding of the cement with the cup and with the bone is insufficient.

b) For the author's own "earlet" cups frequently used even today, the situation is quite different: the earlets are positioned by trimming precisely into the entrance of the acetabulum and reduce the pass by which the excess cement runs out by about 50 %. In this way, when the cup is pressed into place, the cement is forced against the implant and the bone to the required degree.

c) The new Weber cup generation in use since 1987 is characterized by the cup fitting precisely into the reamed cavity in the pelvis, resembling the piston in the cylinder of a syringe. Pressure on the cup leads to the maximum possible bonding between cement, implant, and bone. The excess cement must, however, still be able to escape. For this reason there are cement run-out holes with a diameter of 2.5 mm in the rim of the cup. The cross-section for run-out is about 10 % of that described in Fig. 1a. The disadvantage is that the excess cement can be pressed out only by applying a great pressure, and particularly for larger cups

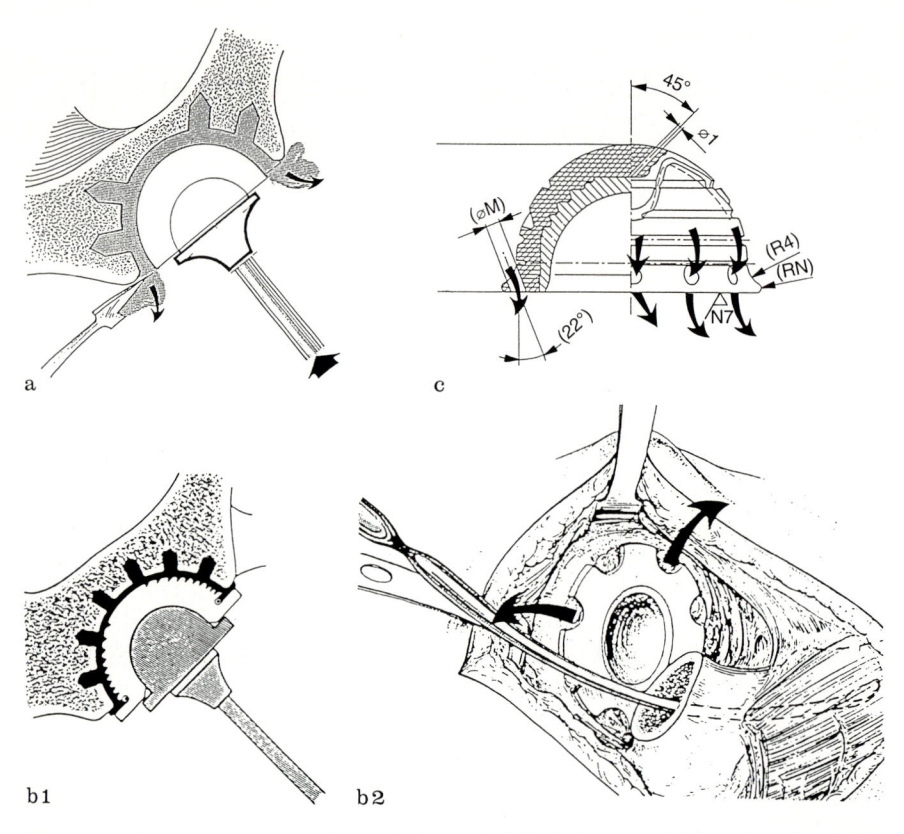

Fig. 1a–c. Cement pressing and cup design. (**a**) Spherical cups without „hat rims." The cement does not undergo any real pressing, since it runs out unhindered when the cup is inserted (*arrow*). (**b**) The „earlet" cup (Weber). *1*, The „earlets" on top prevent the cement from flowing away. There is a certain degree of pressing of the cement; *2*, the cement can flow out only through the gaps between the „earlets" (*arrows*) and in this way undergoes pressing. (**c**) The Weber cup 1987. The „hat rim" is equipped with numerous cement run-out holes. Since the cup fits exactly in the reamed cavity in the acetabulum, the cement can run out only through the holes provided for this purpose (*arrow*). This achieves the best possible pressure on the cement

the strength of the surgeon's own arms may not be sufficient for this. An instrument must therefore be available to help him.

Weber Cups Since 1987

The types of Weber cups available since 1987 include the following (Fig. 2):
a) Polyethylene cups for pairing with ball heads made of aluminium oxide ceramic, inside diameter 28 or 32 mm.

The Cemented Hip Cup 133

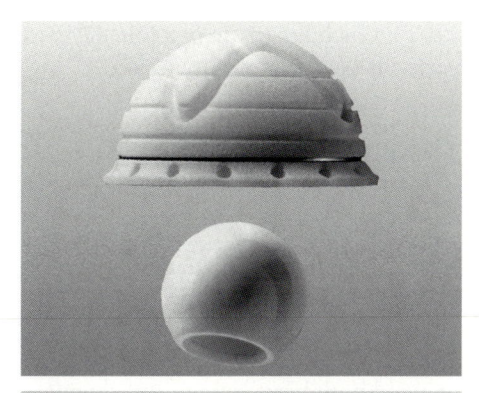

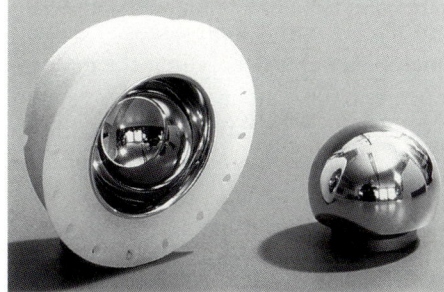

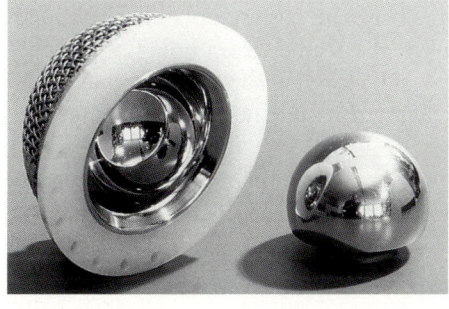

Fig. 2a–c. Weber cups, 1987. (**a**) Cup for polyethylene aluminium oxide ceramic pairing. Optimized outer surface structure. Marking wire round the equator. Cement runout holes; 32 and 28 mm ball heads. (**b**) Cup for Metasul pairing; 32 and 28 mm ball heads. (**c**) Cup for Metasul pairing with Sulmesh surface; 32 and 28 mm ball heads

b) Polyethylene cups for CoCrMo Metasul, i. e. for metal-metal-pairing, inside diameter 28 or 32 mm. The Metasul inlay is irremovably pressed into the polyethylene. In (a) and (b) the surface of the cup is roughened by sand blasting, and the surface is given a new structure. This gives rise to a fivefold improvement in the bonding of the bone cement compared to cups with smooth surfaces.

c) Similar Metasul cups, the outer surfaces of which are made of a four-layered metal grid. This optimizes the bone-cement bonding even tenfold.

High-Pressure Cementing Technique

The aim of cementing is to obtain the most intimate and direct mirror copy possible of the bone seat with the help of the bone cement, that is to say peroperative production of what is the closest possible to the ideal custom-made prosthesis. In doing this, it is necessary to avoid both heat damage and chemical damage to the bone seat, which is easier to achieve with a high-viscosity cement rather than with a low-viscosity one, which penetrates deeply into the biologically sensitive structure of the bone. The demand for high viscosity in cement in the 1960s, by Charnley, is still equally valid today. In this respect the mold-locking ability is the foremost consideration, considerably more important than deep penetration of the cement into the cancelleous bone.

It is not possible to describe the operating technique in detail here. Anyone who is interested in it must see this technique demonstrated. For this reason only the main points are described here:
- Denude the surface slightly with the aid of the largest possible acetabular reamer. Use the centering pin to prevent the reamer from going off course. Sufficient care is required to spare the subchondral supporting bone layer. Prepare 10–15 6-mm anchoring holes. Wash. Brush. Check the bleeding with swab packing (Fig. 3).
- With the help of the silicone disc and the cup test punch, press the medium-viscosity cement into the cup seat. After removal of the silicone plate and the punch, finger packing, as described by Charnley, is strongly recommended in the region of the roof of the cup to improve primary interlock between the cement and the bone (Fig. 4).
- Position the cup exactly and use the seating punch with the rim to align it. In the meantime the cement will have achieved high viscosity (Fig. 5).
- High pressure is now required to press out the remaining excess cement through the cement run-out holes. The pressure lever instrument set is used to achieve this (Fig. 6).

The Hohmann lever with the chain must be inserted into the pelvis immediately after resection of the femoral head. Now, with the help of the chain and the counterpressure lever, press the cup inwards applying a force of about 100 kp. Using the strength of one's arms only, a force of 30 kp at most can be exerted. Spaghettilike strings of high-viscosity cement are extruded through the cement run-out holes. In this way it is always possible to press the cup in as far as required without difficulty even when implanting cups with large diameters.

The Cemented Hip Cup

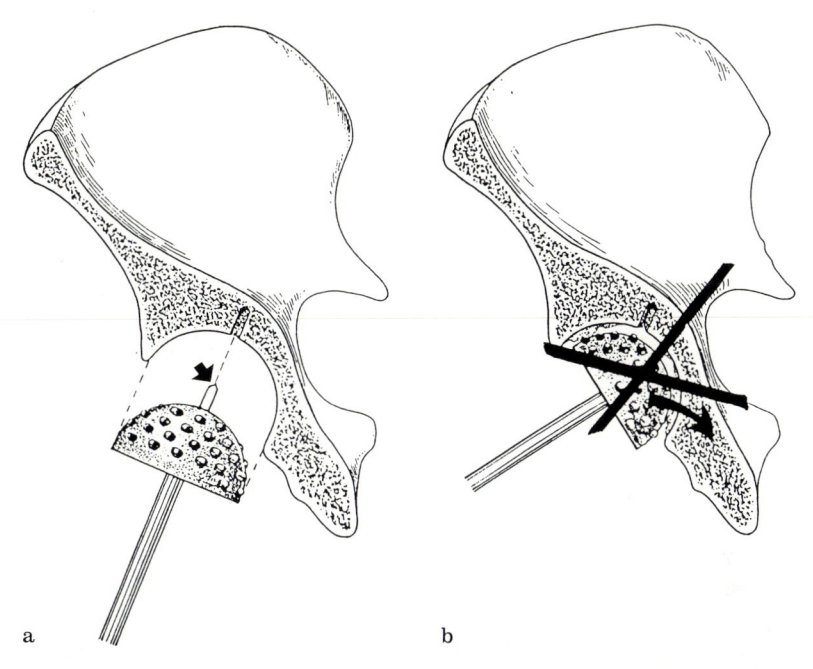

Fig. 3ab. Reaming the acetabulum for hight-pressure cementing. (a) Reaming is performed in one step, with the largest possible acetabular reamer. The reamer remains centered with the help of the centering pin. (b) When reaming without the centering pin, the acetabular reamer diverges uncontrollably (*arrow*). It fails to ream a shape with a correct fit for the high-pressure cementing (*X*)

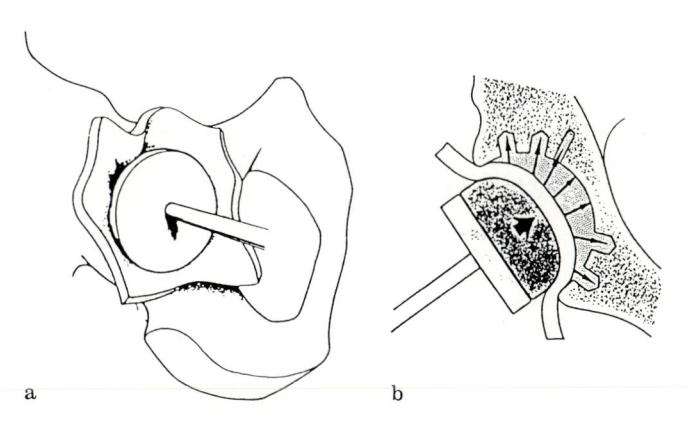

Fig. 4ab. Preliminary pressing of the cement in the acetabulum. (a) The half-soft cement is pressed into the acetabulum with the help of the test cup and the silicone plate. (b) This preliminary pressure already creates an inner dovetailing of the cement in the bony seat

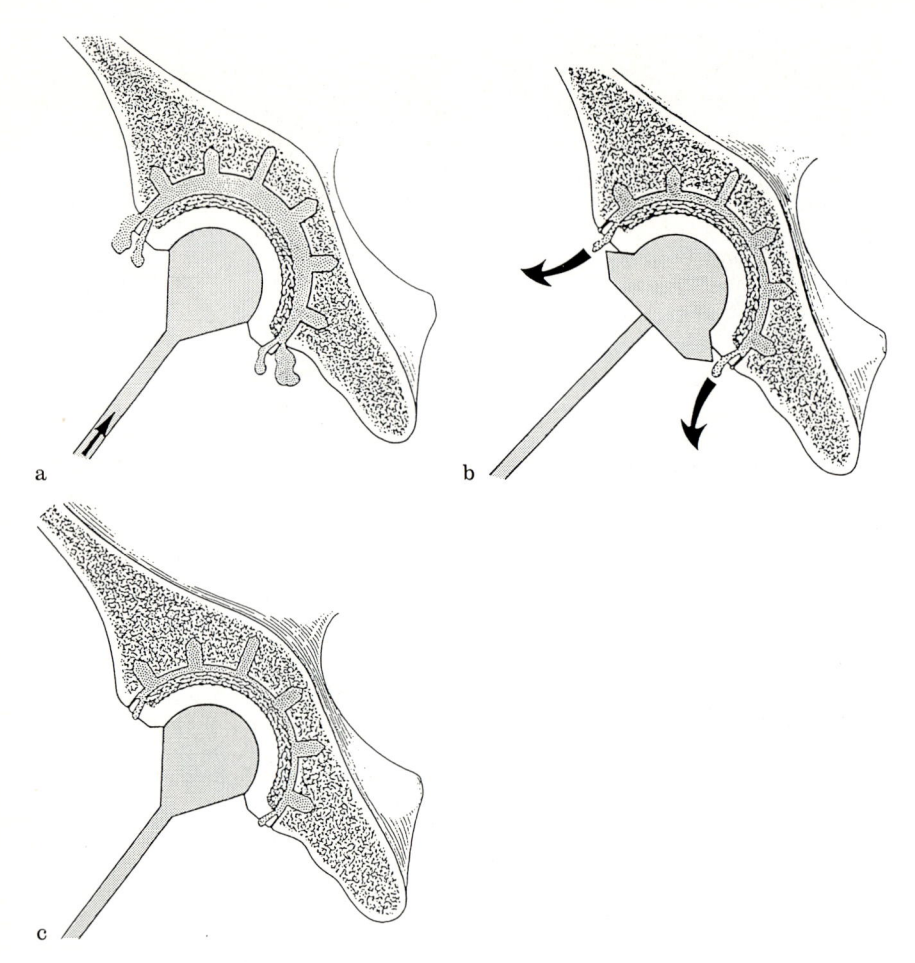

Fig. 5a–c. Positioning of the Weber cup, 1987. (**a**) The preliminary pressurization is followed by the precise seating of the cup in the reamed cavity, with the help of the rimless seating instruments, so as to leave a free view for this delicate step. (**b**) As soon as exact fitting is ensured, the rimmed seating punch is inserted. Orientation of the cup is completed and hight-pressure is carried out with the appropriate instruments, as shown in Fig. 6. Now the cement runs out of only the cement run-out holes (arrows). (**c**) The rimless seating punch must continue to be used until the cement has hardened

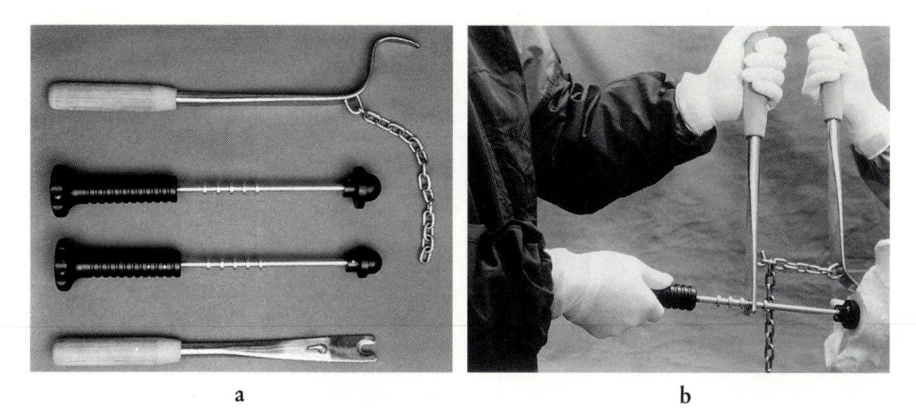

Fig. 6ab. The pressure lever instrument set for the cup. (**a**) From top to bottom: the special Hohmann lever with its chain, the cup seating instrument; 32 and 28 mm. The forked pressing lever with its hook. (**b**) Providing the high pressure: the Hohmann lever is placed under the tendon of the m. psoas opposite the floor of the acetabulum. The forked lever grips the cup seating instrument. The chain is hung into it. The surgeon and his assistant can generate a pressing force of 100 kp or more

Experience with the Weber Metasul Cup and High-Pressure Cementing Technique

Cups inserted

Between 1988 and 1992 110 Weber Metasul cups were implanted. Two cups came loose, one each of 44 and 48 mm diameter, both made of metal. Two more of these cups, together with all the other types described above, have remained stable up to the present day. These were all cups with Sulmesh surface (Fig. 7). Since 1993 only Weber Metasul cups without Sulmesh have been implanted. Both types, all together 150 cups, are still firmly seated.

Cement pressurizing using instruments has been practiced systematically since mid-1992, and makes it possible to work with higher cement viscosities. No disadvantages have been observed, either on the patients' circulation or other locally recognizable phenomena on the site of anchorage.

With the high-pressure cementing technique it is now possible, without failure and in spite of working with even higher viscosity cements, to press the cup in as far as intended, i. e., until the desired thickness of the layer of cement, 4–6 mm, is achieved.

(Note: The high-pressure cementing technique is not only suitable for cups, but also for implanting femur components; (see above).

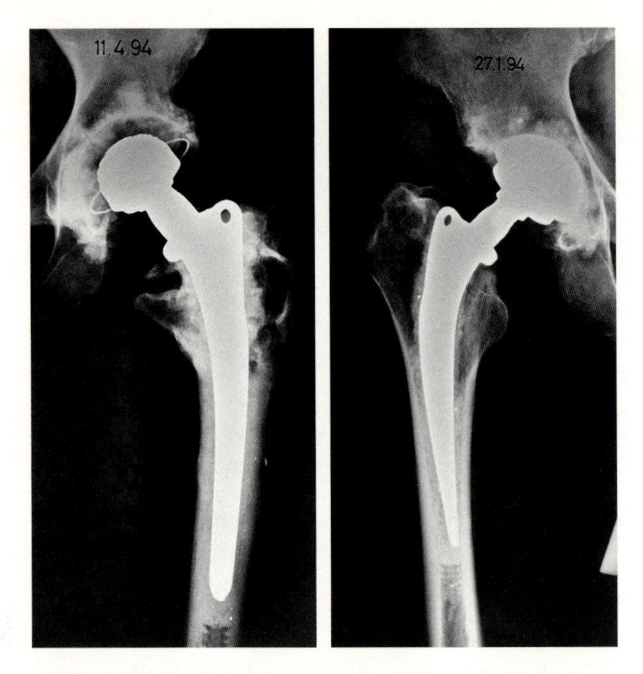

Fig. 7ab. X-raiy of the Weber Metasul cups. (**a**) Example of a Weber polyethylene Metasul cup Status after a valgus-shaping osteotomy with the consequent straight stem. (**b**) Example of a Weber polyethylene Metasul cup with Sulmesh surface. Status after idiopathic necrosis of the head in a „normal hip," with the consequent anatomically curved stem

Summary

Weber polyethylene and Metasul cups are used for the high-viscosity cementing technique described by Charnley. The cementing technique is, made easier with the help of a lever instrument set, so that the procedure can thus be precisely controlled, with no fear that the cup might not be pressed in to a sufficient depth.

Premature loosening following insufficient filling is simply and safely avoidable. With Weber Metasul cups a far higher working life can be foreseen, since with the help of Metasul pairings the abrasion of polyethylene, a harmful substance for the prosthesis has been eliminated.

References

1. Charnley, J (1970) Total hip replacement by low friction arthroplasty. Clin Orthop 72: 7
2. McKee, GK (1982) Total hip replacement. Present and future. Biomaterials 3: 130–135
3. Weber, BG (1988) Pressurized cement fixation in total hip arthroplasty. Clin Orthop 232: 87–95
4. Weber, BG (1993) Total hip joint replacement using a CoCrMo metal-metal sliding pairing. J Jpn Orthop Assoc 67: 391–398
5. Willert, HG (1977) Reactions of the articular capsule to wear products of artificial joint prostheses. J Biomed Mat Res 11: 157–164

Part III

Noncemented Acetabular Fixation

Noncemented Acetabular Fixation in Primary Total Hip Replacement

E. Morscher

Introduction

The main long-term problem with total hip arthroplasty remains aseptic loosening, particularly of the cup. This was pointed out by Charnley in 1979 [31] and is demonstrated by the survivorship analyses of Sutherland et al. [240], Morscher and Schmassmann [170], and others (Fig. 1). Mulroy and Harris [177] found a 20-fold increase in the rate of acetabular loosening between 5 and 11 years. Whereas the rate of loosening for the stem follows a roughly linear course, aseptic loosening of the cup is relatively rare during the first 6–8 years but increases exponentially after the 10th postoperative year [170] (Fig. 1).

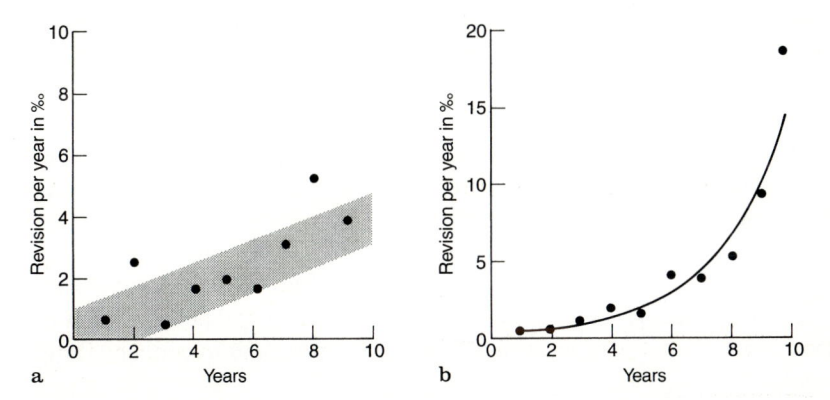

Fig. 1. a Linear loosening (revisions) of femoral stems. **b** Exponential increase in acetabular cup loosening after 8–10 years

Reported rates of loosening of cemented acetabula vary enormously, from 1 % to 29 % [152], but much of this variation depends on how loosening is defined, on component design, on the technique of implantation, and of course on the follow-up period.

Although aseptic loosening of the acetabular component is undoubtedly the major problem in total hip replacement, when loosening is defined radiologically, there is a substantial disparity between radiographic and clinical results. Many patients who radiologically have a definitely loose acetabular component continue to have excellent clinical function and experience no pain [97, 160]. The verdict on an acetabular socket therefore must be based on (a) histomorphological analysis of retrieved implants, (b) analysis of the roentgenograms, (c) clinical results, and (d) on survivorship analysis. Furthermore, it must be remembered that some failures will always occur, and that they can be recognized in the above sequence.

Risk Factors for Aseptic Loosening

Age and Activity

The results of hip arthroplasty in younger patients are generally much less favorable than with older ones [4, 22, 28, 52, 60, 97, 116, 170]. However, the reported higher loosening rates among younger individuals affects most often the femoral component [28, 52, 97]. We have also found an increased rate of cup wear in younger individuals, probably related to increased activity levels [257].

Sex

In the Swedish multicenter study for patients with arthrosis the percentage of men with aseptic loosenings was higher than that among women in all age groups [4]. In our experience, however, the risk of cup loosening is significantly higher for women than for men. We found an increase acetabular failure rate among women with cemented [170] as well as with noncemented [257] acetabular components. On the other hand, stem loosening is more frequent among men [170].

We also found the average acetabular size to be smaller in women, and failure was more common in those with a smaller acetabulum. This may be due to sex-related differences [170]. A marked preponderance of females is evident in rheumatoid arthritis, in complications after hip fracture, and in congenital hip dysplasia [4].

Body Weight

Schurman et al. [224] investigated risk factors associated with mechanical loosening of total hip arthroplastics and found weight ($p < 0.015$) and age ($p < 0.087$) to be important determinants of hip failure. Greater body weight is also associated with increasing volumetric wear of polyethylene [128].

Underlying Pathology of Osteoarthritis

The quality of implant anchorage depends largely on the quality of the host's bone. If the quality is inferior, fixation is basically insufficient, and early loosening must be expected. The etiology of osteoarthritis of the hip therefore correlates directly with the final outcome of the arthroplasty.

Congenital Dislocation of the Hip

The shorter longevity of acetabular fixation in osteoarthritis secondary to congenital dislocation of the hip is at least partially due to the younger age in this group of patients and the increased incidence of previous operations on the affected hip [43]. Our own follow-up study showed that even in acetabulae with a high acetabular angle the survival of an acetabuloplasty with augmented femoral head grafts is not diminished [101].

Protrusio Acetabuli

To prevent the acetabular cup from sinking too deeply in cases of protrusio acetabuli, fresh autologous cancellous bone grafts from the femoral head or solid autogenous femoral head are laid into the depth of the acetabulum [12, 57, 75, 139]. Correction of the anatomic position is vital whether accomplished with cement, mesh, protrusio shell, or bone graft. However, Bayley et al. [12] found a 50 % loosening rate in the cement group with protrusio acetabuli.

Rheumatoid Arthritis

In rheumatoid arthritis the acetabular component is especially at risk for loosening [4, 20, 201, 236, 245, 258]. Gschwend and Siegrist [89] reported in their patients a rate of cup loosening that is increased by a factor of 11 when rheumatoid arthritis patients are compared to cases with primary osteoarthritis. In the Swedish multicenter study there was a significant increase in loosening of the acetabular component in the older rheumatoid group [4].

Out of 14 total hip replacements in patients with rheumatoid arthritis, at a mean age of 16 (12–22 years) and with an average follow-up of 8.5 years (4–11) Learmonth et al. [124] did not have to revise a single hip. However, 57 % showed radiological changes suggestive of impending failure. In a stereophotogrammetric analysis of acetabular prostheses Snorrason and Kärrholm [235] found that the proportion of cemented cups migrating was significantly greater in patients with rheumatoid arthritis than in osteoarthrosis.

Sickle-cell Hemoglobinopathy

In a review of 22 total hip replacements performed in 14 patients at the New York Hospital for Special Surgery Moran et al. [153] and Acurio and Friedman [1] in a retrospective review of 25 hip arthroplasties in 25 patients with sickle-cell hemoglobinopathy found that it carries a high risk of complications and failures, although hip arthroplasty provides the most reliable measure of effective treatment in sickle-cell hemoglobinopathy.

Avascular Necrosis of the Femoral Head

In a follow-up of 54 patients (73 hips) with avascular necrosis of the femoral head at our own institution [60] we found a loosening rate of 10 % after an average of 4.9 years. The revision rate is hence lower than that reported by other authors but is still higher than in patients with osteoarthritis. It must, however, be remembered that the age of patients with avascular necrosis is much lower, and this also may contribute to the higher loosening rate [20]. In a retrospective review of 25 hip arthroplasties in 25 patients with sickle-cell hemoglobinopathy and osteonecrosis at a mean age of 30 years (16–45), Acurio and Friedman [1] found a very high risk-to-benefit ratio. Of these arthroplasties 40 % had been revised at a mean postoperative time of 7.5 years.

Paget's Disease

The results of total hip replacement in Paget's disease [65, 93, 132, 140, 145, 238] are comparable to those in non-Pagetic bone.

Transformation of an Arthrodesis into an Arthroplasty

Under favorable conditions, particularly of the muscular system, an arthrodesis can be successfully converted into a total hip arthroplasty. In a follow-up of 41 fused hips in 38 patients which were converted to total hip replacement, Kilgus et al. [115] found that the quality of the results approached that of primary hip arthroplasty and the probability of survival of the implant was 96 % at 13 years postoperatively!

Sequelae After Fracture of the Femoral Neck

As in rheumatoid patients Snorrason and Kärrholm [234, 236] found the proportion of migrating cemented cups significantly greater in patients with sequelae after fracture of the neck of the femur compared to osteoarthrosis.

Fracture of the Acetabulum

According to a retrospective study of 55 primary total hip arthroplasties with a history of previous acetabular fracture at the Mayo Clinic [34], the incidence of radiographic loosening, symptomatic loosening, and revision was four to five times higher than in routine arthroplasties. The authors conclude that a history of prior acetabular fracture has a significant adverse impact on the longevity of any subsequent total hip arthroplasty.

Acetabular Fixation with Bone Cement

The introduction of bone cement (polymethylmetacrylate PMMA) to hip surgery by Charnley in 1960 [29] revolutionized total arthroplasty. However, the loosening, particularly loosening of the cemented acetabular component, remained a major problem.

Radiological signs of loosening differ when a cup is fixed with or without cement, and therefore proper definitions of loosening must be established [174].

The radiographic criteria for assessing the fixation of a cemented cup are radiolucency, demarcation, migration, and component tilting. Charnley reported in 1979 [31] that after an observation time of 12–15 years 25 % of the cups in his patients showed radiolucency. Radiolucency is evaluated in relation to extent, thickness, progression, and localization. An impending failure is implied by complete radiolucency, that is, a radiolucency of 2 mm or more in all three zones.

In contrast, Gruen's investigation [88] revealed no correlation between biomechanical features and radiographic data. It is also well known that radiographic signs which have been considered to indicate loosening of the cup are frequently seen in patients with no clinical discomfort [242]. This is in contrast to the findings with cemented femoral stems. In a radiographic analysis of 102 revisions of Charnley prostheses Thorén and Hallin [242] found a radiolucent zone at the cup with a width of 2 mm or more in 12/30 loose cups and in only 4/24 firm ones. Migration of the cup of 6 mm or more was seen in 12/34 loose cups but in only 3/33 well-fixed ones ($p < 0.05$). The authors concluded that the criteria for radiographic loosening do not necessarily predict the optimal timing for revision.

Mjöberg [152] defined migration as the only definite sign of loosening in cemented hip replacement. If this definition is applied, the loosening rate following cemented arthroplasty reported by Charnley 12–15 years postoperatively was 11 % [31], by Gudmundsson et al. [91] 10–14 years postoperatively 10 %, and 5–12 years after cementless Ring arthroplasty 7 % [6]. These are the rates of loosening with which other results must subsequently be compared.

There is no question that improved cementing techniques have yielded a marked reduction in the rate of femoral component loosening. The incidence of acetabular loosenings, however, is only slightly reduced or not influenced at all. Nasser et al. [179] found an improvement in the longevity of the acetabular component in the older age group whereas Mulroy and Harris [177] found the incidence of acetabular loosening unchanged. Their incidence of radiographic loosening on the acetabular side was 42 % after an observation time of 11.2 years. According to Philips and Hamilton [194], the predicted survivorship at 18 years is 74 % for the acetabulum but 96 % for the femur.

In 1976 Charnley introduced a flanged socket [32] that offers an advantage in terms of cement pressurization at the time of implantation. With this socket the incidence of radiological demarcation at the cement/bone interface could markedly be reduced [102].

Long Posterior Wall Acetabulum. To prevent dislocation Charnley also introduced sockets with a long posterior wall. However, these implants removed at revision frequently showed erosion indicating impingement. The repetitive torques exerted on these sockets may thus contribute to loosening of these sockets [178].

Metal Backing of Cemented Acetabula. The rationale for metal-backed hemispheric cups has been presented as optimal strength, as minimal bone resection, rigid immobilization, and ease of possible removal [96]. Metal backing helps to avoid peak stresses by spreading stress over a much larger area [40, 188]. Apart from modifying the transmission of forces metal backing acts as a polymer containment and diminishes cold flow of the polyethylene, as was shown in tibial components by Ryd et al. [214]. On the other hand, Cates et al. [27] found a 37 % increase in mean polyethylene wear rates in cemented metal-backed cups, which may partially explain the higher failure rate of these sockets. In a three-dimensional model Dalstra and Huiskes [41] have shown increased stresses within the polyethylene if it is metal-backed. Hernandez et al. [98] found a significant increase in polyethylene wear in uncemented metal backed acetabular components. This was even worse if the femoral component was uncemented as well. Failures have been reported in modular metal-backed acetabular components (fractures of the polyethylene and the metal back, dislocations etc.) [21, 23, 80, 215]. Comparing 100 non-metal-backed polyethylene cups with 138 metal-backed cemented cups Ritter et al. [208] reported 22 % radiolucencies, 2 % loose cups, and 2 % revisions in polyethylene cups in comparison to 41 % radiolucencies, 3 % loose sockets, and 5 % revisions in metal-backed acetabula. Since clinical practice has failed to indicate any improvement in results with metal backing, while results may be even worse, the question of elasticity of the pelvis in combination with a rigid acetabular component becomes an important issue, as discussed below.

Cementless Acetabular Fixation

The implantation of acetabular components without PMMA may improve the long-term results of hip replacement by accomplishing the following six objectives.

Establishing a Better Host/Implant Interface

It is recognized that PMMA has certain potential disadvantages. These include shrinkage on polymerization, thermal injury to adjacent tissues, possible toxicity to adjacent tissues, mechanical weakness in shear, and tension and elastic modulus mismatch between implant and cement and between cement and bone. Bone lysis associated with histiocytic or macrophage activation with PMMA has been reported repeatedly [69, 78, 252–254]. These factors could compromise long-term fixation and ultimately lead to implant failure. If the cemented implant does loosen and the bone lysis proceeds, bone stock can be compromised and reconstruction made difficult. PMMA has also been associated with the potentiation of infection by inhibition of normal host responses to bacteria [191-193]. These disadvantages can be eliminated if the acetabular component is fixed without cement, provided the implant materials are better tolerated than PMMA itself.

Smaller Sized Implant Composite

To implant an acetabular prosthesis with PMMA it is necessary to have a cement mantle of at least 2 mm thickness surrounding the entire prosthesis. In addition, as cement is being pressurized into anchoring holes and cancellous bone, the total size of the implant construct increases. Should fixation fail, this increased volume of cement bone composite is destroyed and reconstruction becomes more difficult. Implantation of an acetabular prosthesis without cement lessens the overall size of the composite and conserves bone stock.

Facilitated Skeletal Augmentation

To reconstruct hips with insufficient bone stock, especially in protrusio or dysplasia, it may be necessary to use autologous or homologous bone grafts [12, 95, 101, 139]. The use of bone grafts in conjunction with PMMA can be difficult. It is necessary to confine the cement to areas which are not grafted so that the graft can be incorporated into the skeleton. If the confinement of the cement is not complete, the graft may be isolated by cement and fail to unite with the host bone. Conversely, bone grafting without PMMA is much easier. The graft is simply placed in the defect and held in place by the acetabulum. It should be noted that whether the prosthesis is fixed with cement or not, the graft itself cannot be used for the transmission of forces at the interface, and there thus seems little point in using cement to fix the prosthesis to the graft itself on purely mechanical grounds.

Simplified Surgical Procedure

Acetabular replacement without cement requires less time because bone preparation and the cleaning steps necessary for cement application are no longer necessary. This shortening of the surgical procedures decreases blood loss and reduces the incidence of postoperative infection.

Clinical Results at Least as Good as or Better with Implants Fixed Without Cement

Cemented arthroplasty of the hip has established a standard of clinical performance which must be at least equalled, if not surpassed, by any new technique. The relief of pain, rapid rehabilitation, and reproducible results to which surgeons and patients are accustomed with cemented replacement must not be sacrificed. The *early* and medium-term results of cementless acetabulum fixation equal those of cemented fixation [96, 161, 162].

Easy and Successful Revision Should Failure Occur

Cementless implants, should they fail, make revision arthroplasty easy if proper precautions are taken. The extensive bone loss associated with cemented acetabula is not present as a rule. After careful removal of the implant the acetabulum can be reamed to a slightly larger size, and any defects can be bone grafted before the new cementless cup is inserted.

Contraindications for the Use of Uncemented Acetabula

The use of uncemented acetabular cups in total hip replacement is contraindicated in cases with poor bone quality, for example, after irradiation of an ovarian carcinoma or in the presence of a malignant tumor of the pelvis. Since press-fit fixation requires a basically intact acetabulum, the use of a "press-fit cup" or "threaded cup" is contraindicated when the acetabular rim is missing. Alternatively, bone grafting might be performed.

Design and Outer Shape of Acetabular Cups

In cementless fixation of acetabular components four main types of cup design are used at present:
1. hemispherical cup (Boutin [18, 19], RM isoelastic joint [155-160], press-fit cup [164, 171] Harris-Galante, PCA etc.)
2. cylindrical socket (Lindenhof prosthesis [85, 86], Judet [111–113],
3. conical cup (Endler [6164], Mittelmeier [148–151], Ring [205, 206, 208], Zweymüller [263])
4. ellipsoidal ring (Lord [130, 131]).

Most of the cylindrical, conical, and ellipsoidal sockets are provided with an outer thread and directly screwed into the acetabulum (threaded cups).

Hemispherical Cups

The normal hip joint is nearly spherical. Therefore compressive forces from the pelvis are transferred harmoniously and evenly to the femur. In a normal hip joint the compressive forces are transferred from the cortex and the subchondral bone plate of the acetabular roof according to the trabecular pattern perpendicular to the surface of the femoral head [104]. The hemisphere therefore appears to be the optimally adapted design for a cup: The subchondral bone can be preserved, adaptation is excellent, and forces can be transmitted in a physiological way from the pelvis to the cup and vice versa. The medial wall is protected, the perioperative defect is minimal, augmentation is facilitated, and revision, if necessary, is feasible.

However, a hemispheric cup in a hemispheric cavity cannot provide intrinsic stability required for primary stability. To achieve stability of a purely hemispheric cup in a hemispheric cavity, additional measures must be taken [141].

Fixation of the Cup with Screws

The evidence of our study with uncoated RM polyethylene cups [257] points to the conclusion that fixation with bone screws makes no difference in the failure rate of the prosthesis. The rate of loosening was even higher when screws had been used (9,5 %) than not (5 %). Where the acetabular cup had been fixed with screws, the occurrence or absence of screw breakage did not make a difference to the loosening rate. Screw fixation therefore appears unnecessary, probably because any stability achieved by bone screws is short lived and does not affect the final stability of the implant. On the contrary, screws may cause additional problems with impingement on the polyethylene insert in case of migration. It has been shown by roentgen stereophotogrammetry that almost all acetabular cups undergo some migration, amounting to about 1–2 mm in the first 2 years [8]. This may not be recognized under normal circumstances [203, 211]. Therefore adequate fixation must be achieved in uncemented hip replacement without the use of bone screws or dowels [71]. Furthermore, Wasielewski et al. [249] Keating et al. [114], and Kirkpatrick et al. [117] performed anatomical and radiographic studies on cadaveric pelvis and clearly showed that venous, arterial, neural, and splanchnic structures are at risk when screws are placed in the acetabulum.

Fixation by Press-Fit

With the development of the press-fit cup we have tried to fulfill the currently understood requirements for successful cementless cup fixation which so far have been covered only partially with other designs [166, 171]. Press-fit (i. e., preload between bone and implant to achieve primary stability) is produced by flattening the hemisphere and using a cup with a size 1.5 mm larger than the corresponding reaming of the acetabulum. The press-fit cup is thus fixed in the acetabulum by a snap fastener mechanism. As a result of this mechanism there are no longer high compression forces concentrated in the dome of the acetabulum, i. e. in zone 2 of DeLee and Charnley [44], but these forces are transmitted to the periphery (zones 1 and 3). As Goodmann and Carter [81] have shown, stress concentrations are developed in zones 1 and 3, with relative sparing of

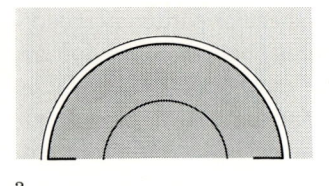

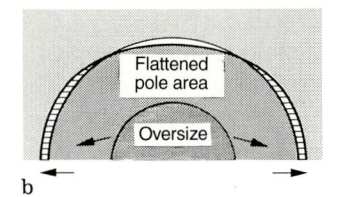

Fig. 2. Snap fastener mechanism. **a** non-stable situation in a hemispheric cup in a hemispheric acetabulum. **b** "intrinsic stability" by an oversized and flattened hemisphere

zone 2 (Fig. 2). When loaded the acetabulum closes in such a manner as to squeeze the cup, creating additional compressive radial stresses superiorly and inferiorly.

Threaded Cups

In laboratory experiments threaded cups provide an excellent primary stability, 2.5 times higher in conical than in spherical cups [246]. No differences in fixation strength attributable to the design of screw ring acetabular components in bone were observed by Kody et al. [120], whereas in foam components with widely spaced, deep threads and minimal thread interruptions offered the strongest initial fixation.

Secondary fixation of threaded and porous-coated acetabular components was evaluated mechanically and histologically in dogs after weight-bearing periods between 2 and 6 months by Tooke et al. [243]. These experiments showed that threaded specimens are significantly more often loose than porous-coated specimens at both 2 and 6 months.

Blum et al. [16] compared 34 PCA cups with 22 threaded (TTAP) cups concerning migration and rotation. Detailed analyses of serial radiographs demonstrated that 35 % of the PCA and 64 % of the TTAP components had migrated more than 3 mm. There was no correlation between the clinical performance and radiographic migration of PCA implants. However, 43 % of the threaded cups with significant (> 3 mm) migration had to be revised. Similarly negative experiences with threaded acetabular components were made by Engh et al. [66] in that an average follow-up of 3.9 years 21 % of the patients with a smooth threaded cup showed radiographic signs of instability and 25 % had clinical symptoms. None of the patients with a porous component had signs of instability (follow-up 4.8 years). At a follow-up of 30 months in 121 patients who had total hip replacement with threaded cups Apel et al. [7] found a 3 % incidence of cup dislodgment, 24 % radiolucencies between 1 and 2 mm, and 22 % with moderate to severe pain. A clinical and radiographic review of 48 total hip arthroplasty patients with threaded acetabular components was undertaken at 24–44 months of follow-up by Shaw et al. [231]. Radiographic analysis revealed stable acetabular components in 88 % of primary and 61 % of revision procedures only. The rate of acetabular component loosening was considered unacceptably high in revision cases and an area of concern in primary cases. The migration of a fully threaded cementless acetabular component (Link V type) was measured by Snorrason and Kärrholm [234] using roentgen stereophotogrammetric analysis. In contrast to the threaded cups, only of 22 cups with press-fit fixation migrated during the observation period.

Many other authors reported similar poor results with threaded acetabular components [25, 33, 81, 82, 133, 233, 235]. Bobyn et al. [17] examined one case in which the threaded titanium ring appeared to be well incorporated with no discernible radiolucency. Microradiography and histology, however, surprisingly showed that the threads were entirely encapsulated in fibrous tissue. In a geometric study of the primary fixation of Lord prosthesis Schimmel and Huiskes [220] showed that threaded designs offer a small contact area between prosthesis and bone, and in a finite element analysis Huiskes [108] found an unfavorable load transfer from cup to bone on a theoretical basis.

Based on these facts threaded cups have been practically abandoned in North America, although it should be recognized that porous-coated threaded cups give significantly superior results over smooth-threaded cups [68, 202].

Reinforcement of the Acetabulum

The principle of reinforcing the acetabulum has been introduced to use intact resistant bone structures of the ilium for distributing the forces over a larger area. There are three means of reinforcement in use: 1. pilot screws [221, 222], 2. the Müller reinforcement ring [2, 181, 193], and 3. the reinforcement cage of Burch-Schneider [218, 221]. In addition to acetabular revision surgery, the use of an acetabular reinforcement ring may be indicated in severe osteoporosis, protrusio acetabuli, total hip replacement following arthrodesis, old fractures of the acetabulum, or congenital dislocation of the hip. According to Rosson and Schatzker [210], the Müller ring is indicated for acetabulae with isolated peripheral segmental defects or cavity defects confined to one or two sectors. The Burch-Schneider cage should be used for medial segmental defects, extensive cavity defects, and combined deficiencies. Defects should be reconstituted with bone grafts rather than cement [210, 218].

Modular Socket Components

Modular socket systems have become increasingly popular. The replaceability of the polyethylene liner seems to be advantageous [97]. In cases where changing of the liner becomes necessary because of the excessive polyethylene wear this could be performed without disrupting the fixation of the metal shell in the bony bed. Revision of the cup, however, is practically never indicated for wear of the polyethylene only. In a review of 1964 primary total hip replacement at the Mayo Clinic none had been revised because of wear of the polyethylene [128]. In contrast, cases have been reported in which removable liners failed either for a design weakness or poor implantation technique [9, 23, 67, 118, 244, 256].

Surface

To ensure a harmonious transmission of forces, the surface of the endoprosthesis must conform closely to the bone and to the contact areas through which forces are transmitted. These areas should be as large as possible to avoid stress concentrations. When the contact surface between implant and bone is enlarged, the fixation of the prosthesis is improved, especially where bony tissue is growing into pores and indentations of the implant surface.

Cup Size

The smaller the cup the more likely loosening is to occur. In our study with noncoated cementless RM polyethylene cups the loosening rate was 8 % with cups of 52 mm diameter and less, compared to a rate of 5.4 % with cups 54 mm and larger [257].

Surface and Surface Structure

Uncoated Cups Made of High-Density Polyethylene

In 1973 a cementless polyacetal acetabular component was developed and used at our institution [155, 159, 167–169], but excessive rates of wear were noted. In 1977 a high-density polyethylene acetabular component was introduced for use in uncemented total hip replacement [156, 165, 173], with the aim of achieving isoelasticity and maintaining sphericity. Early results using this acetabular component were very encouraging [173]. Excellent early results have also been reported by others using polyethylene acetabulae in direct contact with bone [13, 119, 182, 207]. Histological examination from retrieved acetabulae [204], however, has suggested that cementless noncoated polyethylene acetabular replacement does not give such good long-term results as had originally been expected, and we therefore undertook a review of all the patients treated at our clinic with this cup in combination with a cemented stem between the years 1977 and 1982 (i. e., with a follow-up of more than 5 years) [257]. Up to 8 years the results with this cup are excellent, but thereafter increasing numbers of radiological loosenings and, after 9 years, increasing numbers of revisions for loosening become evident. At the time of revision there were almost always abraded areas on the outer surface of the cup where there had been contact areas and movement between bone and the polyethylene of the cup. The study of the histology of 23 cups retrieved postmortem showed that there was rarely bone integration into the grooves of the prosthesis [99, 204]. Conversely, we found that almost all of the cups were surrounded by a layer of fibrous tissue, with bone pseudopodia supporting the cups at certain discrete points, and the fibrous layer contained quiescent polyethylene debris. In direct polyethylene-to-bone contact areas a vicious circle takes place which leads eventually to implant loosening with bone resorption cavities. The contact between the outer surface of the polyethylene cup and bone tissue, which is not extensive but punctuated, induces areas of high pressure in the bone/implant interface. The alternating high loads at these contact areas induce impression of the polyethylene. Bone cannot resist this high specific pressure. Microfractures and resorption are the consequence, and this results in migration of the implant. Friction between bone and polyethylene produces polyethylene debris, inducing the formation of macrophages which cause enzymatic bone resorption (prostaglandin E). The loosening process of a polyethylene implant in direct contact with bone tissue is therefore a biological phenomenon which cannot be reproduced in a purely mechanical way in laboratory.

Charnley [31] was one of the first to implicate polyethylene debris as a cause of loosening of total hip replacements. Wroblewski [259] demonstrated that wear of polyethylene could result in bone resorption of massive proportions clinically, and Goldring et al. [79] reported high levels of prostaglandin E 2, which almost certainly cause the bone resorption secondary to the foreign body type giant cell reaction. It has been suggested that polyethylene should never come into direct contact with bone [13, 204, 227], and Wroblewski et al. [260] have subsequently shown that 32 % of loose acetabular components have a deficient cement layer between the bone and cup, with direct contact of the polyethylene on the bone which is then abraded. Gut et al. [92] found a loosening rate of the conical noncoated threaded polyethylene socket of Endler of 33.3 % (34/102) after an average observation period of 57.4 months. Krugluger and Eyb [121] found 36 Endler cups of 103 only to be stable after 10 years.

The early hopes that this type of implant would result in diminished bone loss and loosening have not been fulfilled, and this type of implant does not appear to offer any significant advantage compared to the results of Charnley and others with cemented acetabular replacements [30,168]. The use of this prosthesis was thus abandoned at our institution in 1983.

Coating for Prosthetic Surfaces

Coating can increase roughening or texturizing of the surface of the cup. Boutin [18, 19] in France was the first in 1969, to use porous ceramic *(alumine frittée)* for attaching a prosthetic cup directly to the acetabular bone. The idea behind macroporosity is to provide a surface of chemically inert pores with diameters greater than 100 µm that are receptive to bony ingrowth. According to Homsy [105, 106], a pore size of around 300 µm with a porosity volume of 40 %–80 % is considered ideal. Pioneer work in this respect has also been carried out by Ducheyne et al. in Belgium [54–56], Galante et al. [72–74] in the United States and Pilliar et al. [195–197] in Canada. These investigations on surface structures were of decisive importance in furthering the progress in cementless fixation of endoprostheses.

Hydroxyapatite Coating

Increasing interest has been shown in hydroxyapatite (HA) coatings [76–78, 125]. Both animal and clinical studies show without doubt that HA enhances in- and ongrowth of bony tissue and also provides strong fixation to bone, presumably by chemical bonding.

We first used HA to coat our polyethylene cups in January 1983. By January 1986, 594 of these cups had been implanted in primary and in revision arthroplasties. Clinical and radiological results remain satisfying to this day. In the follow-up period up to 4 years no cup has had to be removed because of aseptic loosening [163]. Geesink et al. [78] studied 100 consecutive cases of total hip arthroplasty using HA coating and found 97 % of the patients with positive roentgenograph

Table 1. Characteristics of Sulmesh

Materials	C. P. titanium
Surface	Fine blasted
Number of layers	4 ("7535")
Wire diameter (mm) of woven mesh layers	0.7/0.5/0.3/0.5
Interwire spacing (mm) of woven mesh layers	1.4/1.0/0.6/1.0
Heat bonding	Spot welding
Total thickness (mm) of four heat bondet layers	2.3–2.6
Average pore size (µm)	400
Porosity (%)	65

bone. To maximize the bone/implant interface area, the Sulmesh is roughened by corundum blasting.

Implant Material and Device Stiffness

The current choice of materials for use in endoprostheses is large. However, since the earliest days of hip joint arthroplasty, metallic implant materials have dominated.

Strength of the Implant Material

Selection of material with suitable mechanical properties and appropriate prosthetic design are crucial for initial and long-term fixation of the implant to the bone. Loosening of beads from porous-coated implants have been described several times. If progressive, it is not only a sign of insufficient fixation of the implant but may also increase the possibility of macrophage response to metallic debris [134].

Elasticity of the Implant

Fixation of an implant to bone is comparable to the healing of a fracture [160, 161]. Under optimal conditions direct bone formation is possible, comparable to primary bone healing in fracture treatment where close reduction and fixation of the fragments by compression is obtained [99]. Stable fixation thus requires implants of sufficient mechanical strength so that loads do not produce plastic deformation and relative movements between implant and bone. But stable fixation does not necessarily imply rigid implants. Both in fracture treatment and in endoprosthetic surgery the requirements for the implant are sufficient strength for lasting stability and flexibility for functional load.

Using a rigid implant to stiffen the entire bone-implant system is one possibility to achieve an interface free of motion. This, however, raises the question of whether stress protection and stress concentration known from the use of rigid implants in fracture treatment may become a problem. A sizable difference between the elasticity of the implant and the surrounding bone inevitably causes relative motion at the interface, as noted by Homsy et al. [105, 106], Mathys [136], and Sarmiento [216]. Obviously this depends largely on the direction of the forces. Under compressive forces differences in elasticity are of minor importance; under bending forces, however, the implant transmitting the forces to the bone should obviously be more rigid.

Metal Backing

Lord and Bancel [130] have reported good results up to 7 years after surgery using a metal-backed uncemented prosthesis, and others have reported similarly favorable *early* results with metal backed prostheses [6, 95, 136, 207]. It is therefore not surprising that metal backing of polyethylene sockets have found wide acceptance in the orthopedic community.

In sharp contrast to the satisfying short- and medium-term results there is a significant deterioration in clinical performance with time. Harris and Penenberg [97] observed 41 % radiolucencies and 17 % revisions after 11.3 years in 48 metal backed cups. Comparing non-metal-backed components with metal-backed components Mulroy and Harris [177] found 39 % loosening of non-metal-backed and 53 % loosening of metal-backed cups. Although the difference was not significant ($p < 0.133$) there was at least no proven superiority with metal backing!

The questionable properties of stiff implants, especially in porotic bone, is evident in ceramic cups. Sedel et al. [225, 226] reported a significantly increased rate of loosening with these cups in elderly patients. In his opinion the fragile bone in elderly patients does not tolerate the continuing blows of the rigid ceramic.

Wanivenhaus and Zweymüller [248] have reported on the 5- to 10-year results of a hemispherical ceramic acetabular cup with small pegs, which is designed for cementless implantation. At an average follow-up of 89 months the results revealed 60 % loosenings and radiolucencies of more than 2 mm width. The authors concluded that a ceramic cup of this shape is apparently unsuitable for osseointegration: "It would appear that the design favours tilting movements and, due to its high E-module, is unable to compensate for the relative movements of the pelvis." Knahr et al. [119] reported 20 % loosenings after 8 years with the same ceramic cup.

Friction, adherence, and press fit are stronger between two elastic materials than between an elastic and a rigid material. A cup with no metal backing improves press fit and maintains it for a longer time than a metal-backed cup of the same geometry. Mechanical tests with the press-fit cup show a decrease of

50 %–75 % in elasticity due to Sulmesh compared with noncoated polyethylene cups. Preservation of some elasticity also guarantees a shock absorption effect.

Metal backing was introduced not only for better force transmission but also to protect polyethylene from abrasive wear where it comes into direct contact with bone. Freeman and Railton [70] introduced a metal back for their component in 1984 using an uncoated hemispheric polyethylene cup. They showed that the fixation of this component, judged both by the need for revision after aseptic loosening and by migration, was less satisfactory than the identical component without metal back. They concluded that both at the acetabulum and the tibia (knee arthroplasties) increased rigidity reduces the stability of fixation when comparing the migration rates for the plain uncemented polyethylene device, for the same device fixed with cement, for the same device with metal backing, and for one of the two metallic-fit implants. These data suggest that a properly designed press fit device may be more stable in the acetabular cavity than a cemented implant. In their view, theoretically at least there is a case for using a flexible but nonabradable surface to interface with bone at the acetabulum [71, 181].

Judging from the conclusion that cemented metal-backed cups are almost certainly not an improvement, one might ask why cementless metal back cups should be viewed as a better solution! It can be concluded that the preservation of some elasticity of the implant is of outmost importance.

Isoelasticity

By adjusting the physical characteristics of the implant material to that of bone tissue and the design of the endoprosthetic components to the host bone, the entire system could be expected to have the same elasticity as the normal pelvis or femur.

Increased elasticity of endoprosthetic components, which can be achieved by the use of titanium or plastic materials, makes possible a more even, harmonious distribution of the forces transmitted from the implant to the bone and vice versa. If the elasticity of the implant approaches that of the bone in the acetabular area, the artificial cup should adjust to the deformation of the bony pelvis. A more elastic hip endoprosthesis may also act as a shock absorber during walking, particularly in the heel-strike and toe-off phases [164]. This has been the concept for the development of the "isoelastic" hip endoprosthesis manufactured by Mathys (Factory for Surgical Instrumentation, Bettlach, Switzerland).

The natural hip joint has a relatively high elasticity. Since cartilage absorbs only about 10 % of the energy [146], it appears that its main function is the distribution of stress [34]. This function can be better duplicated with an elastic acetabular component which is in close contact with the bone than with a metal backing. The shock-absorbing and stress-distributing properties of high-density polyethylene are based on the high compressibility and the high impact strength.

Brake Drum phenomenon. The force acting from the prosthetic head on the cup can – under unfavorable conditions such as excessive stresses in combination with high elasticity – produce a deformation of the cup, the outer rim of the cup clutching the prosthetic head (Fig. 3). This so-called brake drum phenomenon was thoroughly investigated by Plitz in 1984 [198, 199]. In his experiment even relatively minimal forces (FZ = 1000–2000 N) led to a reduction of some 0.1 mm in the cup diameter in the equatorial region. The play of 0.6 mm in the diameter between prosthetic head (28 mm) and inner bearing surface of the press-fit cup guarantees that there is no locking of the prosthetic head in the cup even under excessive load.

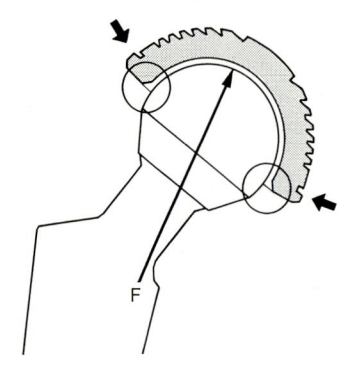

Fig. 3. Brake drum phenomenon. Maximum deformation when impacted, 0.14 mm (in vitro); play between prosthetic head and cup 0.4–0.6 mm

Articulating Surface

Size of the Femoral Head

In respect to the articulating surfaces acetabular cup loosening depends on the friction between the gliding surfaces and on the material wear. Pedersen et al. [188] found a steady increase in stress levels in the bone cement with increasing femoral head diameter from 22 to 44 mm. In their experimental study Hoeltzel et al. [103] quantified the states of stress on the surface of the acetabular cup and proposed the possible existence of an optimum component size to minimize surface stress. The largest absolute strains were recorded when loading with the 22-mm head size. Peak strain values decreased to a minimum with the 26-mm head size and increased steadily with head sizes beyond 26 mm. Furthermore, the results of Pedersen et al. [188] indicate that stresses also depend on the polyethylene wall thickness. Higher stresses are generated in thin-walled cups.

Friction depends on the area of contact and on the amount of pressure. The smaller the head size, the smaller is the contact area, and the higher the pressure per unit surface. Therefore for a given case (body weight, level of activity, etc.) there should be a compromise between smaller and larger head sizes. However, the influence of friction and polyethylene wear is time dependent. With high friction – as is the case in resurfacing arthroplasties (Wagner, Freeman, Capello, Amstutz) – loosening of the components takes place in the short run. Loosening due to polyethylene wear, however, is a long-term phenomenon. Therefore on short-term follow-up better results are demonstrated by endoprostheses with a small head size (Charnley's low friction arthroplasty). The longer the observation time, the more important is the amount of polyethylene wear.

In the Swedish multicenter study [4] 22-mm heads (Charnley) were compared with 32-mm heads (Lubinus). No difference was apparent in the loosening rate with these two head diameters. However, Ritter et al. [208] reported a higher loosening rate for 32-mm head size in Müller total hip replacement (15 %) than for 22-mm Charnley hip arthroplasty (4 %). Morrey and Ilstrup [154] found the following revision rates: 1 % with a 22-mm head (44/4.576) after 9,1 years, 0,4 % with 28-mm heads (2/520) after 5.7 years, and 2.7 % with the 32-mm head diameters (13/487) after 8.2 years. In a 9.5-year radiographic study Livermore et al. [128] found the least amount of wear to be associated with the 28-mm femoral head component and the greatest amount in 22-mm components ($p < 0.01$). Furthermore, radiographic evidence of adverse bone/prosthesis interface characteristics was positively correlated with increased wear debris. This appears to contrast with the results of Frankel et al. [69] who found in a radiographic analysis of 182 hip arthroplasties using modern cement techniques including metal-backed acetabular components a three-zone demarcation of acetabular bone/cement interface in 56 % of the 32-mm group compared to only 5 % of the 22-mm group. These authors emphasize the adverse effects of large femoral head prosthesis on cement/bone interface. However, the observation time in their study was only 19 months for the 32-mm and 24 months for the 22-mm head sizes. During this period the adverse effect of polyethylene debris on the loosening process could not yet become effective.

The conclusion from these mechanical studies and clinical experiences is that stress at the implant-bone and cement/bone interface depends on a variety of factors. Since for the loosening process not only stress but also polyethylene debris plays a decisive role the biological process is very time dependent. For a given case it should theoretically be possible to optimize the geometrical dimensions of the components. However, in daily practice our selection of the acetabular and femoral components is arbitrary, and a compromise for 26- or 28-mm head diameters could be the solution to the problem. This corresponds with experience at the Mayo Clinic where stability, acetabular loosening, and wear with a prosthetic femoral head of intermediate size, such as a 28-mm head, appears to provide the best wear characteristics in total hip arthroplasty.

Materials for the Gliding Surfaces

Low friction between the prosthetic components and minimal abrasion are both fundamental for a long service of an artificial joint replacement.

Metal-Polyacetal

In 1973 we implanted the first cementless acetabular cup made of polyacetal resin designed by Mathys [155, 167-169, 172]. During testing in vitro the elastic values were similar to those of bone, and the friction properties were satisfactory. In vivo, however, there was unexpected, excessive abrasive wear which eliminated this material altogether for further use as a gliding surface in weight bearing joints and thus for acetabular hip replacement.

Mathiesen et al. [135] found that friction in retrieved polyacetal sockets was twice as great as in retrieved polyethylene sockets, and they also found that frictional characteristics of polyacetal change as the material ages in vivo. High friction in the polyacetal socket may therefore well be an explanation for the high incidence of loosening with the Christiansen prosthesis, which has been widely used in Scandinavian countries.

Metal (Stainless Steel, Cobalt-Chrome)-High-Density Polyethylene

Charnley was the first to use plastic material on metal as articulating surface. After his first, catastrophic experiences with Teflon he introduced high-density Polyethylene (HDPE) as gliding surface for the acetabulum in 1962. Although HDPE debris may be one of the main cause of late endoprosthesis loosening this material has withstood the test of time [32].

Increased wear rates and excessive amounts of wear debris can be found where bone and bone cement particles have been found in the articulating surface of explanted hip prostheses [26]. The additives to render PMMA radiopaque cause scratching and deterioration in the surface finish of metallic femoral heads. In experiments performed by the same authors, particles of bone cement with zirconium dioxide and barium sulfate additives and particles of cortical bone scratched the stainless steel surface. The cement particles with zirconium dioxide additive produced significantly greater surface damage.

Cup wear of the articulating surface has been minimal in our study of non coated HDPE sockets in the majority of patients [257], as reported also by other authors [29, 130, 237]. However, in cases with cup loosening the wear was very marked. There are three possible explanations for this. First, polyethylene wear in the acetabulum leads to particles being released; these migrate between the acetabulum and the bone causing a foreign body reaction and bone lysis, leading eventually to loosening. Second, once the cup is loose, deformation of the acetabulum is increased because the polyethylene is no longer supported by the subchondral bone plate due to bone destruction, and as a result friction and wear are increased. Third, wear leads to eccentricity of the head in the socket, which causes increased rotating moment and friction and thus increased shear between the bone and the polyethylene, which results in socket loosening [152].

Ceramic-High-Density Polyethylene

According to Semlitsch et al. [227-229], Gualtieri [90], Schüller and Marti [223], and others [42, 59, 185, 250, 262], a lower longterm rate of wear on the polyethylene socket is provided by a ball head made of extremely pure, high-strength Al_2O_3 ceramic than by a metal HDPE combination. Using a knee prosthesis model, Oonishi et al. [184] found that the wear of polyethylene is ten times less in combination with ceramic than in combination with metal.

Ceramic-Ceramic

Aluminium oxide was introduced in endoprosthesis surgery by Boutin [18, 19] in 1970. Ceramic shows excellent biocompatibility and the combination ceramic-ceramic has also been shown to have excellent tribological properties [49, 83-87, 181]. The investigation of Dorlot et al. [50, 51] on 20 prostheses with a ceramic-ceramic combination removed because of aseptic loosening showed wear to be 400 times less than in metal-polyethylene combination, while the ceramic-polyethylene combination reduced wear only by a factor of 2. Low rate of wear, however, is possible only if the two joint components are perfectly congruent, and if the ceramic cup is not placed in vertical position. Unfavorable conditions as described above induce a remarkable wear and can consequently end in progressive ceramic wear [200]. Mittelmeier and Harms [151], Griss and Heimke [83], Griss et al. [84], Knahr et al. [119], and many others have observed remarkable wear after some years of clinical use. Considerable wear in six Autophor prostheses (Mittelmeier) after an average of 29 months was also observed by Kummer et al. [122]. Most authors have therefore discontinued the use of this combination.

Metal to Metal

Since hemiarthroplasty – at least in osteoarthritis of the hip – revealed unsatisfactory results, the acetabular side as well was replaced and total hip replacement introduced. The first combinations employed were metal (cast CoCrMo alloy) to metal. Since femoral components with large femoral heads already existed, such as the Moore prosthesis, a large acetabular component (35–42 mm) was required as well [142, 175, 205, 232, 250]. With the introduction of Charnley's low-friction arthroplasty using the combination metal-polyethylene, the metal-metal combination was replaced almost completely at the end of the 1960s. Semlitsch et al. [229] and Streicher et al. [239] performed investigations on total hip prostheses with cups and balls made of cast CoCrMo alloy that were implanted 10–20 years before. Their results revealed that metal-metal combinations produced very low wear. In comparison to polyethylene-metal combination the wear was 40–100 times lower. Based on these promising long-term clinical results, the metal-metal combination once again is of great interest for total hip prostheses [251, 252].

Titanium-High-Density Polyethylene

Black et al. [14] reported a case in which pain in the absence of infection or definite loosening led to revision. There was excessive wear of titanium alloy particles. The inflammation appeared to be predominantly phagocytic. McKellop et al. [142–144] observed an especially high wear rate in the presence of cement particles: the wear rate was increased by a factor of 50! From clinical experiences Dobbs and Scales [48] concluded that where titanium (or its alloys) are used as bearing surfaces in combination with polyethylene, they should be used with care, and that contact with acrylic cement should be avoided. Agins et al. [3] described the observation of nine cases of revised total hips with femoral shafts and femoral heads made of Ti6A14V alloy. They concluded that a femoral component made of titanium alloy can undergo severe wear on the head surface and on the stem when it comes loose. Lombardi et al. [129] found in two cases of aseptic loosening that the cause of failure was severe osteolysis induced by metallic debris from the modular head made of Ti6A14V without surface treatment

In summary, the combination surface untreated titanium versus HDPE has shown unsatisfactory results due to wear debris causing osteolysis and ultimately prosthesis failure [152]. Galante and Rostoker [72] concluded as early as in 1973 from the results of their experiments that the use of titanium or titanium alloys as gliding surface is not to be recommended.

Operating Technique

Preservation of the Subchondral Bone

There is little doubt that the subchondral bone is of great importance in supporting the acetabulum and preventing migration [36, 50, 51, 107, 109, 127]. Reaming of the subchondral bone weakens the normal acetabulum [108] and encourages micromovements [5]. Thus a hemispherical acetabular component which allows preservation of the subchondral bone is ideal. The cartilaginous layer and the subchondral bone is thus removed only until bleeding spots appear, so that bone tissue can grow into the porous surface of the uncemented device.

Position of the Acetabular Cup

The orientation of the acetabular component determines the direction of force transmission from the pelvis to the cup, the stability of the cup, and the range of motion.

Rotational Center of the Hip

The biomechanical situation of a given hip joint is determined mainly by the location of the center of rotation. The center of rotation is determined by both the acetabular component position and the outside and inside diameters of the acetabular component [261]. To avoid tilt moments between cup and bony acetabulum both rotational centers must coincide (concentricity; Fig. 4). During reaming the reamer is directed superiorly and medially; this results – especially with cups with a small head size and smaller outer diameter – in a more medial and more superior position than for normal hips. A medial and inferior position of the center of rotation results in a decrease in the forces generated [110]. Yoder et al. [261] found that femoral components with the center of rotation placed in a nearly anatomic location loosened at a statistically significantly lower rate than hips with the center of rotation superior and lateral. The acetabular component loosening rate was not affected by the inclination or anteversion of the cup, and this supports the theoretic evidence that the hip center location indeed affects hip loads. In addition, there are several clinical studies documenting that an anatomic placement of the acetabulum results in lower risk of loosening [24, 31, 123].

In contrast to these experiences, the findings of Russotti and Harris [212] and Russotti et al. [213] suggest that if circumstances dictate, proximal positioning of the acetabular component without lateral displacement can give an acceptable result in cemented total hip replacement procedure.

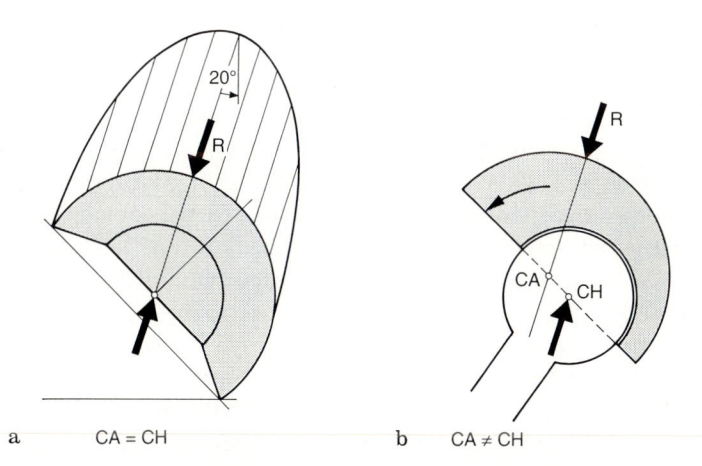

Fig. 4. Concentricity and eccentricity of the acetabular cup. To avoid tilt moments between cup and bony acetabulum both rotational centers must coincide. *CH*, Center of the head; *CA*, center of the acetabular cup

Coronal Orientation of the Cup

Recommendations for the orientation of the cup to the horizontal vary; some authors recommend 30° [93, 141], others 40° [170], and still others 45° [30, 39, 57]. Since the forces should be transmitted over an area as large as possible and mainly as compressive forces, a nearly horizontal position should theoretically be advantageous for longe-vity. A too horizontal position, however, runs the risk of lateral overhang with insufficient bony containment of the cup, with impingement between cup and greater trochanter, with limitation of abduction and cup loosening. Furthermore, Sarmiento et al. [217] propose that when a load on the hip results in forces directed upward and laterally, a horizontal cup is more susceptible to tilting than a vertically orientated one. On the other hand, a vertical position does not increase the risk of dislocation of the femoral head [217]. Dislocations are due mainly to the position of the posterior rim of the cup and the osseous acetabulum which acts as a hypomochlion for the neck in external rotation of the limb. Therefore it is mandatory to remove completely all protruding osteophytes from the posterior part of the acetabulum after the fixation of the socket. This mechanism of dislocation also explains the pitfalls of augmenting the cup rim in recurrent dislocation [180, 255]. This report is in accordance with our own findings [45] and those of Lewinnek [126] that in respect to the orientation of the cup the anteversion is much more relevant.

Several authors have studied the problem whether an unfavourable orientation of the artificial cup would influence the rate of cup loosening. The results of these studies are controversial. A correlation between acetabular cup loosening and cup orientation was found by Cotterill et al. [37] and Beckenbaugh and Ilstrup [11], but Tapadiya et al. [241], Miller [147], and Shaughnessy et al. [230] found no such correlation. The reason for these discrepancies may be that it is not the orientation itself but the containment of the cup in the acetabular cavity that is the determining factor for the loosening process. Sarmiento and coworkers [217] found lower incidences of continuous radiolucent lines and of acetabular wear with completely covered (cemented) cups. This is in accordance with the findings of Pellicci et al. [189, 190], Sutherland et al. [240], McBroom and Müller [138], and Morrey and Ilstrup [154] who associated partial containment with a higher incidence of acetabular loosening. Mechanical tests in cadaver pelves performed by Volz and Wilson [247] showed that less stability is achieved when the prosthetic cup is incompletely seated in the acetabulum.

The good results with vertically orientated cups reported by Russotti et al. [213], Salvati et al. [215], and Sarmiento et al. [217] are in contrast to reports by other authors who found vertical position to be correlated with higher incidences of calcar resorption [100], polyethylene wear [35], loosening of the cup [3, 24, 38, 47, 138, 190], and dislocation [126].

Since full containment of the cup in the acetabular cavity is more relevant than a more vertical position for the stability of the cup, and impingement on the inferior half-circumference of the cup should be avoided under all circumstances, we decided to bevel the press-fit cup.

A variety of devices have been developed to improve the positioning of the acetabular socket during surgery [53]. When, however, full containment of the cup and avoiding impingement of the lower rim of the cup with the neck of the femoral prosthesis is the main objective, the press-fit cup can easily be positioned without an aiming device. With this approach to the solution of various problems associated with the orientation of the acetabular cup only 13 dislocations (1 %) have been observed in 1254 primary total hip replacements performed with the press-fit cup with c. p. titanium Sulmesh coating from October 1985 until December 1992.

Primary and Secondary Stability of Cups Fixed Without Cement

With cemented cups fixation is best at the end of surgery. Overstated, this means that loosening begins when the wound is closed. However, in implants with a porous surface, that is, when final stability is achieved by bony ingrowth, the stability increases postoperatively. Bereiter (this volume), confirmed this hypothesis with experiments in mountain sheep.

Conclusions

The major long-term problem in total hip replacement is aseptic loosening of the cup. Younger age increases risk for the stem more than for the cup. The risk for cup loosening is higher in women than in men. Congenital dislocation of the hip, rheumatoid arthritis, and fractures of the acetabulum are definitive risk factors for cup loosening. Improved cementing techniques have resulted in a marked reduction in the rate of femoral component loosening but have only slightly reduced the rate of acetabular loosening. Even metal backing has failed to improve longer term results of acetabular fixation. The results of various noncemented cups are as good or better than those of cemented cups. Further advantages of cementless acetabular fixation are a better host/implant interface, facilitated skeletal augmentation, simplified and shorter surgical procedure, and easy revision in case of failure.

Hemispherical cups have been shown superior to cylindrical, conical, and ellipsoidal designs. The disadvantages of screws (for example operational risk) far outweigh their benefit, and it has yet to be shown that the results with screw fixation are superior. Since a hemispheric cup provides no stability in a hemispheric acetabulum, an oversized cup with flattened dome results in a snap fastener mechanism of fixation and therefore an intrinsic stability, as is the case with the authors press-fit cup. Threaded cups have been virtually abandoned, at least in North America.

The requirements for the coating are now well known and defined in relation to strength, bonding to the substrate, porosity, porous volume, and biocompatibility. Although there is some enthusiasm about HA a wait-and-see attitude is justified because of the brittleness of the material and its strength of bonding.

Concerning the operation technique a compromise between preservation of the subchondral bone and creating a vital bone bed – which allows bony ingrowth – is crucial. The orientation of the cup and the medial and inferior location of the hip center of rotation also play an important role in decreasing the interface shear forces.

For long-term success a femoral head size of 26–28 mm diameter could be a valuable compromise between low friction (22 mm) and lower HDPE abrasion (32 mm). The combination ceramic-head and HDPE socket has proven successful. Thanks to technological progress the combination of metal to metal once again is of great interest and must be followed carefully in the future.

References

1. Acurio MT, Friedman RJ (1992) Hip arthroplasty in patients with sickle-cell-haemoglobinopathy. J Bone Joint Surg [Br] 74: 367–371
2. Aebi M, Richner L, Ganz R (1989) Langzeitergebnisse der primären Hüfttotalprothese mit Acetabulumabstützring (ARR). Orthopäde 18: 504–510
3. Agins HJ, Alcock NW, Bansal M, Salvati EA, Wilson PD, Pellicci PM, Bullough PG (1988). Metallic wear in failed titanium – alloy total hip replacements. A histological and quantitative analysis. J Bone Joint Surg [Am] 70: 347–356
4. Ahnfelt L, Herberts P, Malchau H, Andersson GB (1990) Prognosis of total hip replacement. A Swedish multicenter study of 4664 revisions. Acta Orthop Scand Suppl 238: 1–26
5. Amstutz H (1982) Restoration of functional biomechanics in reconstructive hip surgery. NIH Consensus Development Conference, Bethesda
6. Andrew TA, Berridge D, Thomas A, Duke RNF (1984) Long-term review of ring total hip arthroplasty. Clin Orthop 201: 111–122
7. Apel DM, Smith DG, Schwartz CM, Paprosky WG (1989) Threaded cup acetabuloplasty. Early Clinical experience. Clin Orthop 241: 183–189
8. Baldursson H, Hansson Ll, Olsson TH, Selvik G (1980) Migration of the acetabular component after total hip replacement determined by roentgen stereophotogrammetry. Acta Orthop Scand 51: 535–540
9. Barrack RL, Burke DW, Cook SD, Skinner HB, Harris WH (1993) Complications related to modularity of total hip components. J Bone Joint Surg [Br] 75: 688–692
10. Bayley JC, Christie MJ, Ewald CF, Kelley K (1987) Long-term-results of total hip arthroplasty in protrusio acetabuli. J Arthroplasty 2: 275–279
11. Beckenbaugh RD, Ilstrup DM (1978) Total hip arthroplasty. A review of three hundred and thirthy-three cases with long-term follow-up. J Bone Joint Surg [Am] 60: 306–313
12. Bereiter H, Morscher E (1982) Spongiosaplastik des Pfannenbodens beim totalprothetischen Ersatz der Protrusionhüfte. Beitr Orthop Traumatol 29: 408–416
13. Bertin KC, Freeman MAR, Morscher E, Oeri A, Ring PA (1985) Cementless acetabular replacement using a pegged polyethylene prosthesis. Arch Orthop Trauma Surg 104: 251–261
14. Black J, Sherk H, Bonini J, Rostoker WR, Schajowicz F, Galante J (1990) Metallosis

associated with a stable titanium-alloy-femoral-component in total hip replacement. J Bone Joint Surg [Am] 72: 126–130
15. Bloebaum RD, Becks D, Dorr LD, Savory CG, DuPont JA, Hofmann AA (1994) Complications with hydroxyapatite particulate separation in total hip arthroplasty. Clin Orthop 298: 19–26
16. Blum HJ, Noble PC, Tullos HS (1990) Migration and rotation of cementless acetabular cups: incidence, etiology and clinical significance. AAOS Meeting, New Orleans
17. Bobyn JD, Engh CA, Glassman AH (1988) Radiography and histology of a threaded acetabular implant. J Bone Joint Surg 70 [Br]: 303–304
18. Boutin P (1972) Arthroplastie totale de la hanche par prothèse en alumine frittée. Rev Chir Orthop 58: 229–246
19. Boutin P (1974) Les prothèses totales de la hanche en alumine. L'ancrage direct sans ciment dans 50 cas. Rev Chir Orthop 60: 223–245
20. Brien W, Natarajan V, Sarmiento A (1989) Long-term results of cemented total hip arthroplasties in patients under and over fifty years of age. AAOS Meeting, Las Vegas
21. Brien WW, Salvati EA, Wright TM, Nelson CL, Hungerford DS, Gilliam DL (1990) Dissociation of acetabular components after total hip arthroplasty, J Bone Joint Surg [Am] 72: 1548–1550
22. Buchholz HW, Heinert K, Wargenau M (1985) Verlaufsbeobachtung von Hüftendoprothesen nach Abschluß realer Belastungsbedingungen von 10 Jahren. Z Orthop 123: 815–820
23. Bueche MJ, Herzenberg JE, Stubbs BT (1989) Dissociation of metal-backed polyethylene acetabular component. A case report. J Arthroplasty 4: 39–41
24. Callaghan JJ, Salvati EA, Pellicci PM, Wilson PD, Ranawat CS (1985) Results of revision for mechanical failure after cemented total hip replacement: 1979–1982. J Bone Joint Surg [Am] 67: 1074–1085
25. Capello WN, Colyer RA, Kernek CB, Carnahan JV, Hess JJ (1993) Failure of the Mecron screw-in ring. J Bone Joint Surg [Br] 75: 835–836
26. Caravia L, Dowson D, Fisher J, Jobbins B (1990) The influence of bone and bone cement debris on counterface roughness in sliding wear tests of ultra-high molecular weight polyethylene on stainless steel. Proc Inst Mech Eng 204: 65–70
27. Cates HE, Faris PM, Keating EM, Ritter MA (1993) Polyethylene wear in cemented metal-backed acetabular cups. J Bone Joint Surg [Br] 75: 249–253
28. Chandler HP, Reineck FT, Wixson RL, McCarthy JC (1981) Total hip replacement in patients younger than thirty years old. A five years follow-up study. J Bone Joint Surg [Am] 63: 1426–1434
29. Charnley J (1960) Anchorage of the femoral head prosthesis to the shaft of the femur. J Bone Joint Surg [Br] 42: 28
30. Charnley J (1972) The long-term results of low-friction arthroplasty of the hip performed as a primary intervention. J Bone Joint Surg [Br] 54: 61–76
31. Charnley J (1979) Low friction arthroplasty of the hip. Theory and practice. Springer, Berlin Heidelberg New York
32. Charnley J, Halley D (1975) Rate of wear in total hip replacement. Clin Orthop 112: 170–179
33. Chauvet JF, Pascarel X, Bosredon J, Honton JL (1992) Cotyles visses: resultats de 72 cas avec un recul moyen de cinq ans. Rev Chir Orthop 78: 340–346
34. Christel P, Derethe P, Sedel L (1980) Periacetabular pressure recording, using a hip simulator. Acta Orthop Belg 46: 647–662
35. Copeland CX, Jr., Caden JG (1988) Long-term results of Charnley total hip arthroplasty. Contrib Orthop 16: 15–18
36. Cornell CN, Ranawat CS (1986) Survivorship analysis of total hip replacements. J Bone Joint Surg [Am] 68: 1430–1434

37. Cotterill P, Hunter GA, Tile M (1982) A radiographic analysis of 166 Charnley-Müller-total hip arthroplasties. Clin Orthop 163: 120–126
38. Coudane H, Fery A. Sommelet J, Lacoste J, Leduc P, Gaucher A (1981) Aseptic loosening of cemented total arthroplasties of the hip in relation to positioning of the prosthesis: new utilization of the Tschuprow Cramer statistical test. Acta Orthop Scand 52: 201–205
39. Coventry MB, Beckenbaugh RD, Nolan DR, Ilstrup DM (1974) 2012 total hip arthroplasties: a study of postoperative course and early complications. J Bone Joint Surg [Am] 56: 273–284
40. Crowninshield RD, Pedersen DR, Brand RA, Johnston RC (1983) Analytical support for acetabular component metal backing. In: The Hip. Proceedings of the Eleventh Open Society Meeting of the Hip Society. Mosby, St. Louis, pp 207–215
41. Dalstra M, Huiskes R (1991) The influence of metal backing in cemented cups. Proc. 37th annual meeting of the Orthopaedic Research Society, Annaheim p 272
42. Davidson JA (1993) Characteristics of metal and ceramic total hip bearing surfaces and their effect on long-term ultra high molecular weight polyethylene wear. Clin Orthop 294: 361–378
43. Davlin LB, Amstutz HC, Tooke SM, Dorey FJ, Nasser S (1990) Treatment of osteoarthrosis secondary to congenital dislocation of the hip. J Bone Joint Surg [Am] 72A: 1035–1042
44. DeLee JG, Charnley J (1976) Radiological demarcation of cemented sockets in hip replacement. Clin Orthop 121: 20–33
45. Dick W, Morscher E (1975) Zur Technik der Pfannen-Implantation bei der Totalprothesennarthroplastik der Hüfte. Arch Orthop Unfallchir 83:215–220
46. Dietschi C (1978) Problematik des künstlichen Hüftgelenkes: Experimentelle Untersuchungen über die Biomechanik des Hüftgelenkes und Langzeitergebnisse nach Hüfttotalendoprothesen. Gentner, Stuttgart
47. Djerf K, Wahiström O, Hammerby S (1986) Loosening 5 years after total hip replacement – a radiological study of the McKee-Farrar-and-Charnley prosthesis. Arch Orthop Trauma Surg 105: 339–342
48. Dobbs HS, Scales JT (1983) Behavior of commercially pure titanium and T-318 (Ti6–A14–V) in orthopaedic implants. In: Luckey HA, Kubli F, jr (eds) Titanium alloy in surgical implants, ASTM STP 796. ASTM, Philadelphia, pp 173–186
49. Dorlot JM, Christel P, Sedel L, Witvoet J, Boutin P (1987) Comportement in vivo du couple alumine-alumine. VIe Réunion scientifique, Dourdan
50. Dorlot JM, Christel P, Meunier A (1989) Wear analysis of retrieved alumina heads and sockets of hip prostheses. J Biomed Mater Res 23: 299–310
51. Dorr LD, Takei GK, Contay JP (1983) Total hip arthroplasties in patients less than forty-five years old. J Bone Joint Surg [Am] 65: 474–479
52. Dörre E, Dawihl W (1978) Mechanische und tribologische Eigenschaften keramischer Endoprothesen. Biomed Tech 23: 305–310
53. Doyle J, Murray P, Mahony PO, Farmer M, Hooper AC (1989) Acetabular cup-siting-device for total hip arthroplasty. Arch Orthop Trauma Surg 108: 317–321
54. Durcheyne P, De Meester P, Aernoudt E, Martens M, Mulier JC (1977) Influence of a functional dynamic loading on bone ingrowth into surface pores of orthopaedic implants. J Biomed Mater Res 11: 811–838
55. Ducheyne P, Aernoudt E, De Meester P (1978). The mechanical behaviour of porous austenitic stainless steel fibre structures. J Mater Sci 13: 2650–2658
56. Ducheyne P, Martens M, De Meester P, Mulier JC (1984) Titanium and titanium alloy prostheses with porous fiber metal coatings. In: Morscher E (ed) The cementless fixation of hip endoprostheses. Springer, Berlin Heidelberg New York, pp 109–117
57. Ebert FR, Hussain S, Krackow KA (1992) Total hip arthroplasty for protrusio acetabuli: a 3- to 9 year follow-up of the Heywood technique. Orthopedics 15: 17–20

58. Eftekhar HS (1978) Principles of total hip arthroplasty. Mosby, St. Louis
59. Egli A, Weber BG, Sieber H, Semlitsch M, Dörre E (1991) Erfahrungen mit der Gleitpaarung Polyethylen/Keramik bei Hüftendoprothesen. In: Willert HG, Buchhorn GH, Eyerer P (Hrsg) Ultra-High Molecular Weight Polyethylene as Biomaterial in Orthopedic Surgery. Hogrefe & Huber, Toronto
60. Elke R, Morscher E (1990) Die Totalprothesenarthroplastik bei Hüftkopfnekrose. Orthopäde 19: 236–241
61. Endler M (1982) Theoretisch-experimentelle Grundlagen und erste klinische Erfahrungen mit einer neuen zementfreien Polyethylenschraubpfanne beim Hüftgelenkersatz. Acta Chir Austr Suppl 45: 1
62. Endler M, Endler F (1982) Erste Erfahrungen mit einer zementfreien Polyethylenschraubpfanne. Orthop Praxis 18: 319–323
63. Endler M, Endler F (1986) Zementfreier Hüftpfannenersatz mit einer konischen Polyethylenschraubpfanne. Med Orthop Techn 106: 2–5
64. Endler M, Endler F, Plenk H, Jr (1984) Experimental and early Clinical experience with an uncemented UHMW polyethylene acetabular prosthesis. In: Morscher E (ed) The cementless fixation of hip endoprostheses. Springer, Berlin Heidelberg New York, pp 191–199
65. Engelhardt P, Bodle A (1988) Prosthetic hip replacement in Paget's disease. Orthopäde 17: 404–406
66. Engh CA, Griffin WL, Marx CL (1990) Cementless acetabular components. J Bone Joint Surg [Br] 72: 53–59
67. Ferenz CC (1988) Polyethylene insert disloction in a screw-in acetabular cup: a case report. J Arthroplasty 3: 201–204
68. Fisher DA (1989) An experience with non-cemented acetabular cups. AAOS Meeting, Las Vegas
69. Frankel A, Balderson RA, Booth RE Jr, Rothman RH (1990) Radiographic demarcation of the acetabular bone-cement interface: the effect of femoral head size. J Arthroplasty [Suppl] 5: 1–3
70. Freeman MAR, Railton GT (1987) Die zementlose Verankerung in der Endoprothetik. Orthopäde 16: 206–219
71. Freeman MAR, McLeod HC, Levai JP (1983) Cementless fixation of prosthetic components in total arthroplasty of the knee and hip. Clin Orthop 176: 88–94
72. Galante J, Rostoker W (1973) Wear in total hip prostheses. An experimental evaluation of candidate materials. Acta Ortrop Scand Suppl 1: 145
73. Galante J, Rostoker W, Lueck R, Ray RD (1971) Sintered fiber metal composite as a basis for attachment of implants to bone. J Bone Joint Surg [Am] 53: 101–114
74. Galante J, Sumner DR, Gächter A (1987) Oberflächenstrukturen und Einwachsen von Knochen bei zementfrei fixierten Prothesen. Orthopäde 16: 197–205
75. Gates HS, McCollum DE, Poletti SC, Nunley JA (1990). Bone-grafting in total hip arthroplasty for protrusio acetabuli. A follow-up note. J Bone Joint Surg [Am] 72: 248–251
76. Geesink RGT (1990) Hydroxyapatite coated total hip prostheses. Clin Orthop 261: 39–58
77. Geesink R, DeGroot K, Klein C (1987) Chemical implant fixation using hydroxyl-apatite coatings. Clin Orthop 225: 147–170
78. Geesink RGT, DeGroot K, Klein CPAT (1987) Bonding of bone to apatite coated implants. J Bone Joint Surd [Br] 79: 17–22
79. Goldring SR, Schiller AL, Roelke M, Rourke CM, O'Neill DA, Harris WH (1983) The synovial-like membrane at the bone-cement interface in loose total hip replacements and its proposed role in bone lysis. J Bone Joint Surg [Am] 65: 575–584
80. Gonzalez MH, Glass RS, Mallory TH (1988) Fracture of a metal backed acetabular component in total hip arthroplasty. A case report. Clin Orthop 232: 156–158

81. Goodman SB, Carter DR (1987) Acetabular lucent lines and mechanical stress in total hip arthroplasty. J Arthroplasty 2: 219–224
82. Gouin F, Fechoz F, Passuti N, Sentucg-Rigal J, Bertrand O, Bainvel JV (1993) Cotyles sans ciment. Résultats à court terme d'une série de 112 cupules vissées. Int Orthop 17: 65–72
83. Griss P, Heimke G (1981) Five years experience with ceramic-metal-composite hip endoprostheses. I. Clinical evaluation. Arch Orthop Trauma Surg 98: 157–164.
84. Griss P, Heimke G, Krempie B, Silber R, Hachner K, Merkle B (1975) Erste Erfahrungen mit der Keramik-Metallverbundprothese. Med Orthop Tech 95: 159–162
85. Griss PG, Heimke G, von Adrian-Werburg H (1975). Die Aluminiumoxidkeramik-Metall-Verbundprothese. Eine neue Hüftgelenktotalendoprothese zur teilweise zementfreien Implantation. Arch Orthop Unfallchir 81: 259–266
86. Griss P, Adrian-Werburg HF von, Heimke G (1975) Ergebnisse der experimentellen Prüfung und klinischen Anwendungsmöglichkeiten der Aluminiumoxydkeramik in der Alloarthroplastik. Z Orthop 113: 756–759
87. Griss P, Werner E, Buchinger R, Heimke G (1977) Die Mannheimer Oxydkeramik-Metall-Verbundendoprothesen. Arch Orthop Unfallchir 87: 73–84
88. Gruen TA, McNiece GM, Amstutz HC (1979). „Modes of failure" of cemented stem-type femoral components. A radiographic analysis of loosening. Clin Orthop 141: 17–27
89. Gschwend N, Siegrist H (1989) Prothesenlockerung an der Hüfte bei der chronischen Polyarthritis rheumatica. Orthopäde 18: 418–427
90. Gualtieri G (1989) Experimental determination of the wear of biomaterials used in the construction of hip arthroprosthesis. Chir Organi Mov 74: 121–125
91. Gudmundsson GH, Hedeboe J, Kjaer J (1985) Mechanical loosening after hip replacement. Incidence after 10 years in 125 patients. Acta Orthop Scand 56: 314–317
92. Gut M, Hilfiker B, Schreiber A (1990) 5 bis 7 Jahresergebnisse der zementfreien Hüftgelenkspfanne nach Endler. Z Orthop 128: 598–605
93. Ha'Eri GB, Schatzker J (1978) Total replacement of the hip joint affected by Paget's disease. Can J Surg 21: 370
94. Harris WH (1978) Total hip replacement for osteoarthritis secondary to congenital dysplasia or congenital dislocation of the hip. Int Orthop 2: 127–138
95. Harris WH (1982) Allografting in total hip arthroplasty in adults with severe acetabular deficiency including a surgical technique for bolting the graft to the ilium. Clin Orthop 162: 150–164
96. Harris WH (1984) Advances in total hip arthroplasty. The metal-backed acetabular component. Clin Orthop 183: 4–12
97. Harris WH, Penenberg BL (1987) Further follow-up on socket fixation using a metal-backed acetabular component for total hip replacement. A minimum ten-year follow-up. J Bone Joint Surg [Am] 67: 1140–1143
98. Hernandez JR, Keating EM, Faris PM, Meding JB, Ritter MA (1994) Polyethylene wear in uncemented acetabular components. J Bone Joint Surg [Br] 76: 263–266
99. Herren T, Remagen W, Schenk R (1987) Histologie der Implantatknochengrenze bei zementierten und nichtzementierten Endoprothesen. Orthopäde 16: 239–251
100. Hierton C, Blomgren G, Lindgren U (1983) Factors leading to rearthroplasty in a material with radiographically loose total hip prostheses. Acta Orthop Scand 54: 562–565
101. Hintermann B, Morscher E (1995) Acetabuloplasty with solid autologous graft for hip dysplasia in total hip replacement. Arch Orthop Trauma Surg 114: 137–144
102. Hodgkinson JP, Maskell AP, Paul A, Wroblewski BM (1993) Flanged acetabular components in cemented Charnley hip arthroplasty. Ten-year follow-up of 350 patients. J Bone Joint Surg [Br] 75: 464–467
103. Hoeltzel DA, Walt MJ, Kyle RF, Simon FD (1989) The effects of femoral head size on the

deformation of utrahigh molecular weight polyethylene acetabular cups. J Biomech 22: 1163–1173
104. Holm NJ (1981) The development of a two-dimensional stress-optical model of the os coxae. Acta Orthop Scand 52: 135–143
105. Homsy CA (1973) Implant stabilization; chemical and biomechanical considerations. Orthop Clin North Am 4: 295–311
106. Homsy CA, Cain TE, Kessler FB, Anderson MS, King JM (1972) Porous implant systems for prosthesis stabilization. Clin Orthop 89: 220–235
107. Huggler AH, Schreiber A, Dietschi C, Jacob H (1974) Experimentelle Untersuchung über das Deformationsverhalten des Hüftacetabulums unter Belastung. Z Orthop 112: 44–50
108. Huiskes R (1987) Finite element analysis of acetabular reconstruction: noncemented threaded cups. Acta Orthop Scand 58: 620–625
109. Jacob H, Huggler AH, Dietschi C, Schreiber A (1976) The mechanical function of subchondral bone as experimentally determined on the acetabulum of the human pelvis. J Biomech 9: 625–627
110. Johnston RC, Crowninshield RD (1983) Roentgenologic results of total hip arthroplasty. A ten year follow-up study. Clin Orthop 181: 92–98
111. Judet R (1975) Total-Hüftendoprothesen aus Porometall ohne Zementverankerung. Z Orthop 113: 828–829
112. Judet J, Judet R (1950) The use of artificial femoral head for arthroplasty of the hip joint. J Bone Joint Surg [Br] 32: 166–173
113. Judet J, Brumpt B, Hamida B (1990) Results of a ten year follow-up of Judet cementless porous metal total hip prostheses. Orthop Trans 14: 209
114. Keating EM, Ritter MA, Faris PM, Czarkowski RA, Brugo G (1989) An anatomic study of structures at risk with acetabular screw fixation of total hip replacement. AAOS Meeting, New Orleans
115. Kilgus DJ, Amstutz HC, Wolgin MA, Dorey FJ (1990) Joint replacement for ankylosed hips. J Bone Joint Surg [Am] 72: 45–54
116. Kim WC, Grogan T, Amstutz HC, Dorey F (1987) Survivorship comparison of Tharies and conventional hip arthroplasty in patients younger than 40 years old. Clin Orthop 214: 269–277
117. Kirkpatrick JS, Callaghan JJ, Vandemark RM, Goldner RD (1990) The relationship of the intrapelvic vasculature to the acetabulum. Implications in screw-fixation acetabular components. Clin Orthop 258: 183–190
118. Kitziger KJ, Delee JC, Evans JA (1990) Disassembly of a modular acetabular component of a total hip replacement. J Bone Joint Surg [Am] 72: 621–623
119. Knahr K, Böhler M, Frank P, Plenk H, Salzer M (1987) Fünf-Jahres-Erfahrungen mit der Polyäthylen-Füsschenpfanne Modell Gerstof. Z Orthop 125 375–381
120. Kody MH, Kabo JM, Markolf KL, Dorey FJ, Amstutz HC (1990) Strength of initial mechanical fixation of screw ring acetabular components. Clin Orthop 257: 146–153
121. Krugluger J, Eyb R (1993) Bone reaction to uncemented threaded polyethylene acetabular components. Int Orthop 17: 259–265
122. Kummer FJ, Stuchin SA, Frankel VH (1990) Analysis of removed autophor ceramic-on-ceramic components. J Arthroplasty 5: 28–33
123. Lachiewicz PF, McCaskill B, Inglis A, Ranawat CS, Rosenstein BD (1986) Total hip arthroplasty in juvenile rheumatoid arthritis. Two to eleven years results. J Bone Joint Surg [Am] 68: 502–508
124. Learmonth ID, Heywood AW, Kaye J, Dall D (1989) Radiological loosening after cemented hip replacement for Juvenile chronic arthritis. J Bone Joint Surg [Br] 71: 2092–2112
125. Lemons JE (1987) Hydroxyapatite coatings. Clin Orthop 235: 220–223

126. Lewinnek GE, Lewis JL, Tarr R, Compere CL, Zimmerman JR (1976) Dislocations after total hip replacement arthroplasties. J Bone Joint Surg [Am] 60: 217–220
127. Lionberger D, Walker PS, Granholm J (1985) Effects of prosthetic acetabular replacement on strains in the pelvis. J Orthop Res 3: 372–379
128. Livermore J, Ilstrup D, Morrey B (1990) Effect of femoral head size on wear of the polyethylene acetabular component. J Bone Joint Surg [Am] 72: 518–528
129. Lombardi AV, Mallory TH, Vaughn BK, Drouillard P (1989) Aseptic loosening in total hip arthroplasty secondary to osteolysis induced by wear debris from titanium-alloy modular femoral heads. J Bone Joint Surg [Am] 71: 1337–1342
130. Lord G, Bancel P (1983) The madreporic cementless total hip arthroplasty. New experimental data and seven-year clinical follow-up study. Clin Orthop 176: 67–76
131. Lord G, Marotte JH, Blanchard JP, Gullamon JL, Gory M (1978) Etude experérimentale de l'ancrage des arthroplasties totales madréporiques de hanche. Rev Chir Orthop 64: 459–470
132. Ludowski P, Wilson-MacDonald J (1990) Total arthroplasty in Paget's disease of the hip. Clin Orthop 255: 160–167
133. Mahoney OM, Dimon JH (1990) Unsatisfactory results with a ceramic total hip prosthesis. J Bone Joint Surg [Am] 72: 663–671
134. Maloney WJ, Davey JR, Harris WH (1992) Bead loosening from a porous-coated acetabular component. A follow-up note. Clin Orthop 281: 112–114
135. Mathiesen EB, Lindgren U, Reinholt FP, Sudmann E (1986) Wear of the acetabular socket. Comparison of polyacetal and polyethylene. Acta Orthop Scand 57: 193–196
136. Mathys R (1973) Stand der Verwendung von Kunststoffen für künstliche Gelenke. Acta Traumatol 3: 253
137. Mattingly DA, Hopson CN, Kahn A, Giannestras NJ (1985) Aseptic loosening in metal-backed acetabular components for total hip replacements. A minimum five year follow-up. J Bone Joint Surg [Am] 67: 387–391
138. McBroom R, Müller M (1984) Aseptic loosening: fifteen years' experience with the Müller total hip arthroplasty. J Bone Joint Surg [Br] 66: 300–301
139. McCollum DE, Nunley JA, Harrelson JM (1980) Bone-grafting in total hip replacement for acetabular protrusion. J Bone Joint Surg [Am] 62: 1065–1073
140. McDonald DJ, Sim FH (1987) Total hip arthroplasty in Paget's disease: a follow up note. J Bone Joint Surg [Am] 69: 766–772
141. McGann WA, Welch RB, Picetti JD (1988) Acetabular preparation in cementless revision total hip arthroplasty. Clin Orthop 235: 35–46
142. McKee GK, Watson-Farrar J (1966) Replacement of arthritic hips by the McKee-Farrar prosthesis. J Bone Joint Surg [Br] 488: 245–259
143. McKellop H, Kirkpatrick J, Markolf K, Amstutz H (1980) Abrasive wear of Ti-6Al-4V prostheses by acrylic cement particles. 26th annual ORS, Atlanta/GA
144. McKellop HA, Sarmiento A, Schwinn CP, Ebramzadeh E (1990) In vivo wear of titanium-alloy hip prostheses. J Bone Joint Surg [Am] 66: 512–517
145. Merkow RL, Pellicci PM, Hely DP, Salvati EA (1984) Total hip replacement for Paget's disease of the hip. J Bone Joint Surg [Am] 66: 752–758
146. Meunier A, Blouet J, Christel P, Sedel L (1978) Etude expérimentale du choc avec frottement d'un contact cartilage/métal. IIIe Congrès de Biomécanique, Paris
147. Miller J (1990) Instructional course lecture. AAOS Meeting, New Orleans
148. Mittelmeier H (1985) Report on the first decennium of clinical experience with a cementless ceramic total hip replacement. Acta Orthop Belg 51: 367–376
149. Mittelmeier H, Harms G (1979) Derzeitiger Stand der zementfreien Verankerung von Keramik-Metall-Verbundprothesen. Z Orthop 117: 478–481
150. Mittelmeier H, Harms J (1979) Hüftalloplastik mit Keramik-Endoprothesen bei traumatischen Hüftschäden unter besonderer Berücksichtigung zementfrei implantierbarer „Autophor"-Tragrippen-Endoprothesen. Unfallheilkunde 82: 67

151. Mittelmeier H, Harms J (1979) Treatment of post-traumatic hip joint disease by total replacement with a ceramic endoprosthesis. Unfallheilkunde 82: 67–75
152. Mjöberg B (1986) Loosening of the cemented hip prosthesis. The importance of heat injury. Acta Orthop Scand 57 221: 1–40
153. Moran MC, Huo MH, Garvin KL, Pellicci PM, Salvati EA (1993) Total hip arthroplasty in sickle cell hemoglobinopathy. Clin Orthop 294: 140–148
154. Morrey BF, Ilstrup D (1989) Size of the femoral head and acetabular revision in total hip replacement arthroplasty. J Bone Joint Surg [Am] 71: 50–55
155. Morscher E (1979) Isoelastische Prothesen. Langenbecks Arch Chir 349: 321–326
156. Morscher E (1982) 4 Jahre zementlose Polyethylenpfannenimplantation an der Hüfte. Z Orthop 120: 486
157. Morscher E (1983) Cementless total hip arthroplasty. Clin Orthop 181: 76–91
158. Morscher E (1983) European experience with cementless total hip replacements. In: Hungerford DS. (ed). The hip. Proc. 11th Open Scientific Meeting of the Hip Society 1983. Mosby, St. Louis pp 190–203
159. Morscher E (1984) The cementless fixation of hip endoprostheses. In: Morscher E (ed) The cementless fixation of hip endoprostheses. Springer, Berlin Heidelberg New York, pp 1–8
160. Morscher E (1987) Current state of cementless fixation of endoprostheses. Swiss Med 9/6: 27–44
161. Morscher E (1989) Endoprosthetic surgery in 1988. Ann Chir Gynaecol 78: 242–253
162. Morscher E (1991) Hydroxyapatite coating of prostheses. Editorial J Bone Joint Surg [Br] 73: 705
163. Morscher E (1992) Current status of acetabular fixation in primary total hip arthroplasty Clin Orthop 274: 172-193
164. Morscher E, Dick W (1983) Cementless fixation of „isoelastic" hip endoprostheses manufactured from plastic materials. Clin Orthop 176: 77–87
165. Morscher E, Dick W (1984) Cementless fixation of a polyethylene acetabular component. In: Morscher E (ed) The cementless fixation of hip endoprostheses. Springer, Berlin Heidelberg New York, pp 200–204
166. Morscher E, Masar Z (1988) Development and first experience with an uncemented press-fit cup. Clin Orthop 232: 16–103
167. Morscher E, Mathys R (1974) La prothèse totale isoélastique de hanche fixée sans ciment. Premiers resultats. Acta Orthop Belg 40: 639–647
168. Morscher E, Mathys R (1975) Erste Erfahrungen mit einer zementlosen isoelastischen Totalprothese der Hüfte. Z Orthop 113: 745–749
169. Morscher E, Mathys R (1976) First experience with a cementless isoelastic total prosthesis of the hip. In: Gschwend N, Debrunner HU (eds) Total hip prosthesis. Huber, Bern pp 289–297
170. Morscher E, Schmassmann A (1983) Failures of total hip arthroplasty and probable incidence of revision surgery in the future. Arch Orthop Trauma Surg 101: 137–143
171. Morscher E, Bereiter H, Lampert C (1989) Cementless press-fit cup. Principles, experimental data and three year follow-up study. Clin Orthop 249: 12–20
172. Morscher E, Henche HR, Mathys R (1976) Isoelastic endoprosthesis – a new concept in artificial joint replacement. In: Schaldach M, Hohmann D (eds) Advances in artificial hip and knee joint technology. Engineering in Medicine, vol 2 Springer, Berlin Heidelberg New York p 403
173. Morscher E, Dick W, Kernen V (1982) Cementless fixation of polyethylene acetabular component in total hip arthroplasty. Arch Orthop Trauma Surg 99: 223–230
174. Morscher E, Graf R, Kohler O, Schmassmann A (1987) Vergleich der Resultate zementierter und nicht zementierter Hüftgelenkspfannen. In: Endo-Klinik (ed) Primär- und Revisionsalloarthroplastik. Springer Berlin Heidelberg New York, pp 124–126
175. Müller ME (1970) Total hip prostheses. Clin Orthop 72: 46–68

176. Müller ME (1981) Acetabular revision. In: Salvati EA (ed) The hip. Proceedings of the 9th open scientific meeting of the Hip Society. Mosby, St. Louis, pp 46–56
177. Mulroy RD, Harris WH (1990) The effect of improved cementing techniques on component loosening in total hip replacement. J Bone Joint Surg [Br] 72: 757–760
178. Murray DW (1992) Impingement and loosening of the long posterior wall acetabular implant. J Bone Joint Surg [Br] 74: 377–379
179. Nasser S, Campbell PA, Nasser S, Campbell PA, Kiligus D, Kossovsky N, Amstutz HC (1990) Cementless total joint arthroplasty prostheses with titanium-alloy articular surfaces. A human retrieval analysis. Clin Orthop 261: 171–185
180. Nicholas RM, Orr JF, Mollan RA, Calderwood JW, Nixon JR, Watson P (1990) Dislocation of total hip replacements. A comparative study of standard, long posterior wall and augmented acetabular components. J Bone Joint Surg [Br] 72: 418–422
181. Nizard RS, Sedel L, Christel P, Meunier A, Soudry M, Witvoet J (1992) Ten-year survivorship of cemented ceramic-ceramic total hip prosthesis. Clin Orthop 282: 53–63
182. Nunn D (1988) The stetring uncemented plastic-on-metal total hip replacement. Five year results. J Bone Joint Surg [Br] 9: 40–44
183. Nunn D, Freeman MA, Hill PF, Evans SJ (1989) The measurement of migration of the acetabular component of hip prostheses. J Bone Joint Surg [Br] 71: 629–631
184. Oonishi H, Hanatate Y, Tsuji E (1987) Comparison of wear test of KOM alumina-to-UHMWPE and metal-to-UHMWPE total knee prostheses by a knee simulator. VIe Réunion scientifique, Dourdan
185. Oonoshi H, Igaki H, Takayama Y (1989) Comparisons of wear of UHMW polyethylene sliding against metal and alumina in total hip prostheses. Bioceramics 1: 272–277
186. Parhofer R, Mönch W (1984) Experience with revision arthroplasties for failed cemented total hip replacements using uncemented Lord and PM prostheses. In: Morscher E (ed) The cementless fixation of hip endoprostheses. Springer, Berlin Heidelberg New York, pp 275–278
187. Pascarel X, Liquois F, Chauveaux D, Le Rebeller A, Honton JL (1993) Utilisation des anneaux endocotyloïdiens de Müller dans la chirurgie de révision des prothèses totales de hanche. A propos de 141 cas avec un recul minimum de 5 ans. Rev Chir Orthop 79: 357–364
188. Pedersen DR, Crowninshield RD, Brand RA, Johnston RC (1982) An axisymmetric model of acetabular components in total hip arthroplasty. J Biomech 15: 305–315; (1987). Orthop Trans 11: 166
189. Pellici PM, Salvati EA, Robinson HJ (1979) Mechanical failures in total hip replacement requiring reoperation. J Bone Joint Surg [Am] 61: 28–36
190. Pellici PM, Wilson PD Jr., Sledge CB, Salvati EA, Ranawat CS, Poss R (1982) Revision total hip arthroplasty. Clin Orthop 170: 34–41
191. Petty W (1978) The effect of methylmethacrylate on chemotaxis of polymorphonuclear leukocytes. J Bone Joint Surg [Am] 60: 492–498
192. Petty W (1978) The effect of methylmethacrylate on bacterial phagocytosis and killing by human polymorphonuclear leukocytes. J Bone Joint Surg [Am] 60: 552–575
193. Petty W, Spanier SS, Silverthorne CA, Shuster JJ (1984) Effect of treatment on infection associated with implantation of bone cement. Trans Orthop Res Soc 9: 375
194. Philips TW, Hamilton H (1990) Hip replacement: the ultimate test. SICOT abstracts. XVIII World Congress, Montreal
195. Pilliar RM, Bratina WJ (1980) Micromechanical bonding at a porous surface structured implant interface. The effect on implant stressing. J Biomed Eng 2: 49–53
196. Pilliar RM, Cameron HU, Macnab I (1975) Porous surfaced layered prosthetic devices. J Biomed Eng 10: 126–131
197. Pilliar RM, Lee JM, Maniatopoulos DDC (1986) Observations on the effect of movement on bone ingrowth into porous-surfaced implants. Clin Orthop 208: 108–113

198. Plitz W (1984) Der Einfluß von Verformung. Spiel und Werkstoffpaarung auf das oszillierende Reibmoment bei künstlichen Hüftgelenkpfannen. Thesis, University Aachen
199. Plitz W (1985) The „Anchorage loading" of the implant bed by the artificial acetabulum. Fortschr Med 93: 103–105
200. Plitz W, Hoss HU (1980) Wear of alumina-ceramic hip joints: home clinical and tribological aspects. Biomaterials. Wiley, New York, p 187
201. Poss R, Maloney JP, Ewald FC, Thomas WH, Batte NJ, Hartnes C, Sledge CB (1984) Six to 11 year results of total hip arthroplasty in rheumatoid arthritis. Clin Orthop 182: 109–116
202. Pupparo F, Engh CA (1990) Comparison of porous threaded and smooth threaded acetabular components of identical design. Two and four year results. SICOT abstracts. XVIII World Congress, Montreal
203. Rapperport DJ, Carter DR, Schurman DJ (1987). Contact finite element stress analysis of porous ingrowth acetabular cup implantation, ingrowth and loosening. J Orthop Res 5: 548–561
204. Remagen W, Morscher E (1984) Histological results with cement-free implanted hip joint sockets of polyethylene. Arch Orthop Trauma Surg 103: 145–151
205. Ring PA (1968) Complete replacement arthroplasty of the hip by the Ring prosthesis. J Bone Joint Surg [Br] 50: 720–731
206. Ring PA (1974) Total replacement of the hip joint. J Bone Joint Surg [Br] 56: 44–5)3
207. Ring PA (1983) Ring UPM total hip arthroplasty. Clin Orthop 176: 115–123
208. Ritter MA, Stringer EA, Littrell DA, Williams JG (1983) Correlation of prosthetic femoral head size and/or design with longevity of total hip arthroplasty. Clin Orthop 176: 252–257
209. Ritter MA, Keating EM, Faris PM, Brugo G (1990) Metal-backed acetabular components of total hip replacement: does it reduce loosening? AAOS Meeting, New Orleans
210. Rosson J, Schatzker J (1992) The use of reinforcement rings to reconstruct deficient acetabula. J Bone Joint Surg [Br] 74: 716–720
211. Russe W, Tschupic IP (1986) Wanderung der isoelastischen RM-Pfanne. Röntgenphotogrammetrische Erfassung. Vortrag Symposium „Ultrahochmolekulares Polyethylen (UHMWPE) als Biomaterial", Göttingen 14./15. 3. 86, pp 170–172
212. Russotti GM, Harris WH (1991) Proximal placement of the acetabular component in total hip arthroplasty. A long-term follow-up study. J Bone Joint Surg [Am] 73: 587–592
213. Russotti GM, Coventry MB, Stauffer RN (1988) Cemented total hip arthroplasty with contemporary techniques: a five year minimum follow-up study. Clin Orthop 235: 141–147
214. Ryd L, Lindstrand A, Stenstrom A, Selvik G (1990) Cold flow reduced by metal backing. An in vivo roentgen stereophotogrammetric analysis of unicompartmental tibial components. Acta Orthop Scand 61: 21–25
215. Salvati EA, Im VC, Aglietti P, Wilson PD jr (1976) Radiology of total hip replacements Clin Orthop 121: 74–82
216. Sarmiento A (1972) Austin Moore prosthesis in the arthritic hip. Clin Orthop 82: 14–23
217. Sarmiento A, Ebramzadeh E, Gogan WJ, McKellop HA (1990) Cup containment and orientation in cemented total hip arthroplasties. J Bone Joint Surg [Br] 72: 996–1002
218. Schatzker J, Glynn MK, Ritter D (1984) A preliminary review of the Müller acetabular and Burch-Schneider antiprotrusio support rings. Arch Orthop Trauma Surg 103: 5–12
219. Schenk RK (1986) Histophysiology of bone remodeling and bone repair. In: Lin and Chao (eds) Perspectives on Biomaterials. Elsevier, Amsterdam, pp 75–94
220. Schimmel JW, Huiskes R (1988) Primary fixation of the Lord cementless total hip. A geometric study in cadavers. Acta Orthop Scand 59 235: 638–642

221. Schneider R (1980) Die Armierung der Pfanne bei der Totalendoprothese der Hüfte. Unfallheilkunde 83: 482
222. Schneider R (1987) Die Totalprothese der Hüfte – ein biomechanisches Konzept und seine Konsequenzen. Huber, Bern (Aktuelle Probleme in Chirurgie und Orthopädie, vol 24)
223. Schüller HM, Marti RK (1990) Ten-year socket wear in 66 arthroplasties. Ceramic versus metal heads. Acta Orthop Scand 61: 240–243
224. Schurman DJ, Bloch DA, Segal MR, Tanner CM (1989) Conventional cemented total hip arthroplasty. Assessment of Clinical factors associated with revision for mechanical failures. Clin Orthop 240: 173–180
225. Sedel L, Christel P, Herman S, Witvoet J (1985) Descellement des cotyles en alumine cimentés. Etiologie et solutions. Rev Chir Orthop 71: 29–32
226. Sedel L, Kerboull L, Christel P, Meunier A, Witvoet J (1990) Alumina-on-alumina hip replacement. Results and survivorship in young patients. J Bone Joint Surg [Br] 72: 658–663
227. Semlitsch M, Willert HG (1981) Biomaterialien für Implantate in der Orthopädischen Chirurgie. Medizintechnik 101 3: 66
228. Semlitsch M, Lehmann M, Weber H, Doerre E, Willert HG (1977) New prospects for a prolonged functional life – span of artificial hip joints by using the material combination polyethylene/aluminium oxide ceramic/metal. J Biomed Mater Res 11: 537
229. Semlitsch M, Streicher RM, Weber H (1989) Wear behaviour of cast CoCrMo cups and balls in long term implanted total hip prostheses. Orthopäde 18: 377–381
230. Shaughnessy WJ, Kavanagh BF, Fitzgerald RH (1990). Effects of acetabular component position on total hip arthroplasty results in patients with congenital dislocation of the hip. AAOS Meeting, New Orleans
231. Shaw JA, Bailey JH, Bruno A, Greer RB (1990) Threaded acetabular components for primary and revision total hip arthroplasty. J Arthroplasty 5: 201–215
232. Sivash KM (1969) The development of a total metal prosthesis for the hip joint from a partial joint replacement. Reconstr Surg Traumatol 11: 53
233. Slätis P, Tallroth K, Paavolainen P, Ylinen P, Paavilainen T (1992) Hip. Loosening of threaded acetabular components. Acta Orthop Scand Suppl 247: 47
234. Snorrason F, Kärrholm J (1990) Primary migration of fully-threaded acetabular prostheses. A roentgen stereophotogrammetric analysis. J Bone Joint Surg [Br] 72: 647–652
235. Snorrason F, Kärrholm J, Holmgren C (1993) Fixation of cemented acetabular prostheses. The influence of preoperative diagnosis. J Arthroplasty 8: 83–90
236. Star MJ, Colwell CW, Jr, Donaldson WFIII, Walker RH (1992) Dissociation of modular hip arthroplasty components after dislocation: a report of three cases at differing dissociation levels. Clin Orthop 278: 111–115
237. Stauffer RN (1982) Ten year follow-up study of total hip replacement. With particular reference to roentgenographic loosening of the components. J Bone Joint Surg [Am] 64: 983–990
238. Stauffer RN, Sim FH (1976) Total hip arthroplasty in Paget's disease of the hip. J Bone Joint Surg [Am] 58: 476–478
239. Streicher RM, Schön R, Semlitsch MF (1990) Untersuchung des tribologischen Verhaltens von Metall/Metall-Kombinationen für künstliche Hüftgelenke. Biomed Tech 35: 107–111
240. Sutherland CJ, Wilde AH, Borden LS, Marks KE (1982) A ten-year follow-up of one hundred consecutive Müller curved-stem total hip replacement arthroplasties. J Bone Joint Surg [Am] 64: 970–982
241. Tapadiya D, Walker RH, Schurman DJ (1984) Prediction of outcome of total hip arthroplasty based on initial postoperative radiographic analysis. Matched paired comparison of failed cersus successful femoral components. Clin Orthop 186: 5–15

242. Thorén B, Hallin G (1989) Loosening of the Charnley hip. Acta Orthop Scand 60: 533–539
243. Tooke SM, Nugent PJ, Chotivichit A, Goodman W, Kabo JM (1988) Comparison of in vivo cementless acetabular fixation. Clin Orthop 235: 253–260
244. Tradonsky S, Postak PD, Froimson AI, Greenwald AS (1993) A comparison of the disassociation strength of modular acetabular components. Clin Orthop 296: 154–160
245. Unger AS, Inglis AE, Ranawat CS, Johanson NA (1987) Total hip arthroplasty in rheumatoid arthritis. A long term follow-up study. J Arthroplasty 2: 191–197
246. Ungethüm M, Blömer W (1986) Biomechanische Aspekte zementfreier Hüftpfannen-Implantate mit Schraubverankerung. Med Orthop Techn 106: 194–197
247. Volz RG, Wilson RJ (1977) Factors affecting the mechanical stability of the cemented acetabular component in total hip replacement. J Bone Joint Surg [Am] 59: 501–504
248. Wanivenhaus A, Zweymüller K (1988). Fünf – 10 Jahresergebnisse mit einer Füßchenpfanne aus Keramik zur knochenzementfreien Implantation. Z Orthop 126: 508–512
249. Wasielewski RC, Kruger MP, Cooperstein LA, Rubash HE (1990) Acetabular anatomy and transacetabular fixation of screws in total hip arthroplasty. J Bone Joint Surg [Am] 72: 501–508
250. Weber GB (1981) Total hip replacement: rotation versus fixed and metal versus ceramic heads. In: Salvati EA (ed) The hip. pp 264–275. Proceedings of the 9th Meeting of the Hip Society. Mosby, St. Louis
251. Weber BG, Fiechter T (1989) Polyethylene wear and late loosening in total hip replacement. Orthopäde 18: 370–376
252. Weber BG, Semlitsch MF, Streicher RM (1993) Total hip joint replacement using a CoCrMo metal-metal sliding pairing. Nippon Seikeigeka Gakkai Zasshi 67: 391–398
253. Willert HG, Ludwig J, Semlitsch M (1974) Reaction of bone to methacrylate after hip arthroplasty. J Bone Joint Surg [Am] 56: 1368–1382
254. Willert HG, Semlitsch M, Buchhorn G, Kriete U (1978) Materialverschleiß und Gewebereaktion bei künstlichen Gelenken. Orthopäde 7: 62–83
255. Williamson JB, Galasko CS, Rowley DI (1989) Failure of acetabular augmentation for recurrent dislocation after hip arthroplasty. Report of 3 cases. Acta Orthop Scand 60: 676–677
256. Wilson AJ, Monsees B, Blair VP (1988) Acetabular cup dislocation: a new complication of total joint arthroplasty. AJR 151: 133–134
257. Wilson-MacDonald J, Morscher E, Masar Z (1990) Cementless uncoated polyethylene acetabular components in total hip replacement. Review of five- to ten-year results. J Bone Joint Surg [Br] 72: 423–430
258. Wood R, Severt R, Cracchiolo A, Amstutz H (1990) Long-term follow-up of cemented total hip arthroplasty in rheumatoid arthritis. AAOS Meeting, New Orleans
259. Wroblewski BM (1979) Wear of high-density polyethylene on bone and cartilage. J Bone Joint Surg [Br] 61: 498–500
260. Wroblewski BM, Lynch M, Atkinson JR, Dowson D, Isaac GH (1987) External wear of the polyethylene socket in cemented total hip arthroplasty. J Bone Joint Surg [Br] 69: 61–63
261. Yoder SA, Brand RA, Pedersen DR, O'Gorman TW (1988) Total hip acetabular component position affects component loosening rates. Clin Orthop 228: 79–87
262. Zichner L, Starker M, Paschen U (1986). In-vivo-Verschleiß der Gleitflächenpaarung A1203-Keramik-Polyäthylen bei Hüftprothesen. Symposium Ultrahochmolekulares Polyäthylen (UHMWPE) als Biomaterial, Göttingen, pp 148–151
263. Zweymüller K (1990) Zehn Jahre Zweymüller-Hüftendoprothese. Huber, Bern

The Saint Nabor Cup: 8 Years of Experience

P. Schuster

Introduction

General Remarks

Aseptic loosening of total hip prostheses is one of the major long-term causes of failure and presents serious reconstruction problems for the surgeon [15]. It has been shown by Sutherland [19] and Morscher and Schmassmamm [13] that femoral loosening increases linearly with time, whereas socket loosening increases exponentially. A rapid acceleration of socket loosening occurs 7 years postoperatively. Orthopedic surgeons therefore rapidly became interested in uncemented fixation by bone ingrowth: press-fit impacted cups: Judet, 1971 [9]; screwed cups: Lord, 1976 [10]; and press-fit cups with additional screw fixation: Harris 1984 [8]. The St. Nabor cup, which belongs to the latter category, and was the first European design of its kind, was first implanted in August 1985 [17].

Biomechanics

The acetabulum deforms elastically under load [20]. The labri of the acetabulum come together when stress is applied and separate at rest. A succession of contractile and relaxing movements therefore occur around the socket horseshoe when walking. Maximum movement occurs in the lower part of the horseshoe; correspondingly, the upper part containing De Lee and Charnley zones I and II [4] is more stable. Elastic deformation of the pelvis remains after implantation of any type of prosthesis. Introduction of a cup by impaction compresses the interface and opens the acetabular fossa. Closure of the acetabulum, when stress is applied, results in temporary release of the static preload [16]. This release is compensated in two areas:
– zone I by press-fit
– zon II, the relatively stable zone.

Because of the deformation occurring in this region, zone III is not suitable for osseointegration.

Role of Screws

Implantation of a press-fit cup and the prestresses which it produces does not offer a solution in all situations. For this reason, and after our vast experience with Müller's acetabular roof rings [18], we selected a cranial anchorage system using two or three screws parallel to the Pauwel's R resultant.

These screws serve three purposes:
- they increase cohesion between bone and implant when tightened and therefore encourage osseointegration by virtue of increased stability;
- they increase rigidity in the roof of the cup as described by Schnieder [16];
- they provide rotatory stability.

Finally, situated in the least mobile zone II of the acetabulum, they guarantee stability over time and allow surgery in difficult situations where press-fit stability alone would be insufficient.

On the other hand, do these cranial screws have adverse effects? Vascular and neurological risks have been reported, but to our knowledge no such reports have ever been published. If socket migration occurs, as we have seen in a few cases, we have invariably found either that the implant had migrated away from the screws, which had remained in a stable postition, or that the screws had fractured, which prevented the screw heads from penetrating into the polyethylene. We have never found major defects of the polyethylene insert itself.

Osseointegration, the biological fixation of the implant, is achieved by the following mechanisms:
- corundum rough-blasted titanium surface, which we feel is sufficient [1], we have very little experience with hydroxyapatite: 50 cases with a follow-up of 3 years;
- the primary stability of the implant, which is obtained by impaction of the implant in the slightly undersized acetabulum, and antirotatory means;
- secondary fixation (the fracture callus);
- late fixation (bone remodeling, Fig. 1).

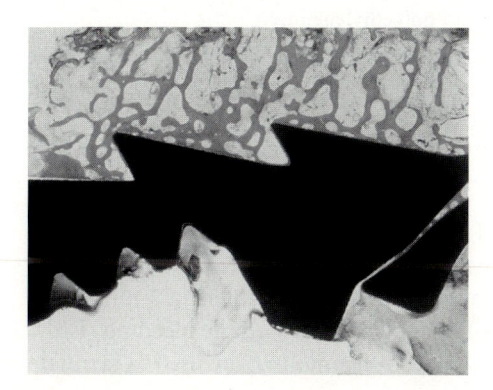

Fig. 1. Extracted prosthesis for recurrent dislocation. Perfect contact between implant and bone ingrowth

Materials and Methods

Implant

The acetabular component consists of a hemispherical cup which is flattened in the pole (Fig. 2). The metal shell has a series of concentric grooves ending abruptly on the external surface and two self-cutting crowns which penetrate into the acetabulum. Depending on the cup size, fixation of the metal shell is enhanced by using two or three screws. The screws are mounted with cone sleeves which have three functions: (a) to solve the problem of the screw head's protrusion into the socket without increasing the thickness of the titanium implant, (b) give the surgeon a choice of direction of approximately 30° from the radial axis, and (c) act as a shock absorber which avoids direct transmission of excess forces from the socket to the screws. The polyethylene insert is screwed into the metal shell. The cup, which is slightly larger than the indicated diameter, is available in nine sizes, ranging from 46 to 62 mm. There are polyethylene inserts for head diameters of 22, 28 and 32 mm (22 mm=cups 46 and 48; 28 mm=cups 46–62; 32 mm=cup 50–62).

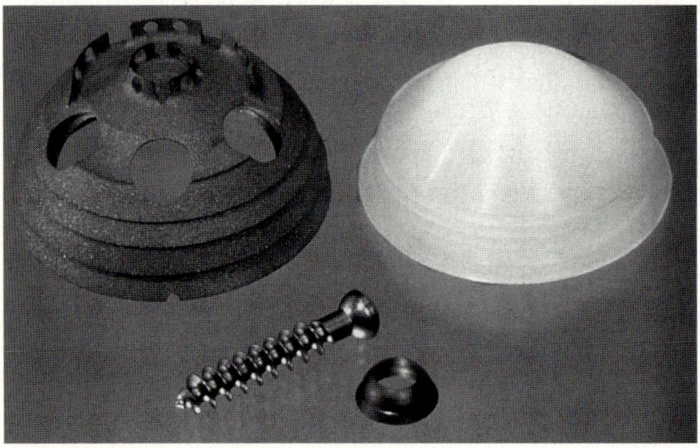

Fig. 2. The Saint Nabor cup, screw, sleeve, and polyethylene insert

Surgical Technique

Standard Approach

We use a posteroexternal approach. The acetabular rim is carefully cleaned of soft tissue and osteophytes, particularly in the lower part. After removing underlying osteophytes the acetabulum is reamed using reamers in 2-mm increments until resistance is reached and the subchondral bone is bleeding. If the bottom of the acetabulum is sclerotic, a 36-mm reamer may be used to facilitate penetration of the "double fond" (double ground). In this case some bone grafts are introduced before impaction of the cup to prevent a gap between the dome of the acetabulum and the implant. The size of the selected implant should correspond with that of the last-used reamer. The cup is impacted (pre-stressed) by hammer blows. Firm seating is confirmed through the screw holes, and the stability is tested with a clamp. The position of the screws is determined, and then with the help of the centering instrument the cone sleeves are introduced. Only then are the screws anchored in their final position, and the polyethylene insert is screwed into place.

Special Situations

In our opinion, screws increase the primary stability and allow the St. Nabor cup to be used in cases of acetabular cysts and protrusion (Fig. 3). If the acetabu-

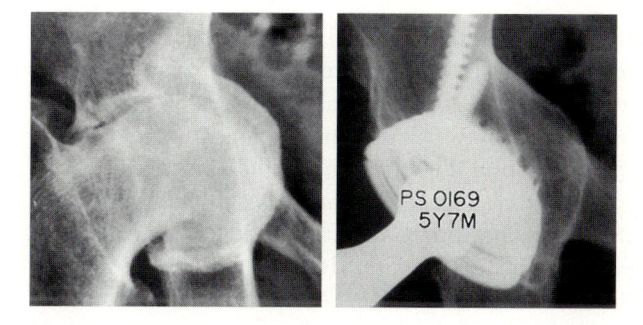

Fig. 3 Protruded coxarthritis. Sclerosis of roof and bottom of the acetabulum. Disappearance of sclerosis and perfect graft integration after 5 years and 7 months

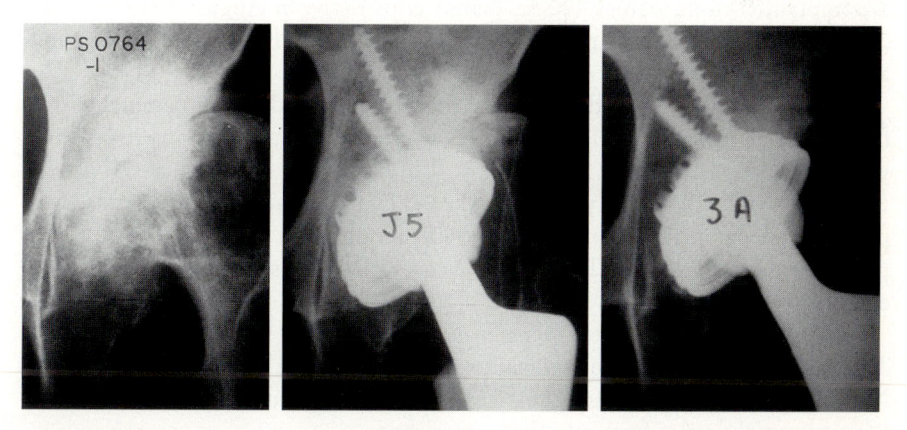

Fig. 4 Dysplastic hip. Perfect integration of the monobloc bone inlay and disappearance of the sclerosis

lum is small and dysplastic, bone grafts may be used to increase superior coverage. Grafts always integrate with the bone. In cases of congenital dislocation (Fig. 4), the cup is impacted into the site of the true acetabulum which has been reamed. Primary stability is confirmed and the superior defect is filled with either bone chips or large bone grafts. In all cases the press-fit between the cup and the patient's acetabulum must be sufficient to guarantee perfect primary stability.

Postopeartive Care

Intraoperative antibiotic prophylaxis (cephalosporin) is used in all cases together with anticoagulant treatment (enoxaparine). Weight bearing is allowed immediately, and patients are kept in hospital for approximately 2 weeks. We find 62 % of patients returning home without requiring rehabilitation.

Indications and Contraindications

In our experience the indication range for this implant is extremely broad and includes approximately 95 % of the cases of inflammatory arthritis of primary and secondary degenerative arthritis. Primary instability of the implant is an absolute containdication: instability prevents osseointegration, and the clinician can never rely upon secondary fixation. Relative contraindications are the need for large grafts, either autografts or allografts. These may only be used to fill bony defects. The implant must be positioned directly in the patient's acetabulum. Contact must be made over at least two thirds of the acetabular surface. Most of our failures in the beginning of our series resulted from not observing essential rules.

Patient Series

We implanted more than 1 400 St. Nabor cups between August 1985 and December 1993. These cases are documented at the Müller foundation in Bern and are followed regularly.

Overall results on 1 314 documented prostheses include 1 092 patients with a follow-up of more than 1 year and 504 cases with a follow-up from 5–8 years.

Mean patient age was 58 years (range: 18–82 years). The underlying cause was primary osteoarthritis in most cases (940), reoperation in only 76 cases, and polyarthritis in 39 cases. There were 92 cases of dysplastic hip (defect or high dislocation).

We have used noncemented stems in 12 % of our cases since 1989 (CLS stem). This series therefore consists of approximately 1 275 hybrid prostheses (St. Nabor cup and cemented straight stem) and 125 totally noncemented prostheses with extremely strict femoral selection criteria.

Results

Complications

There were 25 intraoperative complications (2 %), principally femoral fracture or fissures. No vascular or neurogical complications resulting from the use of screws have occurred. We observed 59 local complications (4 %): hematomas (13), dislocations (32: 2,4 %), sciatic nerve paralyses (6, of whom 4 recovered completely), 8 infections (0,6 %). There were 81 general complications (6 %), primarily thrombophlebitis, embolism, cardiovascular or urological complications, etc. One death during the stay at the hospital was due to a severe pulmonary embolism. Regarding ossifications 143 cases (11 %) were observed. Graded by the Brooker classification [2], these cases could be divided into 80 patients in stage I or II, 61 in stage II, and 2 in stage IV, which required reoperation and radiotherapy. Since January 1993, in about 200 patients, we have used 75 mg indomethacine for 8 days, which has reduced the ossification rate to almost zero [7]. Surgical reinterventions included 20 cups that were revised (1,5 % of cases). Six cases were revised for sepsis; of these, we were able to provide four with a revision component. Five cases were revised for recurrent dislocation and eight for migration. The latter were treated with Müller acetabular reinforcement rings. One case was revised for pain (nonintegration). We currently have 11 cases of migration which are followed regularly, and which have not yet undergone revision. We included these in our poor results.

Clinical Results

Method

Patients were reviewed at 2 months, 1 year, and then every 2 years after operation. Results are sent together with the X-rays to the Müller documentation center in Bern. Results were evaluated from clinical examination (pain, walking, mobility) using the Merle d'Aubigné score [11]. The evaluation was conducted on 1 092 patients with a follow-up of more than 1 year.

Results

Pain. 1 015 hips wich are completely painless (93 %); 77 are graded 4 or 5 (7 %).

Walking. 960 patients have no limp and can walk for more than 1 h (88 %).

Mobility. Among these patients 983 (90 %) have mobility which is either unchanged or better than before operation; 58 have markedly reduced mobility: 2 have become completely ankylosed.

Radiographic Results

Method

We paid particular attention to X-ray films. It is difficult to confirm that noncemented implants have integrated. We have been able to establish three criteria for failed anchorage:
- adverse changes in neighboring bone: appearance of sclerosis or cysts;
- radiolucent lines in zones I and II, the areas where bone integration should occur;
- migration or tilting as described by Sutherland [19] and changes in the orientation of the implant (Fig. 5).

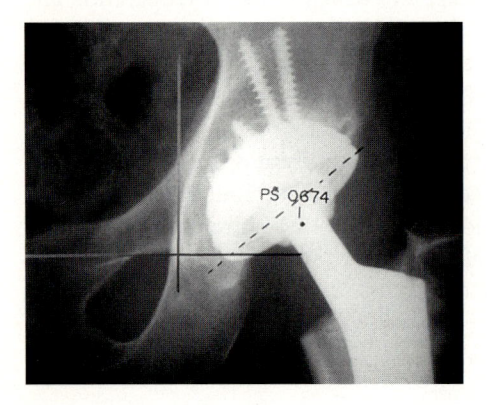

Fig. 5 Sutherland diagram. The axis and the center of the implant are marked

Changes in Bone Structure

We have *never* found areas of sclerosis around the screws or around the implant. In all cases where significant acetabular sclerosis was present (particularly in cases of protrusion), newly formed bone appeared to be healthy. Similarly, grafts used to fill cysts and to create superior coverage (apposition or monobloc ridges) have integrated in most cases.

Radiolucent Lines

We observed the development of 87 radiolucent lines (8 %). In 79 cases these were thin and in 8 cases wide lines; all of them were found in zone III. We find that these lines indicate deformation of the acetabular rim and failure to integrate in this area, consistent with biomechanical theory.

Migration

In this group, consisting of 19 cases (1,7 %), we include internal, superior, and tilting movement of the cup. Eight occurred in 1 047 primary prostheses (0,8 %) and 11 in 45 revisions where large homografts were used (24 %). Due to the latter finding we totally changed our methods in such cases of revision. Eight screws had broken in six of the cases of migration. In the remaining cases the implant had tilted around the plane formed by the two or three screws, without braking the screws themselves.

Long-Term Results

We reviewed 504 St. Nabor cups implanted before August 1988 in detail over a period of 5-8 years: 28 were implanted in revisions and 476 in primary surgery (Fig. 6).

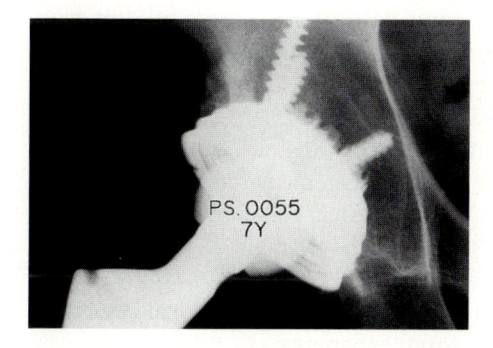

Fig. 6 Result after 7 years. Neither bone sclerosis, migration, nor radiolucent line

Results of Revisions

Depending on the lack of bone stock, the results were more or less good or poor. Results were satisfactory in light revisions (16 cases). On the other hand, in the 12 severe revisions where the socket was built up with homologous grafts we found 11 failures due to migration or variable extent. The St. Nabor cup can in no way be thought of as a traditional roof reinforcement ring to rely on massive allografts. Where necessary (e. g., in the case of septic antecedents), we currently prefer to ream the acetabulum generously, even if this means reaming higher and deeper. A large implant is then used. Bone grafts are inserted only to fill cavities.

Results of Primary Interventions

Of the 476 primary prostheses, 42 patients died, 38 were lost to follow-up or refused to show up, and 396 were reviewed, Four hips were painful (1 %). Pain was present only on changing position in three cases, but one particularly painful hip underwent revision. Osseointegration had not occurred in that case, but an intervening fibrous membrane had developed. We found five cases of migration 1,2 %); all of them underwent revision. Of these five cases three developed due to a large bone graft which had not integrated because of direct contact between the cup and the graft.

Conclusion

Do noncemented sockets produce better long-term results than their cemented counterparts? We cannot confirm this yet. Macrostructured impacted sockets have been abandoned because of their high failure rates. Results of screwed sockets vary. Lord [10] and Mittelmeier [12] found migration rates of approximately 3–4 % after 5 years, whereas Duparc [5], Engh [6], and Honton [3] published much higher failure rates and recommended that their use be either abandoned, or at least that their indication be restricted. Press-fit cups have produced satisfactory results [14], although we prefer the option of additional screw fixation because of their greater stability. Our statistics demonstrate a migration rate of 1,2 % between 5 and 8 years after primary surgery. In other cases the excellent appearances of the contact bone, the lack of migration and, particularily, the absence of pain give us encouragement for the future. Our implant, a congruence of forms combined with perfect stability, provided by the use of screws and excellent surface treatment of the titanium, lies at the foot of the Sutherland curve. We will see in future years whether the poor results remain low, and whether this concept is genuinely preferable to traditional cemented implants, with which we now have 30 years' experience.

References

1. Alberktsson T, Branemark PI, Hansson HA, Lindstrom J (1981) Osseointegrated titanium implants. Acta Orthop Scand 52: 155 1981
2. Brooker AF, Bowermann JW, Robinson RA, Riley LH (1973) Ectopic ossification following total hip replacement = incidence and a method of classification. J Bone Joint Surg [AM] 55: 1629
3. Chauvet JF, Pascarel X, Bosredon J, Honton JL (1992) Cotyles vissés – résultat de 72 cas avec un recul moyen de 5 ans. Rev Chir Orthop 78: 340–346
4. De Lee JG, Charnley J (1976) Radiological demarcation of cemented sockets in total hip replacement. Clin Orthop 121: 20–32
5. Duparc J, Massin P (1991) Prothèses totales de hanche avec des anneaux vissés. Rev Chir Orthop 77: 221–231
6. Engh CA, Griffin WL, Marx C (1990). Cementless acetabular components. J Bone Joint Surg [BR] 72: 53
7. Goutailler D, Colmar M, Penot P (1993) Les ossifications périprothétiques de hanche. Rev Chir Orthop 79: 22–28

8. Harris WH, Krushell RJ, Galante JO (1988) Results of cementless revision of total hip arthroplasties using the Harris-Galante prosthesis. Clin Orthop 235: 120 – 126
9. Judet R, Siguier M, Brumpt B, Judet T (1978) A non cemented total hip prosthesis. Clin Orthop 137: 76–84
10. Lord G, Marotte JH, Blanchard JP (1988) Arthroplasties totales de hanche madréporiques. A propos de 2688 cas. Rev Chir Orthop 74: 3–14
11. Merle D' Aubigne R (1970) Cotation chiffrée de la hanche. Rev Chir Orthop 56: 481–486
12. Mittelmeier H (1985) Report of the first decinium of clinical experimentation with a cementless ceramic hip replacement. Acta Orthop Belg 2/3: 367–377
13. Morscher E, Schmassmann A (1983) Failures of total hip arthroplasty and probable incidence of revision surgery in the future. Calculations according to a mathematical model based on a ten years' experience in total hip arthroplasty. Arch Orthop Trauma Surg 101 (2): 137–143
14 Morscher E, Bereiter H, Lampert C (1989) Cementless press fit cup. Principles, experimental data, and three years follow-up study. Clin Orthop 249: 12–20
15. Müller ME (1992) Lessons of 30 years of total hip arthroplasty. Clin Orthop 274: 12–22
16. Schneider R (1989) Total prosthetic replacement of the hip. Huber, Bern
17. Schuster P (1993) La cupule cotyloïdienne non cimentée Saint Nabor. A propos de 7 ans d'expérience et plus de 1100 implantations. Acta Orthop Belg (Suppl) 1: 248-252
18. Schuster P, Vergnat C, Abisset-Bouvier C (1989) L'anneau de soutien endocotyloïdien MEM. Pierron, Sarreguemines
19. Sutherland CJ, Wilde AH, Borden LS, Marks KE (1982) A ten years follow-up on one hundred consecutive
    Muller curved stem total hip arthroplasties. J Bone Joint Surg [AM] 54: 970–982
20. Teinturier P, Terver S, Jaramillo CV, Besse JP (1984) La biomécanique du cotyle. Rev Chir Orthop (Suppl) 11: 41–46

Rationale of the Press-Fit Cup

E. Morscher

Introduction

The hitherto known main problems with acetabular fixation include aseptic loosening, compromise between mobility and stability of the joint, problems with threaded cups, modular cups, screw fixation, wear, stiffness (metal backing, ceramic), osteolysis, and loss of bone stock in cases of revision.

Experience with cementless hip endoprostheses over the past two decades has shown that a number of requirements must be fulfilled for successful osseointegration. The quality of fixation and the differences between cups fixed with and without bone cement lie mainly in the design, nature of the implant surface, mechanical properties of the cup materials and operative technique [18]. Based on clinical experiences with both cemented and uncemented components, on histological observations of retrieved sockets, and on laboratory investigations, an acetabular cup, the Press-Fit Cup (see Fig. 1), was developed that respects the following basic principles and requirements [16-20]:
- intrinsic stability by press-fit (snap-fastener mechanism)
- close contact between implant and bone
- no screw fixation
- porous surface for bony ingrowth
- full bony containment of the cup
- preservation of the subchondral bone

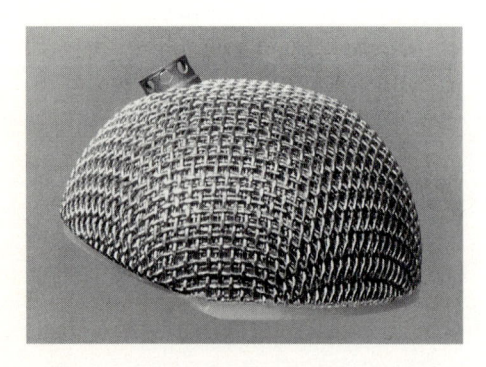

Fig. 1. Press-Fit Cup with Sulmesh coating

- preservation of elasticity (no rigid metal backing)
- no compromise in cup orientation
- optimum range of motion.

The key problem in achieving long lasting reliable fixation of a component is stress distribution between host bone and implant. With the implantation of a cup the "flow" of the forces from the prosthetic head into the acetabulum changes in magnitude and direction and a new equilibrium must be achieved. This adaptation is a biomechanical problem and can take place only on the biological side, i. e., by remodeling of the bony tissue. Fixation and loosening of an implant are two superimposed, opposite processes. The first consists in the apposition and the second in the resorption of bone. Bony ingrowth is only the first step in the whole process. With the achievement of bony ingrowth the goal of a lasting fixation is still far from achieved. Osseointegration, as the goal of a noncemented implant fixation, means not only that bone adheres directly to the implant surface without the interference of fibrous tissue, but also that force transmission between implant and bone occurs through bone structures which are adapted to the mechanical demand, and a biomechanical balance of bone apposition and resorption is achieved [23]. Design, surface, material, and operative technique must therefore not only result in good fixation but also prevent secondary loosening of the implant.

Press-Fit by Intrinsic Stability (Snap-Fastener Mechanism)

A hemisphere seems to represent the ideal design for a cup. The subchondral bone can be preserved, adaptation is excellent, and forces can be transmitted in a physiological manner from the cup to the pelvis and vice versa. The medial wall is protected, the perioperative defect is minimal, augmentation is facilitated, and revision, if necessary, is feasible. However, a hemispheric cup in a hemispheric cavity of the same diameter cannot provide intrinsic stability by press fit. To achieve stability of a purely hemispheric cup, additional measures must be used, such as screw or dowel fixation. Primary stability, however, is best realized by press fit. With the Press-Fit Cup, press-fit (i. e., preload between bone and implant) is produced by flattening the hemisphere and using a cup with a size 1, 5 mm larger than the corresponding reaming of the acetabulum. The Press-Fit Cup is fixed in the acetabulum by a snap-fastener mechanism.

As a result of the snap-fastener mechanism there are no longer high-pressure forces concentrated in the dome of the acetabulum as these forces are transmitted to the periphery. In other words, the forces are transmitted at almost a right-angle to the direction of a potential migration of the implant. As Goodman and Carter [8] have shown, stress concentrations are developed in zones 1 and 3, with relative sparing of zone 2. When loaded, the acetabulum closes in such a manner as to squeeze the cup, creating additional compressive radial stresses superiorly and inferiorly. The cup is secured against rotation and tilting by an eccentrically located single spigot in the form of a perforated hollow cylinder.

Close Contact

Primary stability and close contact between bone and implant are the most important requirements for extensive osseointegration of a non cemented implant. Press-fit generated by an oversize has been shown to be most effective and is more effective than screw fixation [4]. With an oversized pure hemisphere in a hemispherical cavity, however, the contact between the acetabulum and the surface of the cup may be insufficient (Fig. 2a). Since gaps of 0,5 mm [11] to 1 mm [9] cannot be bridged primarily by bony tissue and osseointegration may be compromised, a hemispheric design of the Press-Fit Cup was chosen where oversize and thus press-fit is created without loosing "line-to-line" i. e., close contact. This goal is achieved by the cup having the same outer radius as the acetabulum corresponding to the last reaming. Oversize, however, is created by an eccentricity of the centres of the radius by 1,5 mm. Furthermore, to assure transmission of the forces to the periphery the dome of the cup is flattened. This

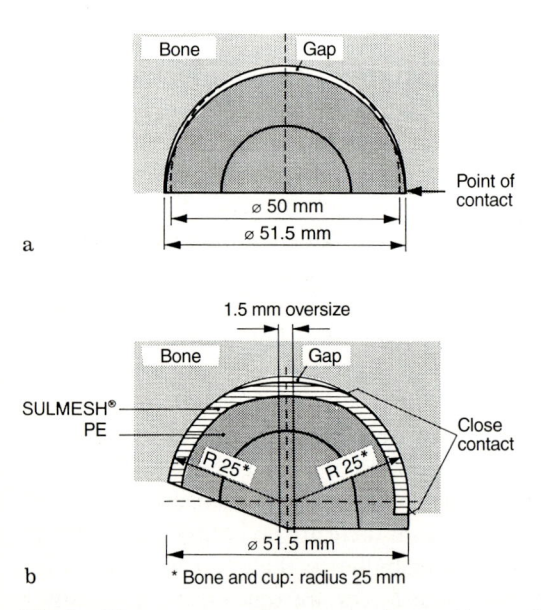

Fig. 2a. The contact area between implant and bone of a purely hemispheric cup consists in point or linear contact only. **b** The press-fit cup has the same outer radius as the acetabulum corresponding to the last reaming. Oversize is created by an eccentricity of the centers of the radius ba 1, 5 mm. With the press-fit cup 80 % of the surface area is in close implant-bone contact

achieves close contact of 80 % between cup surface and bony acetabulum (Fig. 2b).

No Screw Fixation

As a rule the most obvious means to create press-fit in orthopedic surgery is by using screws. However, in our series of noncoated RM polyethylene cups a higher loosening rate was observed when screws were used for fixation than when screws were not used: 9,5 % versus 5 % [26]. It may be that the screws prevent the settling process and increase tilting moments of the cups thus enhancing loosening rather than avoiding it.

Mechanical testing of acetabular stability shows; that the addition of screws gives a modest improvement only to the fixation of hemispheric cups, and that pegs are superior to screws [4, 24]. As can be shown in radiological follow-ups and histological studies, pegs seem to stimulate bone formation, thus increasing stability. Furthermore Wasielewski et al. [25], Keating et al. [12], and Kirkpatrick et al. [13] have demonstrated that venous, arterial, neural, and splanchnic structures are at risk when screws are placed in the acetabulum. In addition, with screws inserted through the border of the cup the metallic surface of the femoral head can be damaged in case of screw loosening. Screws seated in a metallic shell are prone to create fretting and wear problems.

Porous Coating SULMESH for Bony Ingrowth

To ensure a harmonious transmission of forces the surface of the endoprosthesis must conform to the bone and to the contact areas through which forces are transmitted. These areas should be as large as possible to avoid stress concentrations. Enlarging the contact surface between implant and bone improves the fixation of the prosthesis, especially where bony tissue is growing into pores and indentations of the implant surface. Coating increases roughening or texturing of the surface of the cup. The requirements for such a coating are well known today [2, 3, 5-7]: biocompatibility (hydroxyapatite, c.p. titanium), pore size between 100 and 500 μm, porosity volume of 30 % to 70 %, and mechanical stability against shear and preserved elasticity. As a coating of the Press-Fit Cup a fiber mesh with orderly oriented wires manufactured from chemically pure titanium has been developed by Sulzer Medical Technology (Fig. 1).

The aim was to have a porous structure which allows bonding of its inner surface with the outer surface of the polyethylene cup while having half of its porous thickness available for the ingrowth of bone tissue. Consideration of both these requirements led to the decision to develop a multilayered, thermally bonded wire mesh from unalloyed titanium ISO 5832-2, grade 1. Sulmesh is built up from multiple layers of wire mesh using wire diameters 0,3/0,5/0,7 mm with a pitch of 0,6/1,0/1,4 mm. The finished Sulmesh consists of three to five layers, with the outer layers always being of wire diameter 0,5 or 0,7 mm. The one or two inner mesh layers have a diameter equal to (0,5 mm) or smaller (0,3 mm) than the outer layers. Mesh combinations 535, 5335, 75335, and 7757 were produced during the course of development work. The Sulmesh surface for the Press-Fit Cup consists of four layers of titanium mesh.

Full Bony Containment

The more completely the cup is contained within the acetabulum, the better is the fixation [22]. An overhang at the superolateral part of the acetabulum may lead to impingement with the greater trochanter in abduction and increase the incidence of early loosening. On the other hand the cup containment below the equator cannot contribute to the stability of the joint. The press-fit cup therefore has a 20° bevel at the equator along one-half of its circumference, preventing the formation of a fulcrum inferoposteriorly against the neck of the femur (Fig. 3). This allows a compromise between the best anatomic position (inclined 30°–45° to the horizontal plane) and optimal freedom of movement by counteracting impingement between cup and greater trochanter as well as the tendency to dislocate. With this approach to the solution of various problems associated with the orientation of the acetabular cup only four dislocations have been observed in 535 total hip replacements performed with the Press-Fit Cup with c. p. titanium Sulmesh coating from January 1988 until December 1990 (= 0,7 %).

A variety of devices have been developed to improve the positioning of the acetabular socket. If, however, full containment of the cup and avoiding impingement of the lower rim of the cup with the neck of the femoral prosthesis are the main objectives, the press-fit cup can easily be positioned without an aiming device.

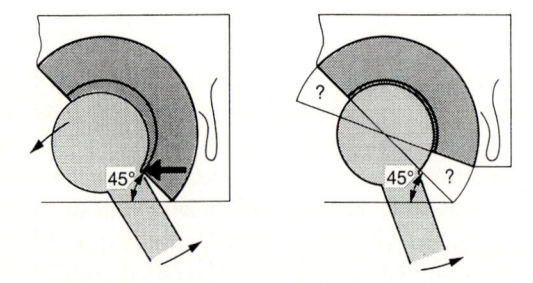

Fig. 3. The rationale of the bevel of the press-fit cup. The bevel of the acetabular component diminishes the risk of dislocation

Preservation of Subchondral Bone

It has been shown that the forces between the pelvis and the femur are transmitted through the cortical and subchondral bone rather than through cancellous structures [10], and that migration of a cup is increased when the subchondral bone is removed [14]. Preservation of the subchondral bone at least partially – seems to be important. With a hemispheric design, of course, the subchondral bone can best be preserved. Bony tissue must be well vascularized if it is to grow into a structure. The acetabulum must therefore be reamed until bleeding spots appear at the bone surface.

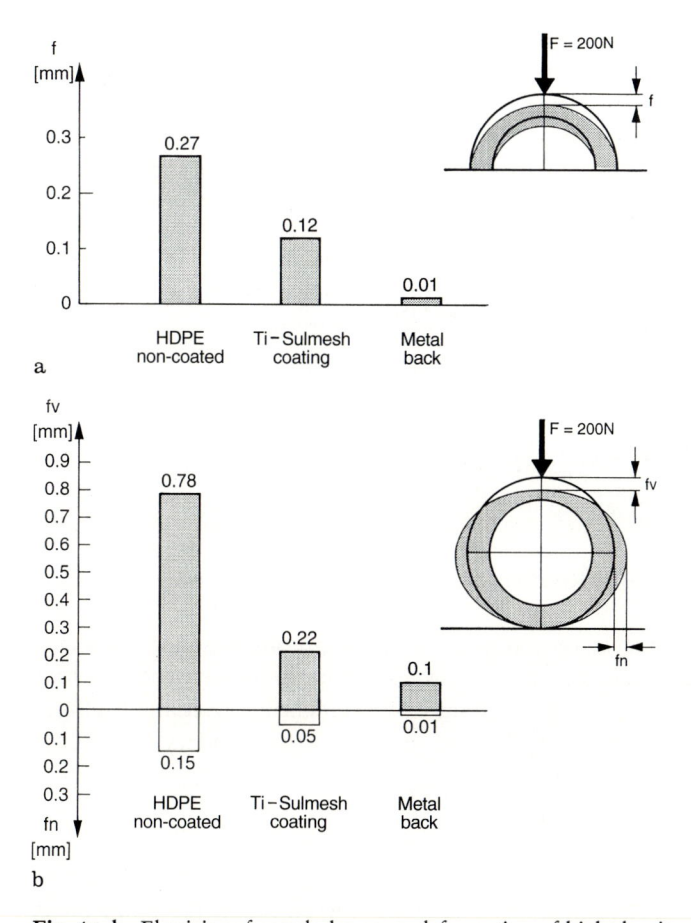

Fig. 4a, b. Elasticity of acetabular cups: deformation of high-density polyethylene (HDPE) noncoated, Sulmesh-coated, and metal-backed cups under 200-N loads. fv, fn directional components of deformation. **a** Elasticity test results with mouth of cup parallel to force (F). **b** Elasticity test results with mouth of cup perpendicular to force (F)

Preservation of Elasticity (no metal backing)

As has been previously demonstrated councerning osseointegration, remodeling of the bony structure around the cup is decisive for the longevity of its fixation. Remodeling with preservation and reinforcement of the bony tissue is possible only if there is no stress shielding and if the bone is able to adapt to the forces transmitted to the surface of the implant. Therefore it is unlikely that metal backing, i. e. stiffening of the cup, improves the longevity of its fixation. Clinical experience with both cemented and uncemented metal-backed cups confirms this [21].

With the Sulmesh fixed directly to the polyethylene the elasticity of the Press-Fit Cup is decreased in comparison to a polyethylene cup but is still higher than in metal-backed cups (Fig. 4).

The fixation of cemented cups is at its best from the time of the operation. However, uncemented implants with porous surfaces develop an increasing (secondary) stability during the postoperative weeks. This has been shown in experiments with mountain sheep. After 8 weeks the bone-implant interface proved to be stronger than the connection between mesh coating and polyethylene or the trabecular bone itself [1,26] (see contribution by Bereiter, this volume).

No Compromise in Cup Orientation

The position of the cup, in combination with the angles and the diameter and length of the femoral neck, determines the range of motion and the stability of the hip joint. The possibility of a uncompromised positioning during the implantation of a cup is therefore of utmost importance. This is achieved most easily with a hemispherical cup in a hemispherical acetabulum.

Optimum Range of Motion

The bevel (Fig. 3) increases the range of motion in comparison to ordinary hemispherical cups. Thus the bevel allows a compromise between the best anatomic position and optimum freedom of movement by avoiding impingement between cup and greater trochanter as well as the tendency to dislocation.

Results

From October 1985 to December 1993, 1432 press-fit cups have been implanted at our institution.

A cohort of 102 primary total hip replacements performed in 1988/ 89 was analyzed clinically and radiologically 1 and 5 years postoperatively. Of the 102 patients 51 were women and 42 men. In 9 patients both hips were operated on. In 92 cases the Press-Fit Cup was combined with a cemented femoral component and in 10 cases with an uncemented femoral component. The mean age of the patients was 67. 2 years (35-87).

All patients had a 6-week postoperative assessment. Two women died within the first postoperative year and were therefore excluded. Eleven patients (six women, five men, 13 hips) died between the 1 and the 5-year follow-up. All patients not having a minimum follow-up of 54 months were excluded from the second follow-up.

97 total hip replacements were available for the 1-year follow-up; 80 patients (88 hips) were available for the 5-year follow-up. The mean observation time for the first follow-up was 15,1 months (8–27) and for the second follow-up 61.0 months (54–73). No patients were lost for follow-up.

The clinical result (according to Merle d'Aubigné) at the 1- and 5-year follow-ups was excellent or good in 94 % and 96 %, moderate in 4 % and 3 % and poor in 2 % and 1 %. There were no cases of infection. An ectopic ossification grade IV (Brooker) occured in only one case (poor result at 1 year). One revision had to be done 41 months postoperatively for loosening of the cup after a fall on the operated hip. This was a female rheumatoid patient and counted as the second poor result.

The radiological analysis showed complete osseointegration in all three zones (according to DeLee and Charnley) in 97 % after 1 year and in 98 % after 5 years (Fig. 5). On the X-rays there was no damage to the Sulmesh coating, no impending or definitive loosening. In particular there was no progressive radiolucency between the 1 and the 5-year follow-up. Between the two follow-ups no new radiolucency appeared.

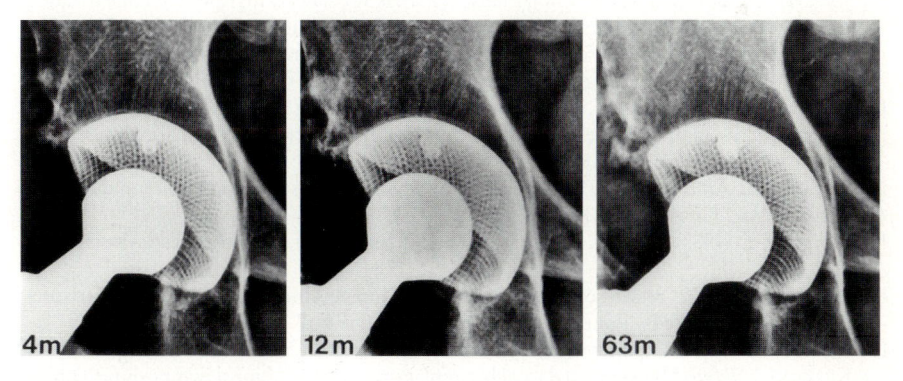

Fig. 5 X-ray series of a press-fit cup 4, 12 and 63 months after implantation

There was one case with a migration of less than 5 mm seen 14 months postoperatively, with no further progression up to 68 months.

The dome gap (due to the flattening of the dome of the cup) was visible in the postoperative X-ray in 28 %. It was still visible in 3 % at the 1-year follow-up. At the 5-year follow-up the dome gap could be detected in only one case.

References

1. Bereiter H, Bürgi M, Rahn BA (1992) Das zeitliche Verhalten der Verankerung einer zementfrei implantierten Hüftpfanne im Tierversuch. Orthopäde 21:63–70
2. Bobyn JD, Pilliar RM, Cameron HU, Weatherly GC (1980) The optimum pore size for the fixation of porous surface metal implants by the ingrowth of bone. Clin Orthop 150:263–268
3. Cameron HU (1982) The results of early clinical trials with a microporous coated metal hip prosthesis. Clin Orthop 165:188–190
4. Clarke HJ, Jinnah RH, Warden KE, Cox QGN, Curtis MJ (1991) Evalation of acetabular stability in uncemented prostheses. J Arthroplasty 6:335–340
5. Ducheyne P, Martens M, De Meester P, Mulier JC (1984) Titanium and titanium alloy prostheses with porous fiber metal coatings. In: Morscher E (ed) The cementless fixation of hip endoprostheses. Springer, Berlin Heidelberg New York, pp109–117
6. Galante J, Rostoker W, Lueck R, Ray RD (1971) Sintered fiber metal composite as a basis for attachment of implants to bone. J Bone Joint Surg [Am] 53: 101–114
7. Galante J, Summer DR, Gächter A (1987) Oberflächenstrukturen und Einwachsen von Knochen bei zementfrei fixierten Prothesen. Orthopäde 16:197–205
8. Goodman SB, Carter DR (1987) Acetabular lucent lines and mechanical stress in total hip arthroplasty. J Arthroplasty 2:219–224
9. Harris WH (1982) Allografting in total hip arthroplasty in adults with severe acetabular deficiency including a surgical technique for bolting the graft to the ilium. Clin Orthop 162:150–164
10. Huggler AH, Schreiber A, Dietschi C, Jacob H (1974) Experimentelle Untersuchung über das Deformationsverhalten des Hüftacetabulums unter Belastung. Z Orthop 112:44–50
11. Jasty M, Bragdon CR, Maloney WJ, Haire T, Harris WH (1991) Ingrowth of bone in failed fixation of porous coated femoral components. J Bone Joint Surg [Am] 73: 1331–1337
12. Keating EM, Ritter MA, Faris PM (1990) Structures at risk from medially placed acetabular screws. J Bone Joint Surg [Am] 72: 672–677
13. Kirkpatrick JS, Callaghan JJ, Vandemark RM, Goldner RD (1990) The relationship of the intrapelvic vasculature to the acetabulum. Implications in screw-fixation acetabular components. Clin Orthop 258:183–190
14. Markolf KL, Amstutz HC (1983) Compressive deformations of the acetabulum during in vitro loading. Clin Orthop 173:284–292
15. Morscher E (1987) Current state of cementless fixation of endoprostheses. Swiss Med 9:27–44
16. Morscher E (1990) Press-fit cementless fixation of hip prostheses. In: Coombs R, Gristina A, Hungerford D (eds) Joint replacement „state of the art". Mosby, St. Louis
17. Morscher E (1991) Experience with the press-fit cup and the press-fit gliding stem. In: Küsswetter W (ed) Noncemented total hip replacement, International Symposium, Tübingen 1990. Thieme, Stuttgart, pp 221–231
18. Morscher E (1992) Current status of acetabular fixation in primary total hip arthroplasty. Clin Orthop 274:172–193
19. Morscher E, Masar Z (1988) Development and first experience with an uncemented press-fit cup. Clin Orthop 232:96–103

20. Morscher E, Bereiter H, Lampert C (1989) Cementless press-fit cup. Principles, experimental data and three year follow-up study. Clin Orthop 249:12-20
21. Ritter MA, Faris PM, Keating EM, Brugo G (1992) Influential factors in cemented acetabular cup loosening. J Arthroplasty Suppl. 7:365-367
22. Sarmiento A, Ebramzadeh E, Gogan WJ, McKellop HA (1990) Cup containment and orientation in cemented total hip arthroplasties. J Bone Joint Surg [Bv] 72:996-1002
23. Schenk R, Morscher E (in press) Histomorphology of the implant/bone interface of the press-fit-cup with the orderly orientated fiber mesh Sulmesh. 5th Biomaterial Symposium, Göttingen, 1992
24. Stiehl JB, MacMillan E, Skrade DA (1991) Mechanical stability of porous-coated acetabular components in total hip arthroplasty. J Arthroplasty 6:295-300
25. Wasielewski RC, Cooperstein LA, Kruger MP, Rubash HE (1990) Acetabular anatomy and transacetabular screw fixation in total hip arthsoplasty. AAOS Meeting, Las Vegas. J Bone Joint Surg [Am] 72:501-508
26. Wilson-MacDonald J, Morscher E, Masar Z (1990) Cementless uncoated polyethylene acetabular components in total hip replacement. Review of five- to ten-year results. J Bone Joint Surg [Bn] 72:423-430

Part IV

Cemented Femoral Stem

The Weber Stem and the High-Pressure Cementing Technique

B. G. WEBER

History

The stem described here [1] was proposed by the author and produced in 1968, in cooperation with Otto Frei, engineer with Sulzer Brothers Ltd., Winterthur, Switzerland (Fig. 1). It consists of three straight and three curved stems, at first made from CoCrMo cast alloy but since 1973 from CoCrMo hot forged alloy. Fatigue fractures, which were a problem with earlier cast alloy stems, have occurred only twice in more than 100 000 forged stems. The first ball heads for the rotation cylinder were made of polyester. The rate of wear of this material was too high an loosening too frequent. Since 1971 the stem cylinder has been

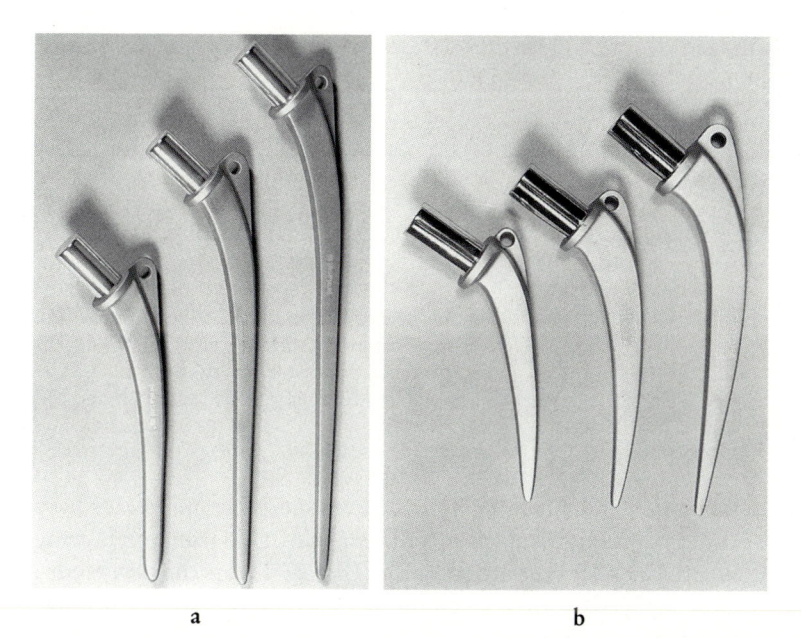

Fig. 1a, b. *The Weber stem for rotating prosthetic heads.* **a** Three straight stems. **b** Three curved stems. First generation stems since 1968 with cylindrical bolt for rotating CoCrMo heads, or for ceramic heads mounted on a CoCrMo rotating cylinder or for hemiarthroplasty heads

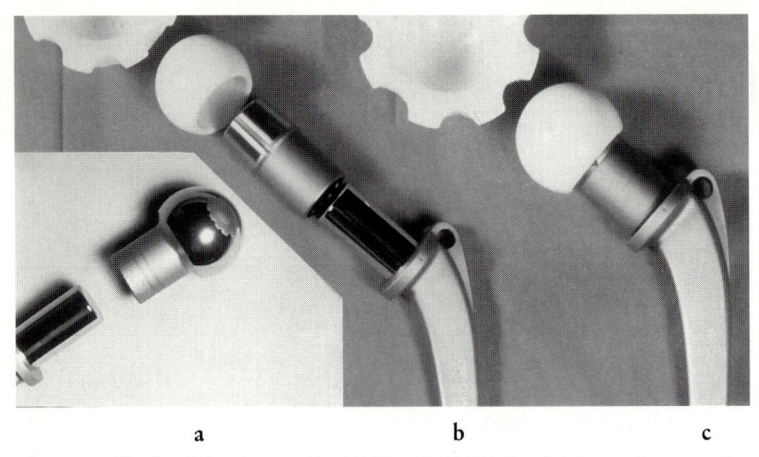

Fig. 2a–c. *The heads for the rotation THP.* **a** CoCrMo head, 32 mm diameter, 3 neck lengths. **b** CoCrMo rotating cylinder of 3 lengths, aluminum oxide-ceramic head to be fixes on the conus of the rotating cylinder. **c** Ceramic head version put together

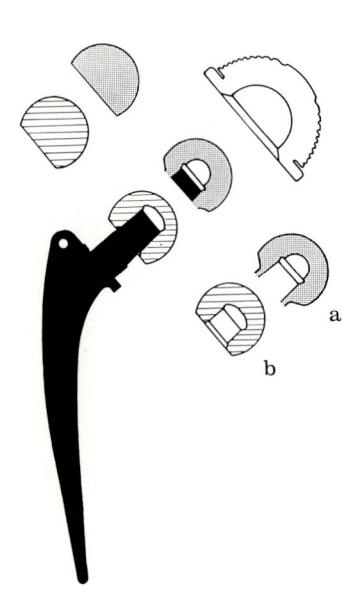

Fig. 3a, b. *The Weber stem with fixed heads.* The heads are producing different neck lengths depending on the depth of the conical boring. **a** CoCrMo heads. **b** Aluminum oxide ceramic heads

fitted with metal heads [6, 8]. Since 1974 aluminium oxide ceramic heads have also been used. Both types represent the metal-metal CoCrMo trunnion bearing prosthesis, of which 4 000 per year are produced (Fig 2). This is the first modular prosthesis allowing heads with different neck lengths and heads for hemiarthroplasty to be fitted.

For the first time since McKee's prosthesis [3–5] a metal-metal bearing is incorporated. This has stood the test of time for over 20 years, disproving the initial criticism, which resulted from unfortunate experiences with the McKee prosthesis. Also since 1974 the same stem, but with a conical bolt 16 mm in diameter, has been made to fix firmly onto modular heads of CoCrMo or of aluminum oxide ceramic. The best pattern in our own experience, with regard to wear, gliding properties (low friction), loosening rate, and longevity, is the rotation trunnion bearing THP with a ceramic head. It seems that due to the movement between bolt and head the wear of the polyethylene of the cup is substantially reduced [6–8]. Since 1988 the conical bolt has been made smaller in diameter, only 14 mm, to allow smaller metal or ceramic heads of 28 mm diameter to be fitted. About 5 000 of these stems are produced per year (Fig. 3). Also since 1988 the cups have been refined for high-pressure cementing anchorage. They are either paired with metal or ceramic heads or supplemented with a CoCrMo inlay, which is paired with a corresponding metal head (METASUL) [9].

Stem Design

The geometry of the six standard stems has remained unchanged since 1968. It consists of a flat medial surface and a flat and larger lateral surface, the cross-section being wedged with rounded edges (Fig. 4). The metal volume increases from the tip to the upper end, so that the stem is wedge-shaped on all faces. A strong collar provides direct buttressing against the cement mantle. A fin on the lateral surface of the stem proximally in the direction of the greater trochanter adds rotational control. It has a 4.5 mm hole for the extraction

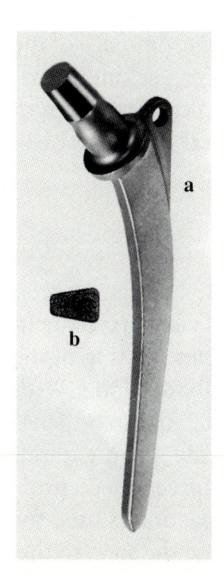

Fig. 4a, b. *Stem design.* **a** Wedge-shaped stem with fin and collar; **b** cross-section, also wedge-shaped

instrument. During its insertion the stem generates an effective impaction of cement into the bonebed by "hydraulic" displacement. The stem is finally secured in the cement mantle and is buttressed against the cement by its collar. The stem, once seated in the cement mantle, loses all cement splittingcracking property since the wedge-shaped stem is now resting with the collar on the upper end of the cement mantle. The result is a compound stem-cement complex, which is stable in itself with no mechanical reasons for debonding.

The flow of forces is undisturbed and uninterrupted from the implant (stem-cement compound) to the bone at all levels, avoiding stress shielding and avoiding stress-void areas. Design, instruments, and surgical technique are a linked trias. The most vulnerable of these is the surgical technique, i. e. the surgeon's performance.

Operation technique: High-Pressure Cementing Technique
General

The use of high viscosity cement and finger packing in the critical proximal femoral cavity, adopted from Charnley, are, for us, of utmost importance. The reaming of the femoral cavity must preserve not only the cancelleous bone structure but also provide a circumferential cement mantle 4 mm thick, particularly in the upper proximal part. All reamed and devitalized bone particles are removed by irrigation and brushing. This provides direct interlocking of the high viscosity cement with the vital bone and allows for penetration of the cement into the cancelleous bone meshwork to a depth of 2–4 mm. The following procedures assist in providing a perfect cement filling, which is not more and not less than the best possible custom made prosthetic fit (Fig. 5): medullary plug; filling of the cement from proximal to distal with a syringe, drainage of the medullary cavity (in the sterile enclosure using succion); finger packing proximally to "inject" the cement into the cancelleous bone; backflow limitation of the cement by means of a silicone-rubber collar. These general quality control prerequisites may be refined as follows.

High-Pressure Cementing

For manual impaction-insertion of the femoral component [1, 2, 7] the surgeon can generate a force of only 25 kg by pushing. Using high viscosity cement, there is always the risk that 25 kg is not sufficient for a complete seating of the stem. If the stem is not properly seated, the leg may be finally too long. With high-pressure instrumentation, however, a pushing force of 100 kg can be generated with ease (Fig. 6). In spite of the high viscosity of the cement and without risk of half-way insertion of the stem, instrumentation allows precisely controlled and trouble-free cementing. The instrumentation for impaction is used for only the last 2–3 cm of stem insertion, as the surgeon has seated the stem to this

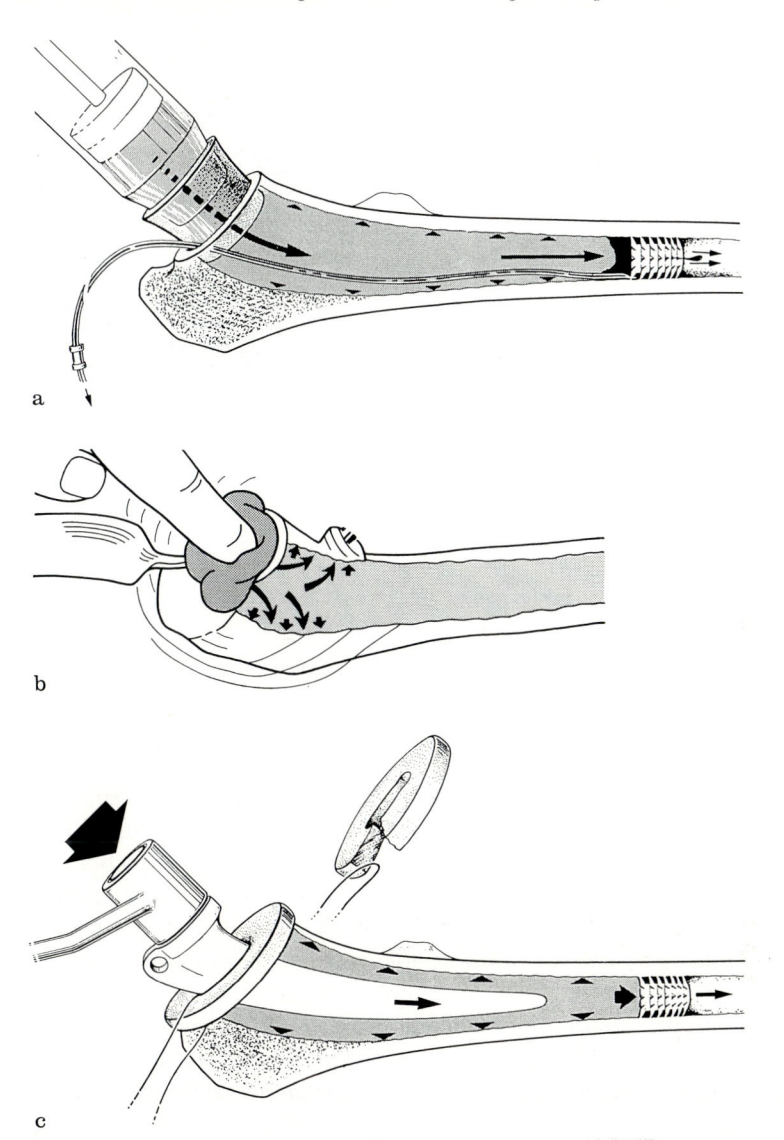

Fig. 5a–c. *Cementing technique.* **a** Filling from proximal to distal, plug, drainage of medullary cavity. **b** Finger packing: digital massage-filling of superficial cancelleous bone structure *(arrows).* **c** Backflow limitation with collar of silicone rubber

point with the seating piece by hand. High-pressure instrumentation is used only for the last critical phase of polymerization, at the point when pure manual impaction would fail.

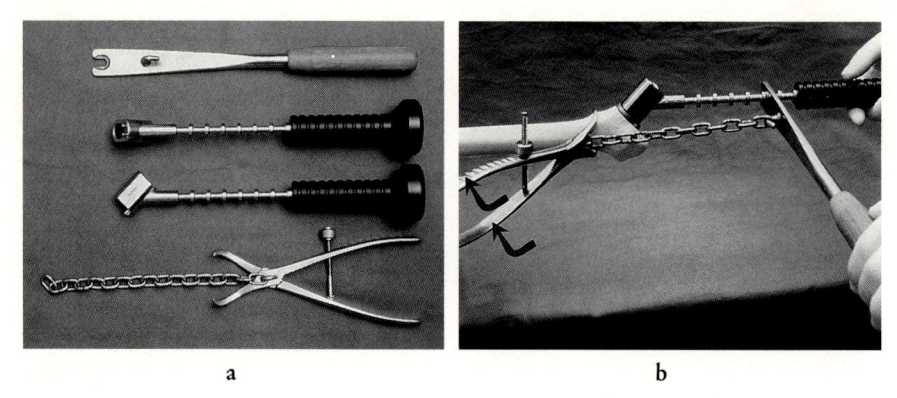

Fig. 6a, b. *High-pressure cementing instrumentation.* **a** Forked lever with hook; stem seating piece (in two views); bone clamp with chain. **b** Generation of high pressure: the bone clamp is connected by the chain with the forked lever, which is engaged to the stem seating piece. A pushing force of 100 kg is easily generated

Discussion, Summary, Prospects

The Weber stem is layed out along the principles as a compound construction: as a metal wedge resisting with its collar on a circumferential cement mantle. An adapted operation technique is most important. Technical mistakes are possible at each step of the procedure. Cementless anchorage is less sensitive in this respect and therefore meets with more acceptance from surgeons. Defective cementing shows up quickly as early or even instant loosening. In contrast, late loosening, after 10 years or more, proves the efficiency of cement anchorage. Late loosening can only be the result of polyethylene particle disease. Metal-metal pairing eliminates harmful polyethylene waste disease. The new metal-metal total hip replacement is promising longevity of 30 years or more, as Müller-McKee THP's from the 1960's have already shown. The Weber stem, in use since 1968, and particularly since being hot forged (1974), has served for 20 years with full satisfaction. It is hoped that in the metal-metal pairing pattern the THP will significantly reduce the number of revision operations required in the future.

References

1. Charnley, J (1970) Total hip replacement by low friction arthroplasty. Clin Orthop 72: 7
2. Charnley, J (1977) Low friction arthroplasty of the hip. Springer, Berlin Heidelberg New York
3. McKee, GK, Watson-Farrar, J (1966) Replacement of arthritic hips by the McKee-Farrar-Prosthesis. J Bone Joint Surg [Br] 48: 245–259

4. McKee, GK (1970) Development of total prosthetic replacement of the hip. Clin Orthop 72: 85–103
5. McKee, GK (1982) Total hip replacement. Present and future. Biomaterials 3: 130–135
6. Weber, BG (1981) Total hip replacement: Rotating versus fixed and metal versus ceramic heads. In: Proc. 9th Open Scientific Meeting of the Hip Society. Mosby, St. Louis, pp 264–275
7. Weber, BG (1988) Pressurized cement fixation in total hip arthroplasty. Clin Orthop 232: 87–95
8. Weber, BG, Fiechter, T (1989) Polyethylen-Verschleiß und Spätlockerungen der Totalprothese des Hüftgelenkes. Neue Perspektiven für die Metall-Metall-Paarung für Pfanne und Kugel. Orthopäde 18: 370–376
9. Weber, BG, Semlitsch, M, Streicher, R (1993) Total hip joint replacement using a CoCrMo metal-metal sliding pairing. J Jpn Orthop Ass 67: 391–398

The Cemented MS-30 Stem

E. Morscher, L. Spotorno, A. Mumenthaler, W. Frick

Introduction

The majority of orthopedists today prefer to treat patients aged over 60 years old by a hybrid arthroplasty, implanting a cementless cup combined with a cemented stem [7, 22, 30]. Cementless fixation of the stem can also be considered in younger and active patients. Improvements in cementation technique have undoubtedly led to a significant improvement in the long-term fixation of implants [3]. The refined cementation technique comprises in particular the cleaning of the medullary cavity by rinsing and drying, and the pressurization of the bone cement. Various authors [23, 25] have pointed out the importance of the prosthesis stem being completely surrounded by a mantle of cement and the danger of direct contact between metal and bone [8].

A study conducted by the Basle University Orthopedic Clinic [29] compared the cemented stem prostheses used in the early 1980s (Müller straight stem, curved stem, and the 130 stem). Survivorship analysis showed the collarless

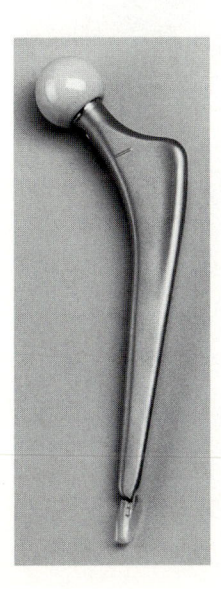

Fig. 1. The MS-30 femoral stem with modular ceramic head and centralizer

straight stem to have the best results after 5–10 years; however, this model exhibited the most subsidence. Despite the excellent clinical results with the straigth stem, there is some concern about its future, and therefore began development of the MS-30 stem (Fig. 1).

Form and cementation technique must undergo further improvement to achieve even better results with cemented prosthesis stems. The most important thing is to obtain a cement mantle able to withstand the mechanical forces. A cement mantle that is too thin results in contact between metal and bone in certain locations, and in fragmentation there. Bone cement has poor resistance to bending forces. The aim is to use an appropriate design and improved cementation technique to achieve a morphologically and qualitatively impeccable cement mantle around the prosthesis which can transfer the stresses from the bone onto the implant and vice versa as mainly compressive forces without impairment of the cement. The most important prerequisites for this are met by the all-round-tapered form of the prosthesis stem, its neutral positioning, and an optimized cementation technique (Fig. 2). These are the three main principles that led to the cemented prosthesis stem MS-30, named after its designers Morscher and Spotorno. The number 30 refers to the special metal alloy used for

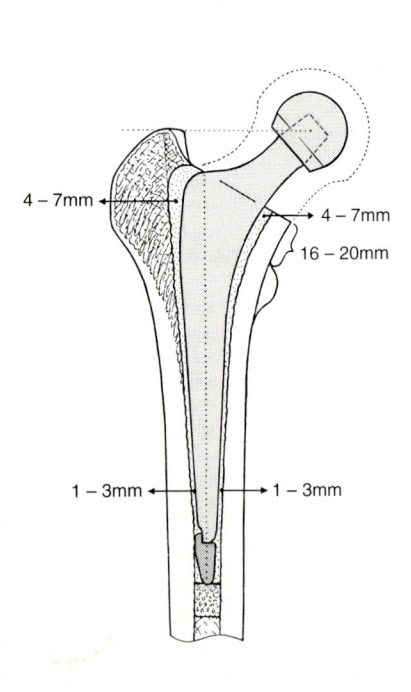

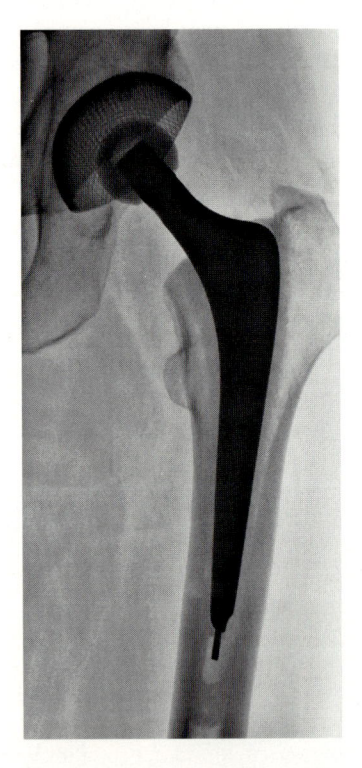

Fig. 2a, b. Schematic drawing and X-ray of the MS-30 stem with optimum cement mantle

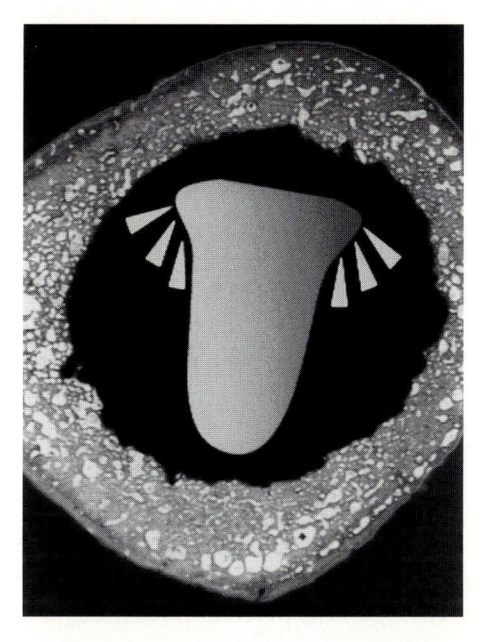

Fig. 3. Anterolateral and posterolateral wings in the proximal part of the MS-30 stem to increase rotational stability and decrease the load to the calcar

this stem, the wrought high nitrogen stainless steel Protasul 30 (FeCrNiMn-MoNbN ISO 5832-9).

The MS-30 stem is tapered on all sides, leading to a uniform distribution of the forces acting on the cement mantle. The tapered form also ensures that the stem wedges itself again upon the slightest subsidence, and that the stresses are transferred as compressive forces. The rounded corners avoid stress concentrations at the implant/cement interface. The principal load transfer occurs medially in the area of the calcar femorale. Anterolateral and posterolateral rounded protrusions in the proximal area of the stem absorb forces acting on the calcar from the implant. This reduces the loading of the calcar area and increases the area of contact and the rotational stability of the stem (Fig. 3). The shape of the stem cross-section is that shown by Crowninshield et al. [5] to subject the bone cement to the least stresses (Fig. 4). The stem neck angle (CCD) depends on the size, being 130° for the smallest prosthesis and 135° for the largest. The stem has a 12/14 taper spigot. Protasul-1 or Protek ceramic ballheads with differing neck lengths can be mounted as appropriate.

The MS-30 stem is manufactured in six sizes, from 6 to 16. An integral part of the MS-30 stem is the centralizer, which is mounted on the distal end and makes possible the neutral positioning of the prosthesis in the femoral cavity. The centralizer is made from polymethylmethacrylate and has the form of a three-

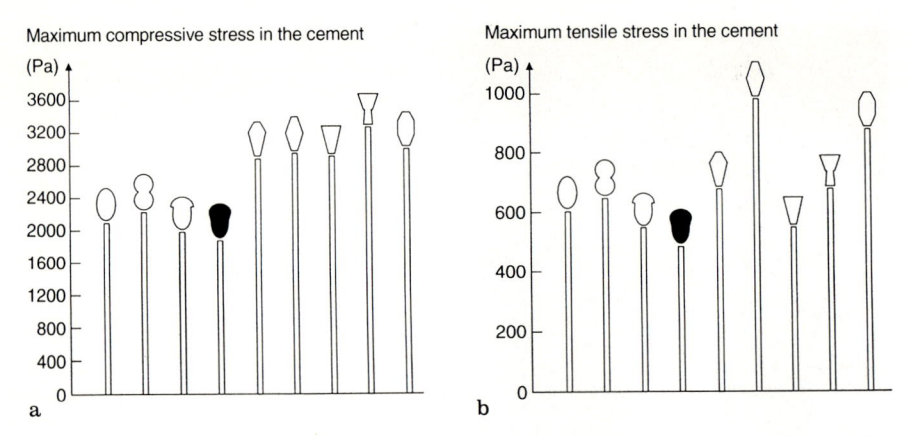

Fig. 4. Maximum compressive (**a**) and tensile (**b**) stress in the cement according to the geometry (transsection) of the femoral stem. (From [5])

sided pyramid with an equilateral triangle as its base, which helps insertion through bone cement. One corner of the base triangle points laterally and thus achieves the defined cement thickness. The tip of the pyramid is rounded, and the sides are concave. This enables cement flow around the centralizer without disturbing its homogenicity. The pin protruding from the centralizer is slightly conical to improve the friction fit. It is inserted into a matching bore in the stem. The centralizer is supported on the lateral side of the stem to ensure its correct positioning. The centralizer is available in six sizes from 8 to 18 mm. The size to be used is determined by measuring the medullary cavity. The best fit is achieved with the largest possible centralizer.

To achieve an optimum cement mantle, preoperative planning and the operative technique are based on the selection of a prosthesis size which provides the necessary space between the implant and the prepared medullary cavity. This space can be achieved by using a rasp that is one or even two sizes larger than the selected stem. Another way to achieve the same result is deliberately to insert the rasp with the same size as the prosthesis stem deeper, bearing in mind that the insertion depth determines the thickness of the resulting cement mantle.

Significance of Cement Mantle Thickness for Long-Term Fixation of a Cemented Femoral Stem

Investigations have shown a direct relationship between the durability of the stem fixation and the properties of the cement mantle and its thickness at various femoral locations and zones. There is thus a direct relationship to the position of the stem prosthesis in the medullary cavity. A neutral or slightly valgus position is seen as advantageous and a varus position as unsuitable. Especially important is the central position of the prosthesis tip, as can be achieved by the use of a centralizer [10]. Investigations by Harrigan and Harris [16] and Harrigan et al. [17] have shown that the separation of bone cement and metal occurs mostly at the medial edge of the distal prosthesis tip, and that the greatest cement mantle loading occurs at that location. Using finite element analyses, Estok et al. [11] showed that the greatest axial compression forces occur medially close to the stem tip, that the loading of the cement mantle is considerably reduced when the thickness of the mantle is increased from 2,5 to 5 mm, and that an increase in cement mantle thickness reduces the axial compression loading by 46 %. These experimental investigations were confirmed in a clinical follow-up study by Star et al. [27], in which there were significantly more cases of prosthesis loosening with a thin cement mantle in zones 5 and 6 of Gruen. Discriminate analysis showed further that a thin cement layer in zone 5 is the best predictor of prosthesis loosening. This ist initially applicable of course only to the prosthesis stem used by the authors. Further investigations are necessary to determine whether this has general applicability. In any case, a varus position of the prosthesis stem in the medullary cavity has always been considered to have an unfavorable effect on long-term fixation [4]. In addition, Embramzadeh et al. [9] has shown that the thickness of the cement mantle between the calcar and the medial prosthesis stem is a useful predictor of long-term fixation. Centering of the prosthesis tip and a thick cement layer in the medial calcar area are the most important operative measures for avoiding a varus position.

Smooth and Rough Prosthesis Surfaces

Until 1975 Ling and Exeter [12] used a tapered stem with a smooth surface (Exeter stem). Since then the same has been used but with a rough surface. Between 1980 and 1985 the results with this stem were not as good as with the smooth stem beginning in 1986. The material of both stems is stainless steel (EN58J).

Two things were responsible for the poorer performance of the stem with the rough surface. Friction between the rough surface and the inner surface of the cement mantle causes wear [2, 15, 19]. In addition, there is a negative effect on load transfer, in that there is an increase in the shear forces and a reduction in compression [21] compared with the polished surface. Subsidence of the rough Exeter stem occurs almost without exception together with the cement mantle, loosening the cement/bone interface. On the other hand, however, the subsidence of the polished stem occurs within the cement mantle. This corresponds to the objective of a tapered stem [28], as needed for load transfer with a smooth surface. This type of subsidence does not compromise the cement/bone interface.

The combination of an incomplete cement mantle, generally caused by too large a stem diameter, and the production of wear products due to movement of the rough surface against the inner surface of the cement mantle has serious consequences [2]. These are increased due to incorrect cementation technique, particularly by improper handling of low viscosity bone cement. In both of the authors' clinics (Basle, Switzerland and Pietra Ligure, Italy) Palacos, a viscous cement with better endurance properties than low viscosity cement, is used on a regular basis.

The Swedish multicenter study of Malchau et al. [20] confirmed the difference between rough and smooth surfaces with the Exeter stem observed by Ling and colleagues. Dall et al. [6] noted a significant difference in the aseptic loosening rate between the polished Charnley flat-back stem and later generations of Charnley stems, all of which have a rough surface. Excellent long-term results were achieved with the polished Charnley flat-back described by Schulte et al. [26] in 1983. The questions for surface finish and wear will probably be considered as more important in the future than to date.

The higher the stress at the implant/cement interface, the sooner loosening occurs with break-up of the cement and the formation of cement particles. The formation of cement particles is greater when the implant surface is rougher (if there is micromotion), and when the material is more elastic (titanium stems). For cement particles to lead to bone resorption there must be a way through to the cement/bone interface. This is the case when the cement mantle is incomplete or fractured. On the other hand, the stronger the implant/bone plus cement bond, the higher the stress is at the cement/bone interface [13].

The whole loosening process can be affected positively or negatively by the surface condition of the implant and thus also by the strength of the bond between the implant surface and the cement mantle. It must be assumed that this bond is always mechanical and not chemical. There is a simple friction fit which is stronger with a larger surface area (fine blasted or structured) than with a smooth (polished) surface.

A smooth surface probably leads sooner to debonding between the implant and the bone cement than with a rough surface. On the other hand, the risk of producing cement wear particles is lower. The stiffness of the implant also plays a role, with increasing stiffness leading to less movement and thus to less wear. The fine blasting of the MS-30 stem increases its bending and fatigue strength and compresses its surface, so that relative movement is reduced.

From investigations on cadaveric specimens with histologically loosened prostheses, Harris and colleagues also found a debonding at the implant cement interface in nearly all cases. They found fractured cement through which particles from the implant/cement interface were able to penetrate through to the bone/cement interface. On the other hand, debonding between a smooth implant surface and the cement must not necessarily lead to wear, and not at all to fracture of the cement mantle. With no cement mantle fracture, wear particles cannot reach the bone/cement interface directly. In other words, debonding of the implant/cement interface cannot in itself be equated with prosthesis loosening.

Points of Initiation of Implant Loosening

Amstutz et al. [1] and Gruen et al. [14] established that 11,1 % of cases of "prosthesis failure" initiate at the bone/cement interface and 10,3 % at the prosthesis/cement interface. This observation indicates that the loosening process can initiate "at the scene of the crime," i. e. at the cement/bone interface, but also that, as postulated by Harris, at the implant/cement interface.

Suggestions have been made as to how to prevent initiation of the loosening process at the implant/cement interface, based on improving the mechanical stability of this connection. Park et al. (1982) [24] showed that precoating results in fewer cell reactions and increases the cement thickness, which improves the mechanical properties of the cement. Measurements of the tensile bond strength between the implant surface and the cement show that this is higher for steel (316LSS) than for CoCrMo or titanium alloys. After about 1 week, however, there are no significant differences in the tensile bond strength. Keller et al. [18] stated that "poor cement coverage generally occurred with titanium alloy at short running times."

Conclusions

On the basis of presently available data it cannot be determined definitively whether a tapered stem with polished or rough surface reduces the likelihood of

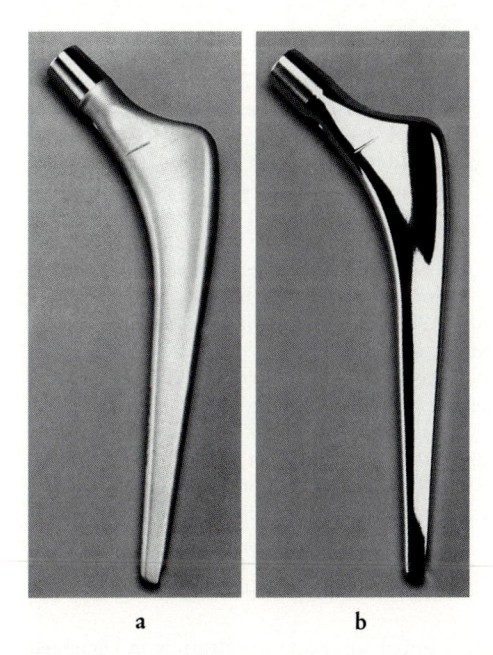

Fig. 5. MS-30 stem with matt (**a**) and smooth (**b**) surface.

loosening. The MS-30 stem makes a compromise between the two in that there is a stable bond between the stem and the bone cement. The final answer will be provided by the long-term clinical results. A prospective randomized study in the clinics of the present authors using MS-30 stems with smooth and fine blasted surfaces (Fig. 5) will contribute to resolving the question of the surface condition for prosthesis stems.

References

1. Amstutz HC, Markolf KL, McNiece GM, Gruen TA (1976) Loosening of total hip components: Cause and prevention. In: Weber BG (ed) The Total Hip. Mosby, St. Louis, pp 102–116
2. Anthony PP, Gie GA, Howie CR, Ling RSM (1990) Localised endosteal bone lysis in relation to the femoral components of cemented total hip arthroplasties. J Bone Joint Surg [Br] 72: 971–979
3. Ballard WT, Callaghan JJ, Sullivan PM, Johnston RC (1994) The results of improved cementing techniques for total hip arthroplasty in patients less than fifty years old. Bone Joint Surg [Am] 76: 959–964
4. Calandruccio RA (1980) Arthroplasty. In: Edmonson AS, Crenshaw AH (eds) Campbell's Operative Orthopaedics, Mosby, St. Louis, p 2192
5. Crowninshield RD, Brand RA, Johnston RC, Milroy JC (1980) The effect of femoral stem cross-sectional geometry on cement stresses in total hip reconstruction. Clin Orthop 146: 71–77
6. Dall DM, Learmonth ID, Solomon MI, Miles AW, Davenport JM (1993) Fracture and loosening of Charnley femoral stems: comparison between first-generation and subsequent designs. J Bone Joint Surg [Br] 75: 259–265
7. Davey JR, Harris WH (1989) A preliminary report of the use of a cementless acetabular component with a cemented femoral component. Clin Orthop 245: 150–155
8. Dorr LD, Takei GK, Conaty JP (1983) Total hip arthroplasties in patients less than forty-five years old. J Bone Joint Surg [Am] 65: 474–479
9. Ebramzadeh E, Sarmiento A, McKellop HA, Llinas A, Gogan W (1994) The cement mantle in total hip arthroplasty. J Bone Joint Surg [Am] 76: 77–87
10. Eglund N, Lidgren L, Onnerfalt R (1990) Improved positioning of the femoral stem with a centralizing device. Acta Orthop Scand 61: 236–239
11. Estok DM, Harrigan TP, Harris WH (1991) Finite element analysis of cement strains at the tip of an idealized cemented femoral component. Trans Orthop Res Soc 16: 504
12. Fowler JL, Gie GA, Lee AJC, Ling RSM (1988) Experience with the Exeter total hip replacement since 1970. Orthop Clin North Am 19: 477–489
13. Gardiner RC, Hozack WJ (1994) Failure of the cement-bone interface. A consequence of strengthening the cement prosthesis interface? J Bone Joint Surg [Br] 76: 49–52
14. Gruen TA, McNeice GM, Amstutz HC (1979) „Modes of failure" of cemented stem-type femoral components. A radiographic analysis of loosening. Clin Orthop 141: 17–27
15. Hale D, Lee AJC, Hooper RM, Ling RSM (1990) The production of acrylic cement and metal debris by the femoral component in cemented total hip replacement. J Bone Joint Surg [Br] 72: 1090
16. Harrigan TP, Harris WH (1991) Mechanical consequences of cement-metal interface disruption (debonding) at the distal tip of femoral total hip prosthesis. Trans Orthop Res Soc 16: 503
17. Harrigan TP, Kareh J, Harris WH (1991) Initial loosening mechanisms in cemented femoral stems: debonding at the cement-metal interface. Trans Orthop Res Soc 16: 520

18. Keller JC, Lautenschlager EP, Marshall GW Jr, Meyer PR Jr (1980) Factors affecting surgical alloy/bone cement interface adhesion. J Biomed Mater Res 14: 639–651
19. Lee AJC, Hooper RM, Ling RSM, Brooks R, Gie GA, Hale D (1993) Fretting as a source of particulate debris in total joint arthroplasty. In: Turner-Smith AR (ed) Micromovement in orthopaedics. Oxford University Press, Oxford
20. Malchau H, Herberts P, Ahnfelt L (1993) Prognosis of total hip replacement in Sweden: follow-up of 92 675 operations performed 1978–90. Acta Orthop Scand 64: 497–506
21. Miles AW, Clift SE, Bannister GC (1990) The effect of the surface finish of the femoral component on lead transmission in total hip replacement. J Bone Joint Surg [Br] 72: 736
22. Morscher E (1993) Current status of acetabular fixation in primary total hip arthroplasty. Clin Orthop 274: 172–193
23. Mulroy RD Jr, Harris WH (1990) The effect of improved cementing techniques on component loosening in total hip replacement. An 11-year radiographic review. Bone Joint Surg [Br] 72: 757–760
24. Park JB, Barb W, Kenner GH, Recum von AF (1982) Intramedullary fixation of artificial hip joints with bone cement-precoated implants. II. Density and histological study. J Biomed Mater Res 16: 459–469
25. Russotti GM, Coventry MB, Stauffer RN (1988) Cemented total hip arthroplasty with contemporary techniques. A five-year minimum follow-up study. Clin Orthop 235: 141–147
26. Schulte KR, Callaghan JJ, Kelly SS, Johnston RC (1993) The outcome of Charnley total hip arthroplasty with cement after a minimum twenty-year follow-up. J Bone Joint Surg [Am] 75: 961–975
27. Star MJ, Colwell CW Jr, Kelman GJ, Ballock RT, Walker RH (1994) Suboptimal (thin) distal cement mantle thickness as a contributory factor in total hip arthroplasty femoral component failure. J Arthroplasty 9: 143–149
28. Timperley AJ, Gie GA, Lee AJC, Ling RSM (1993) The femoral component as a taper in cemented total hip arthroplasty. J Bone Joint Surg [Br] 75 [Suppl]: 33
29. Wilson-MacDonald J, Morscher E (1989) Comparison between straight- and curved-stem Müller femoral prostheses; 5- to 10-year results of 545 total hip replacements. Arch Orthop Trauma Surg 109: 14–20
30. Wixson RL, Stulberg SD, Mehlhoff M (1991) Total hip replacement with cemented, uncemented and hybrid prostheses. J Bone Joint Surg [Am] 73: 257–270

The Cement-Fixed (CF) Hip Replacement System

H. G. Willert, G. Köster, H. P. Köhler

Introduction

One of the most important factors causing loosening and failure of cemented artificial hip joints is deterioration of the polymethylmethacrylate (PMMA) bone cement. The process of bone cement fragmentation develops slowly, but cracks, having once being started, propagate continuously [3, 11, 13, 14, 16]. Irregularities and defects of the cement cuff, eccentric placement of the implants, and direct contact between implant and bone promote fragmentation of the bone cement [1, 4, 8, 10, 12, 15]. Fragmentation of bone cement produces PMMA particles[4]. The particles induce granulomatous tissue reactions which subsequently give rise to the development of endosteal osteolyses [14, 15, 27, 28]. To avoid these disadvantages of cement fixation a cemented artificial hip joint should fulfill the following requirements:
- the cement mantle should be as complete and homogeneous as possible
- the implants should be well centered within the cement
- the bone cement should be pressurized even during insertion of the endoprosthetic components, and
- a good connection between implant and bone cement should be achieved.

These objectives led to a new design of a cementable artifical hip joint: the cement-fixed (CF) endoprosthetic system.

Characteristic Features of the CF Endoprosthetic System

Sockets

At present two types of CF sockets are available.
   The CFPS (cement-fixed-polyethylene-sulmesh) socket has a core of Ultra high molecular weight (UHMW) polyethylene RCH 1000 (Chirulen) which is surrounded by a Sulmesh grid. The grid is made of four layers of a meshed, forged steel alloy (Protasul-S-30) wire. The layers are arranged at 45° angles to each other; they are spot welded and securely anchored in the polyethylene. This metal backing reduces the contact between polyethylene and cement to

minimum, improves the mechanical fixation of the socket in the cement, and increases the stiffness of the polyethylene core.

The all-polyethylene CFP (cement-fixed-polyethylene) socket has exactly the same shape but no Sulmesh mantle. A new type of oval-shaped recesses provide good conditions for a firm anchorage in the bone cement (Fig. 1a,b).

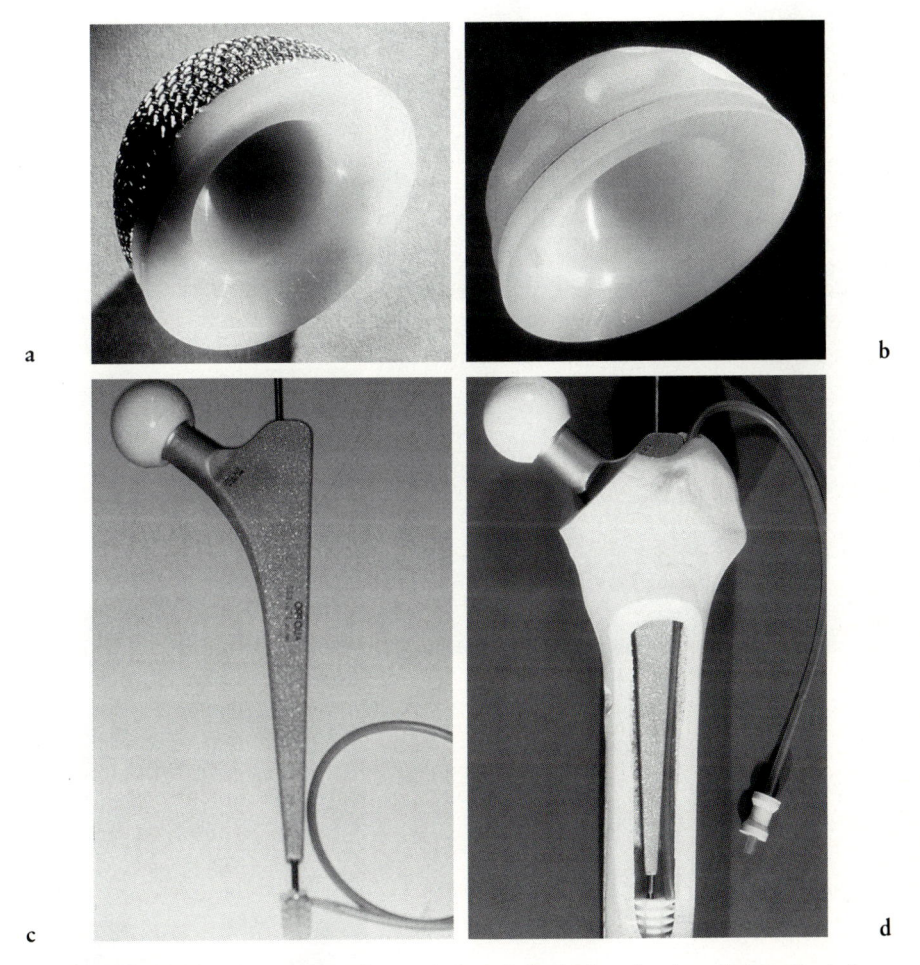

Fig. 1. a The CFPS socket with an inlet consisting of ultrahigh molecular weight polyethylene is surrounded by Sulmesh made out of Protasul S 30. **b** The CFP socket is made completely of ultrahigh molecular weight polyethylene. It has the same shape as the CFPS socket, but instead of the Sulmesh grid there are oval-shaped recesses for the anchorage of the cement. **c** CF-30 stem made of the forged-steel alloy Protasul-S-30, with the guide wire which is attached to the cement stopper. **d** The guidewire is positioned in the marrow cavity and directs the stem into a central position

To achieve a complete bone cement mantle of about 2–5 mm thickness, the reamer for the acetabulum is somewhat larger than the implant. The space thus created can be explored through a window in the testing socket. Nevertheless, the bone resection can be performed conservatively because of the elliptical shape of the socket. The bone cement should be injected through a syringe. For

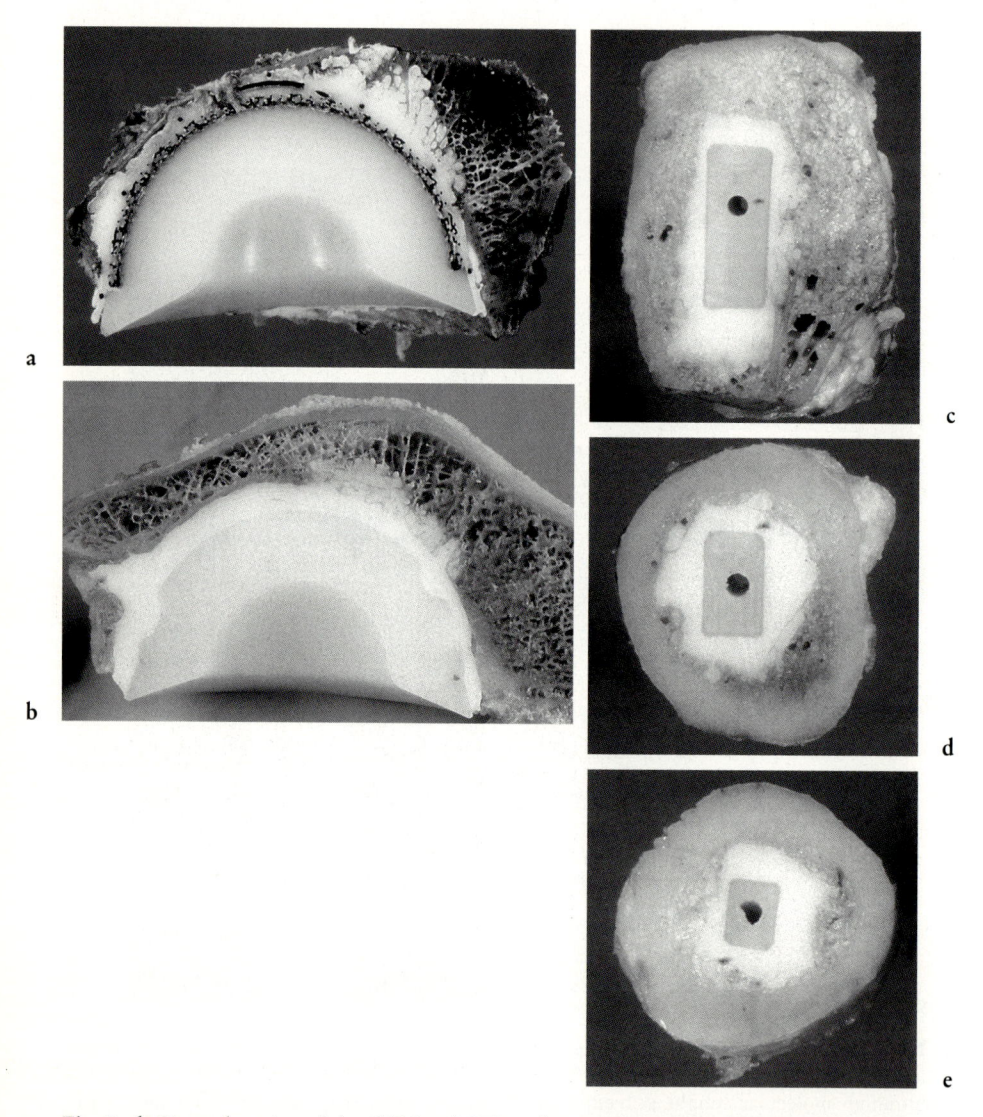

Fig. 2a, b Coronal section of the CFPS and CFP sockets, each implanted in a specimen of the pelvis. The protruding edges centralize the components. The cement layers are homogeneous, and the firm anchorage between cement and implants becomes visible. **c–e** Cross-sections show the central position of the prosthesis in a specimen of the femur

The Cement-Fixed (CF) Hip Replacement System

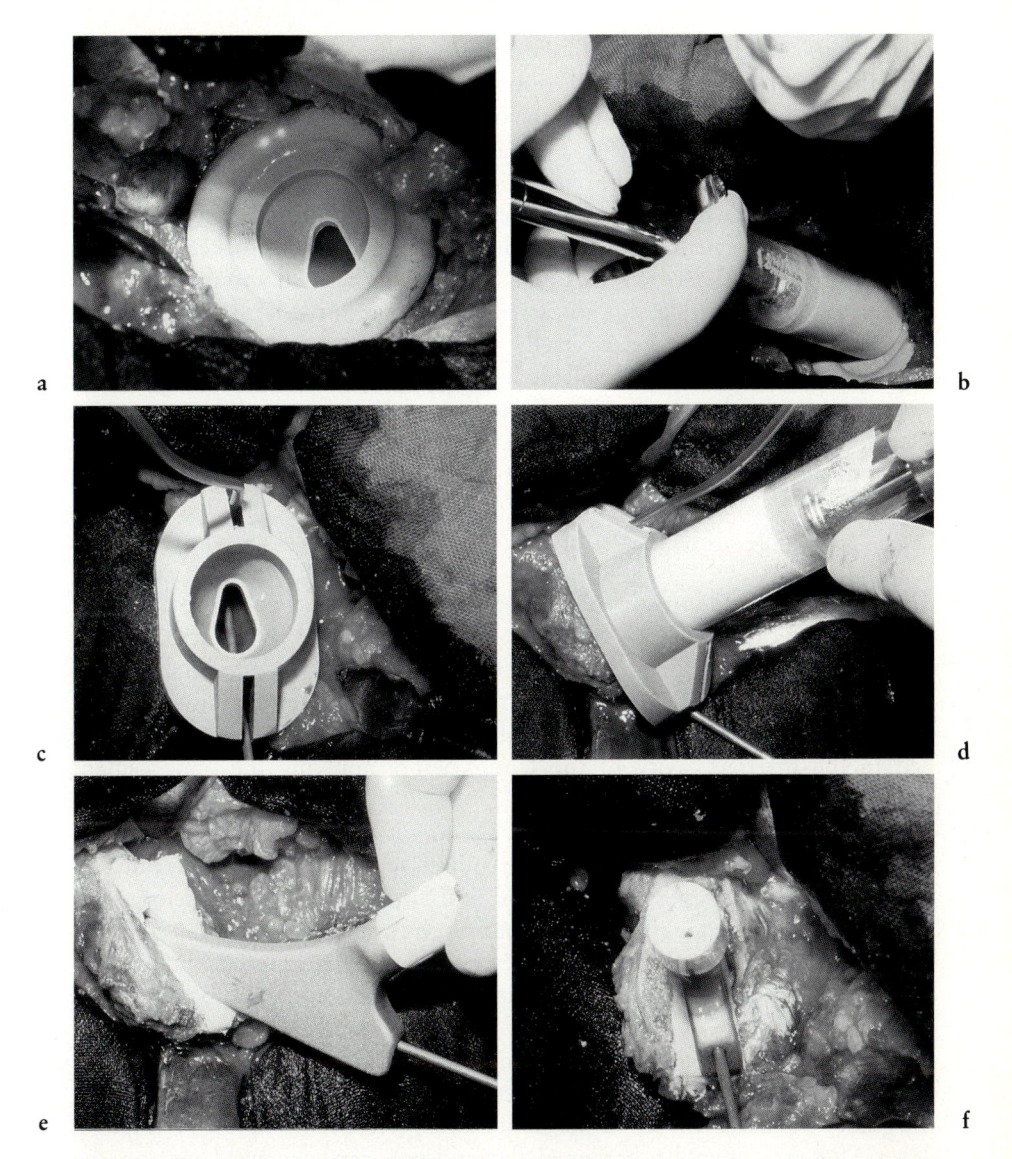

Fig. 3a, b Seal for the acetabulum. The cement-syringe mounted on the seal. The cement is pressurized in the acetabular bone and a clean and dry cement layer can be preformed. **c,d** Seal for the femur. The cement, applicated with a syringe which is mounted on the seal, can be pressurized into the bone. **e,f** Insertion of the CF-30 stem into the bone cement. Distally the guidewire directs the tip of the stem into a perfect central position. Proximally correct orientation can be monitored by vision. After the cement has hardened, the guide-wire can be screwed out from the cement stopper

this purpose we developed an applicator especially for the acetabulum which seals the rim of the acetabulum, pressurizes the cement and directs its spreading within the acetabular bed and into the bone. It also keeps the blood away from the outer surface of the cement (Fig. 3a, b).

The slightly protruding edge of the socket contributes to cement compression and centering of the implant; if it fits snuggly into the acetabular rim it also cuts off excess bone cement (Fig. 2a, b). The entry plane of the socket is slightly inwardly inclined. This facilitates repositioning of the head and in the case of subluxation, for example, due to extreme movements, the head may fall back into the cavity of the socket by itself.

Both types of sockets are available in six different sizes, graduated in 4-mm steps. This means that they can be adapted practically to most of the anatomical situations. For the preparation of the acetabular bed it is advisable to use reamers in 2-mm steps.

Stem

The stem of this endoprosthesis is made of the forged-steel alloy Protasul-S-30 and therefore called the CF-30 stem. It is straight and has a rectangular cross-section and a tapered shape. In the center the stem has a longitudinal channel that takes up a guidewire which directs the stem during insertion into the center of the cement. The guidewire is attached to the cement stopper which is positioned in the marrow cavity of the femur before applying the bone cement (Fig. 1c,d).

As a prerequisite for a complete cement cuff with sufficient wall thickness on all sides, such as in the acetabulum, the required space in the femur is created by a reamer somewhat larger than the stem. To fill this space even in differing sizes of marrow cavities enough bone cement must be available. At least 60 g should be used in every procedure. While the cement is being injected, the marrow cavity is closed proximally by a seal in order to pressurize the bone cement dough (Fig. 3c,d).

While inserting the stem into the cement-filled marrow cavity of the femur, its correct orientation must be monitored proximally by vision (Fig. 3e); distally the guidewire directs the tip of the stem into a perfect central position (Fig. 1d, 2c–e). After the cement has hardened, the guidewire can be screwed out from the cement stopper and removed (Fig. 3f).

The conical shape of the prosthetic stem pressurizes the bone cement dough and causes it to protrude into the bone. The result is a better fixation of the cement in the bone. To achieve an intimate bond between metal and cement the surface of the stem is coarse blasted. The rectangular cross-section of the stem protects the femoral prosthesis and the cement against rotational forces. The stem's rounded edges prevent unfavorable stress raising in the cement.

Five sizes of CF-30 stems are availble, depending on the different sizes of the femora and their marrow cavities.

Preliminary Results

From August 1988 to January 1992 we implanted 186 total hip endoprostheses of this new design in 180 patients. Of these, 168 (90 %) have been in function for more than 3 months and could be followed-up. The observation period ranged between 3 months and 4 years, with an average of 21 months. Because we are currently implanting cemented hip endoprostheses only in patients over 70 years old, the average age of the patients was 75.5 years (ranging between 61 and 90). The indications for the joint replacement were osteoarthritis (165 hips), rheumatoid arthritis (11 hips), femoral neck fracture (7 hips), and aseptic necrosis of the femoral head (3 hips).

We have recorded 22 complications (11.8 %), 3 classified as intraoperative and 19 as perioperative. There were: one trochanter tear off, one femoral fracture, one transient femoral nerve lesion, three joint dislocations, six delayed wound healings. two deep infections, and eight deep vein thromboses with five pulmonary embolisms. The quality of the cement mantle and the position of the implants were assessed by means of immediate postoperative radiographs. The patients were followed up and examined clinically and radiologically 3, 6, and 12 months postoperatively and then in yearly intervals. The clinical outcome was assessed according to the rating scale of Merle D'Aubigne on the basis of the criteria pain, walking ability and range of motion and according to the Harris hip score. In addition, the patients were asked after their opinion regarding the effect of the operation. Clinical results revealed a marked improvement from preoperatively to postoperatively in all criteria. In the Merle D'Aubigne score the change was from 2.3 to 5.8 for pain, from 2.7 to 5.1 for walking ability, and from 3.5 to 5.0 for joint mobility. It is obvious that the most impressive improvement was in pain conditions. The Harris hip score showed an impressive increase, from 22.2 to 79.8 (Fig. 4).

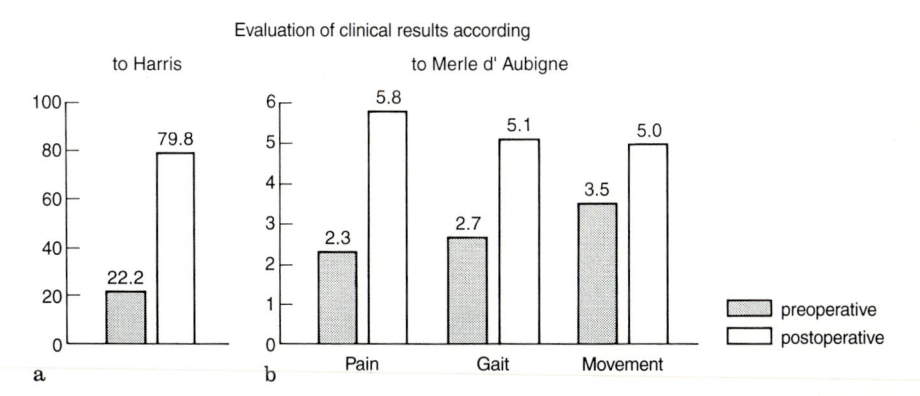

Fig. 4a, b. The evaluation of the clinical results according to the hip scores of a Harris and b Merle d'Aubigne reveals a marked improvement from preoperatively to postoperatively in all criteria

Subjectively, 52 % of the patients were very satisfied, 44 % satisfied, and 4 % not satisfied with the results of surgery. This means that 96 % of the patients stated that they were very satisfied or satisfied. The seven patients who were not satisfied experienced the complications mentioned above. In the radiological assessment of the results we devoted particular attention to the orientation of the implants and the state of the bone-cement cuff in the acetabulum as well as in the femoral shaft. The implant bed therefore was classified into four zones (Fig. 5).

Dimensions of the cement covering in the four sectors of the acetabulum

	< 2 mm	2 - 5 mm	> 5 mm
I	9.2 %	84.9 %	5.9 %
II	7.0 %	84.9 %	8.1 %
III	5.4 %	84.9 %	9.7 %
IV	-	76.9 %	23.1 %

Dimensions of the cement covering in the four sectors of the shaft

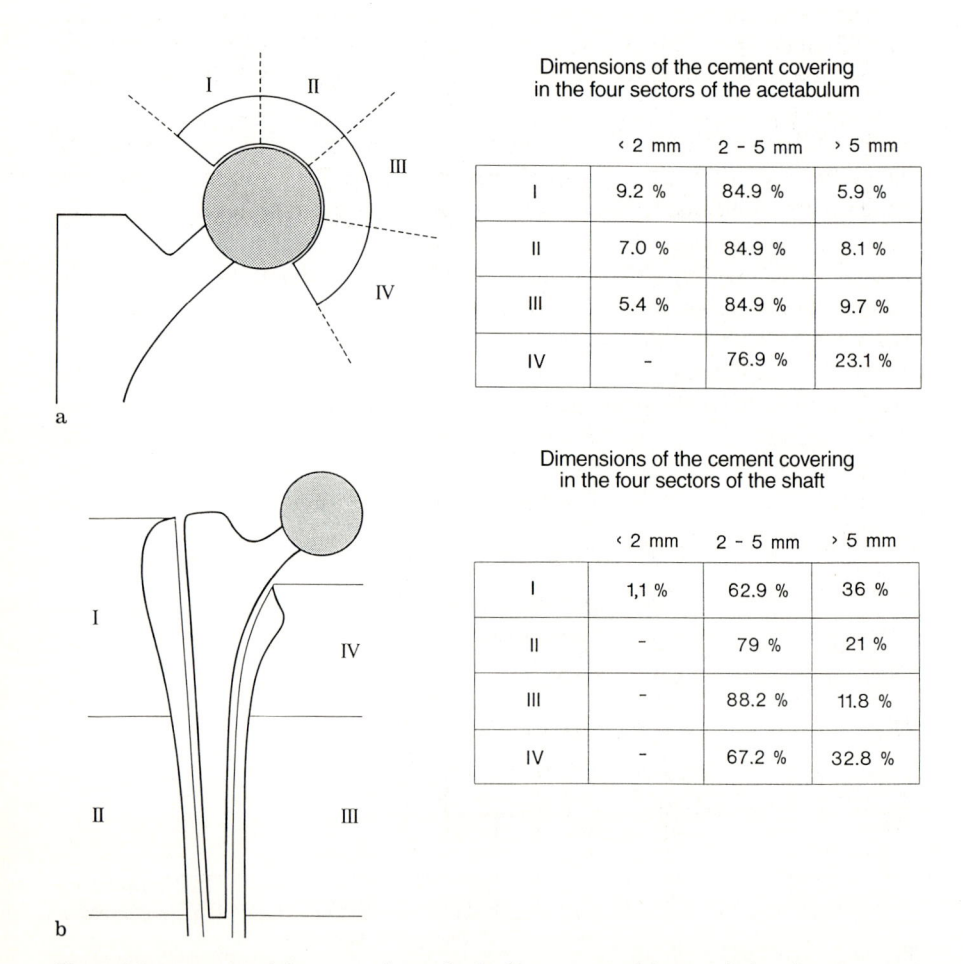

	< 2 mm	2 - 5 mm	> 5 mm
I	1,1 %	62.9 %	36 %
II	-	79 %	21 %
III	-	88.2 %	11.8 %
IV	-	67.2 %	32.8 %

Fig. 5a Measurement of the cement layers in the four sectors of the acetabulum in most cases shows a layer of between 2 and 5 mm thickness. Only in a few cases were the layers less than 2 mm. **b** The cement covering in the four sectors of the stem usually evenly measures between 2 and 5 mm

The Cement-Fixed (CF) Hip Replacement System

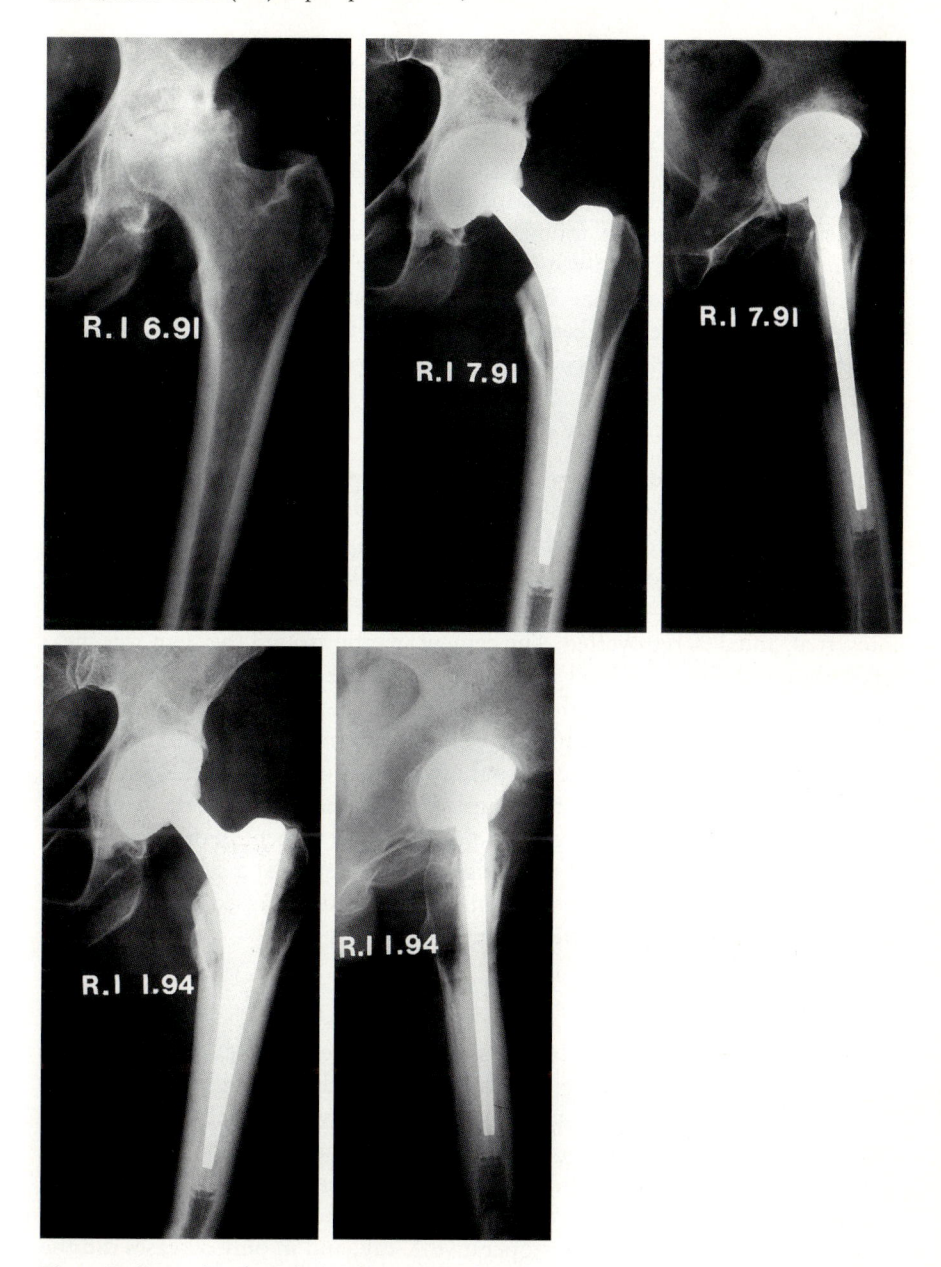

Fig. 6. Radiographs of a right hip joint in AP and lateral view, taken preoperatively, postoperatively and 2.6 years after implantation of a CF prosthesis in a 72-year-old man with osteoarthritis

Position and Cement Mantle of the Socket

The inclination of the cup ranged between 40° and 70° (mean of 48.2°); the anteversion ranged between 0° and 30° (mean 15°). There was a congruence between the acetabular rim and the entry level of the socket in 154 hips, while the socket was lateralized in 11 and medialized in 21 cases. Excess of cement at the acetabular rim was not found at all. The thickness of the cement layer surrounding the socket was always measured at the same spot in each of the four zones averaged 3.5 mm (range 0–20 mm). In around 83 % of the sockets the cement layer in all zones was between 2 and 5 mm thick; it was 2 mm or thinner in zone 1 only in 9.2 %, in zone 2 in 7 %, and in zone 3 in 5.4 % (fig. 5).

Position and Cement Mantle of the Stem

We found 80 % of the stems to be ideally centered proximally and distally in the AP view of the marrow cavity of the femur. Only two stems were distally not centered because of a dislocated cement stopper. A slight varus position was found in 11 % and moderate valgus position in 9 %, never exceeding 10°. From the lateral view 67 % of the stems were ideally centered, 30 % moderately anteverted, and 3 % retroverted. The cement mantle around the stem was measured always at the same level in each of the four zones: proximal-lateral (I), distal-lateral (II), distal-medial (III), and proximal-medial (IV). Overall, the mean thickness of the cement mantle was 4. 8 mm (range 0–15 mm). In 74.3 % of the cement cuffs around the stem the wall measured between 2 and 5 mm (Fig. 5). In only two cases was the mantle thinner than 2 mm in the proximal-lateral zone I, and in another case a complete lack of cement in this area was to be seen. In one case a primary debonding between stem and cement appeared proximal-lateral right after the implantation, obviously caused by moving the stem intraoperatively before the cement hardened.

Radiological Follow-Up

The radiological follow-up of 168 hips was performed to reveal changes of the implant bed, the cement mantle, and the position of the implants (Figs. 6 and 7). At the site of the cup only a few changes were observed. Radiolucent lines, not exceeding 1 mm in thickness, were observed in 58 cases. The radiolucent lines occured 46 times in zone I, 12 times in zone II, 17 times in zone III, and 15 times in zone IV, but only 6 times in all four zones. In 19 cases the radiolucent lines were visible even on the first postoperative X-ray, and in only 39 cases did the lines thus develop during the phase of tissue repair [25, 26].

Fig. 7. Radiographic course of an 83-years-old woman with a bilateral implantation of a CF prosthesis after femoral neck fracture because of severe osteoporosis

The Cement-Fixed (CF) Hip Replacement System

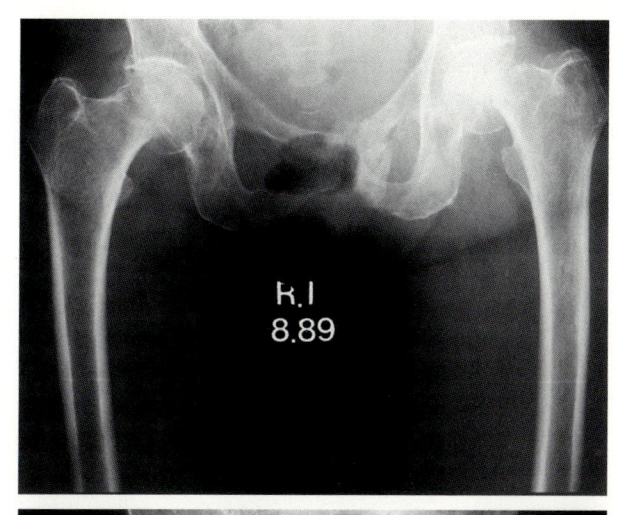

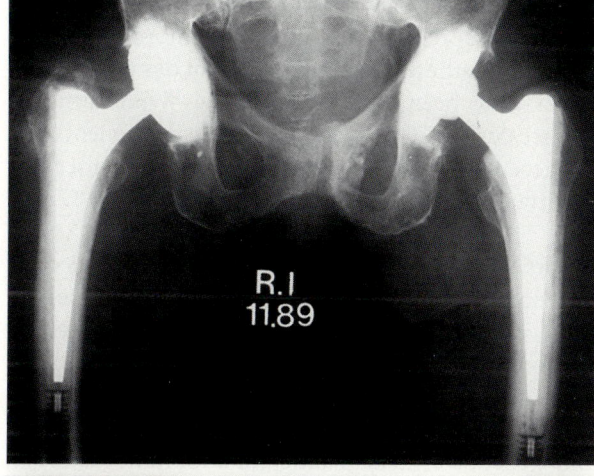

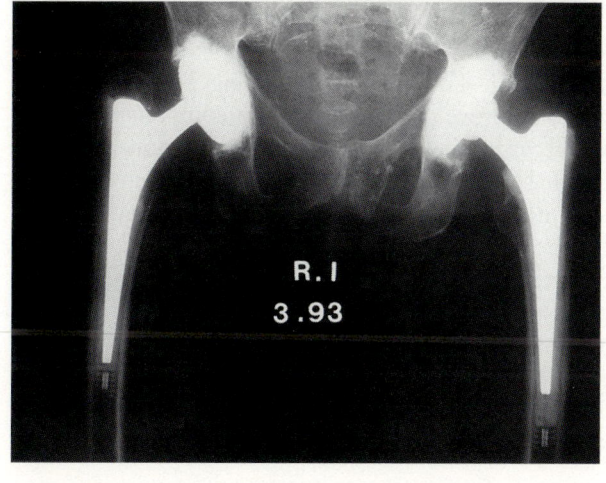

The changes around the stem indicated by the radiographs comprised the following phenomena: Radiolucent lines occurred in 18 cases, all were thinner than 2 mm. In addition two sclerotic lines were found. Six femoral stems showed pedestal formation around their tips and five stems subsidence of less than 5 mm; except of one, all of the pedestal formations were combined with subsidence. Two cement fractures occurred due to wrong cementing technique: one because of debonding between cement and implant, as mentioned above, and the other because of a greater cement defect due to insufficient pressurizing.

Heterotopic ossifications were quantified according to the Brooker index. In 86 % of hips there were no ossification or only small islands; 12 % were classified as Brooker II and 2 % as Brooker III. No ankylosis was seen.

Discussion

Since Charnley [5] introduced PMMA 34 years ago to anchor the components of artificial joints to the bone, many efforts have been made to improve the long term durability of cemented endoprostheses. Not only different designs but also varying cementing techniques have been utilized clinically. While different biomaterials, shapes, and surface designs of the endoprosthetic components still compete, it is now generally accepted that the quality of the cementing technique is one of the most important factors influencing durability [2, 8, 17, 20, 21].

Especially in elderly patients, where a revision is less likely to be expected, and primary stability is necessary for immediate weight bearing, a cemented endoprosthesis seems favorable. Nevertheless, the remaining risk of loosening because of cement deterioration and subsequent osteolysis should be minimized.

It is also widely accepted now that a central position of the implants within the bone cement and a homogeneous cement mantle are important factors in preventing early failures [4, 8, 12, 21]. Most often the area of osteolysis corresponds to either a focal defect in the cement mantle, a cement fracture, or an area of very thin cement [10, 15]. The aim in developing a new cemented endoprosthetic system was to improve positioning of the components within the cement mantle and to improve its quality. Radiological evaluation of the new CF hip replacement system has confirmed ideal centering of the components and good quality of the cement mantle on the acetabular and the femoral site in the majority of cases. The percentage of neutral positioning of the stem is comparatively high [21]. Very few femoral components have had significant cement defects, and the thickness of the cement mantle shows an equal thickness between 2 and 5 mm in most of the implants.

Radiological follow-up on the acetabular site shows very few changes. Radiolucent lines smaller than 1 mm were found, localized in most cases only in zone I. This phenomenon was often seen even on the first postoperative X-rays and was never combined with migration or clinical symptoms. Such signs of demarcation are quite common around cemented cups; their incidence varies between 21 % and 88 % [6, 9, 21]. Radiological analyses of revised sockets have shown that only these radiolucent lines are to be regarded as significant which were not apparent on the initial radiographs but appear newly and grow. Hodgkinson et al. [9] found only very few sockets intraoperatively loose if the radiolucent lines were localized in the outer third.

At the femoral site the number of radiolucent lines at the bone/cement interface are comparatively rare. They are well described with higher incidence for the femoral components (Gruen et al. [7]: Charnley stems 11.1 %; Salvati et al. [22]: Charnley stems 50 %), even when using modern cementing techniques (Rusotti et al. [21]: Harris II stem 15 %). Although it is not clear yet what these lines mean [6, 21], they must be observed closely during the further follow-up. The sclerotic lines were seen in the two cases between the bone and the radiolucent line. The few pedestal formations at the tip of some stems occured in combination with a subsidence of the stem, which never exceeded 5 mm. Pedestal formation and subsidence were not related to clinical symptoms and are known as signs without clinical relevance for the long-term result.

The heterotopic ossifications showed no remarkable difference in quantity and extension compared to other endoprostheses [21, 22, 23]. The rate of complications must be assessed considering the age profile. Especially for thromboembolic complications the average age of 75.5 years is relevant [18, 19]. Two cement fractures were seen – one due to moving the stem while the cement was not yet hard enough and the other developing in a defective cement mantle – but none of them caused clinical symptoms. Cement fractures are known from other prostheses [22] in which the incidence of local osteolyses seem to be higher in the affected areas [10]. Such cement defects could have been avoided by better cementing technique.

Although the follow-up period in this study is comparatively short, the results demonstrate that the desired effects could be achieved clinically and radiologically.

References

1. Anthony PP, Gie GA, Howie CR, Ling RSM (1990) Localized endosteal bone lysis in relation to the femoral component of cemented total hip arthroplasties. J Bone Joint [Br] 72: 971–979
2. Barrack RL, Mulroy RD, Jr, Harris WH (1992) Improved cement techniques and femoral component loosening in young patients with hip arthroplasty. A 12-year radiographic review. J Bone Joint Surg [Br] 74: 385–389
3. Beaumont PWR, Young RJ (1975) Slow crack in acrylic bone cement. J Biomed Mater Res 9: 423
4. Carlsson AS, Gentz CF, Lindern L (1983) Localized bone resorption in the femur in

mechanical failure of cemented total hip arthroplasties. Acta Orthop Scand 54: 396–402
5. Charnley J (1961) Arthroplasty of the hip. A new operation. Lancet 1: 1129
6. DeLee JG, Charnley J (1976) Radiological demarcation of cemented sockets in total hip replacement. Clin Orthop 121: 20–32
7. Gruen TA, McNeice GM, Amstutz HC (1979) Modes of failure of cemented stem-type femoral components: A radiographic analysis of loosening. Clin Orthop 141: 17–26
8. Harris WH, Davies JP (1988) Modern use of modern cement for total hip replacement. Orthop Clin North Am 19: 581–589
9. Hodgkinson JP, Shelly P, Wroblewski BM (1988) The correlation between roentgenographic appearance and operative findings at the bone-cement junction of the socket in Charnley low-friction arthroplasties. Clin Orthop 228: 105–109
10. Huddlestone HD (1988) Femoral lysis after cemented hip arthroplasty. J Arthroplasty 3: 285–297
11. Kusy RP, Turner DT (1974) Intergranular cracking of a weak two-phase polymethyl methacrylate. J Biomed Mater Res 8: 185
12. Lee ALC (1991) Can cementing technique affect long-term results of total hip replacement. Orthop Rel Sci 2: 208–214
13. Lewis JL (1988) The mechanical state of the bone-implant interface. In: Fitzgerald R (ed) Non-cemented total hip arthroplasty. Raven, New York, pp 23–30
14. Maloney WJ, Jasty M, Burke DW, O'Connor DO, Zalenski EB, Bragdon C, Harris WH (1989) Biomechanical and histologic investigation of cemented total hip arthroplasties. A study of autopsy-retrieved femura after in vivo cycling. Clin Orthop 249: 129–140
15. Maloney WJ, Jasty M, Rosenberg A, Harris WH (1990) Bone lysis in well fixed cemented femoral components. J Bone Joint Surg [Br] Vol 72: 966–970
16. Miller ML (1966) The structure of polymers, New York. Quoted in Homsy CA (1973) Some mechanical aspects of methylmethacrylate prosthesis seating compound. In: The Hip. The Hip Society, Saint Louis 1973.
17. Müller KH (1981) Lokale Komplikationen nach totalem Hüftgelenkersatz. Unfallheilkunde 84: 444
18. Müller KH (1984) Ergebnisse und Perspektiven des künstlichen Hüftgelenkersatzes in der Traumatologie. Unfallheilkunde 87: 89
19. Mulroy RD, Jr, Harris WH (1990) The effect of improved cementing techniques on component loosening in total hip replacement. An 11-year radiographic review. J Bone Joint Surg [Br] 72: 757–760
20. Roberts DW, Poss R, Kelly K (1986) Radiographic comparison of cementing techniques in total hip arthroplasty. J Arthroplasty 1: 241–247
21. Rusotti GM, Coventry MB, Stauffer RB (1988) Cemented total hip arthroplasty with contemporary techniques. A five-year minimum follow-up study. Clin Orthop 235: 141–147
22. Salvati EA, Wilson PD, Jr, Jolley MN, Vakili F, Aglietti P, Brown GC (1981) A ten year follow-up of our first one hundred consecutive Charnley total hip replacements. J Bone Joint Surg [Am] 63: 753–766
23. Sutherland CJ, Wilde AH, Borden LS, Marks KE (1982) A ten year follow-up of one hundred consecutive Muller curved-stem total hip replacement arthroplasties. J Bone Joint Surg [Am] 64: 970–982
24. Willert HG (1987) Die Zerrüttung des Zementköchers. In: Willert HG, Buchhorn G (Hrsg) Knochenzement. Werkstoff, klinische Erfahrungen, Weiterentwicklungen, vol 31, Huber, Bern, Aktuelle Prob Chir u. Orthop pp. 326–333
25. Willert HG, Puls P (1972) Die Reaktion des Knochens auf Knochenzement bei der Allo-Arthroplastik der Hüfte. Arch Orthop Unfallchir 72: 33–71
26. Willert HG, Ludwig J, Semlitsch M (1974) Reactions of bone to methacrylate after hip

arthroplasty: a long-term gross, light microscopic, and scanning electron microscopic study. J Bone Joint Surg [Am] 56: 1368–1382
27. Willert HG, Buchhorn G, Hess T (1989) Die Bedeutung von Abrieb und Materialermüdung bei der Prothesenlockerung an der Hüfte. Orthopäde 18: 350–369
28. Willert HG, Bertram H, Buchhorn G (1990) Osteolysis in alloarthroplasty of the hip – The role of bone cement fragmentation. Clin Orthop Relat Res 258: 108–121

Part V

Noncemented Femoral Stem

The Cementless Femoral Stem

E. Morscher

Introduction

Charnley's introduction of bone cement to hip arthroplasty in 1960 [12] made it possible for the procedure to be carried out worldwide to the extent it is today. With increasing numbers of procedures and increasing implantation time, however, the numbers of failures have also increased. The principal cause of failure is aseptic loosening of the implant [40]. Somewhat too prematurely, bone cement was considered responsible, causing a trend for direct (or biological) cementless implantation to develop worldwide. At the same time attempts were being made to improve the cement and, in particular, the cementing technique.

There are great differences between the acetabulum and the femoral stem with regard to the incidence and time of failure, and the consequent need for revision of cemented implants. While the rate of loosening of the femoral stem is linear, loosening of the acetabulum is rare during the first 6–8 years, but then increases exponentially [10, 31, 34].

While advances in cementing technique, especially the introduction of pressurization, have led to a significant improvement in fixation of the prosthetic stem [3], the incidence of acetabular loosening has decreased only slightly [33, 34]. As a result, many orthopedic surgeons have chosen to use a cementless acetabulum combined with a cemented femoral stem prosthesis, a so-called hybrid system, especially for patients over 55–60 years of age. Cementless fixation of the stem, on the other hand, is desirable for younger patients and revisions.

Goal of Cementless Fixation: Osseointegration

The goal of every cementless implantation of an endoprosthesis is its osseointegration. We take this to mean direct contact between bone and implant, i. e., fixation of the implant in bone without interposition of connective tissue [1]. This definition has been expanded and completed by Schenk, in that the bone tissues not only have contact with the implant without interposed connective tissue but should also be structured functionally to meet the direction and magnitude of the transmitted forces [39] (see contribution, this volume).

Primary stability is the most important requirement for lasting fixation of an implant. Dispensing with bone cement requires special measures to ensure primary stability. This is the main problem with cementless fixation.

The differences in prostheses which are fixed with or without bone cement are in (a) design of the implant, (b) characteristics of the implant surface, (c) material properties of the implant, and (d) operating technique.

Design of Implant

The way in which force is transmitted from bone to implant and vice versa is determined largely by the design of the implant. The most reliable fixation and stability between bone and implant would be achieved if it were possible to transmit all the forces between the two in the form of pressure. Not least because of the function of movement which an endoprosthesis must fulfill, it is impossible to have the forces constantly striking at a right angle to the implant surface. The relative movements between bone and implant due to shearing forces have to be eliminated as far as possible by an increase in friction and/or by production of a pressure preload between the two. The pressure to compensate the harmful shearing forces is called precompression, or press-fit. Various techniques such as screw fixation or wedging have been adopted to achieve this kind of precompression in cementless endoprostheses. The precompression should be maintained for at least the period required for primary fixation by ingrowth of bone onto or into the implant surface, i. e., for about 6 weeks.

The problems in cementless fixation of the femoral stem derive particularly from (a) the achievement of primary stability of the implant adequate for osseointegration, (b) pain in the thigh, (c) so-called stress shielding, which leads to absorbent bone remodelling in the proximal femur, (d) femoral fractures occurring intraoperatively during the generation of press-fit (which is important for osseointegration) or later near the tip of the femoral stem, and (e) osteolysis.

Since spongy bone is not suitable for transmission of force and the femoral stem endoprosthesis must be supported by cortical bone, it is hardly possible to provide all the anatomical variations of the femur with a single model [35]. It is therefore obvious that the use of different designs, modular systems, or custom-made endoprostheses must be considered.

One way of adapting the implant to the inner shape of the proximal femur consists in pressing metal or plastic wedges between the prosthesis and the cortical bone, thus generating the required pressure (press-fit gliding stem, Pegasus prosthesis, etc.).

Whether custom-made femoral stems will have a firm place in the armamentarium of hip prostheses in future remains to be seen and would seem doubtful not only because of the cost but also because of experimental and clinical experience hitherto. Gebauer et al., for example, found no advantages in their measurements of primary stability in five individual prostheses constructed with computer assistance compared to measurements involving conventional cementless prosthetic stems [19,20]. Thomas et al. found an increased incidence of proximal femoral atrophy in 100 patients having a total of 114 arthroplasties using a computer-assisted design endoprosthesis, which, however, was cemented [44]. Bone damage due to stress shielding of the proximal femur is a problem associated with all computer-assisted design femoral stems.

A problem with cementless stem fixation which is being studied particularly intensively at present is loss of bone in the proximal femur, which is explained as a consequence of the stress shielding or decreased stress on the bone tissue as a result of the implantation of the femoral stem. In etiology and pathogenesis the rigidity of the implant and its adherence to bone are the decisive factors (see below).

As a result of clinical and experimental investigations, there is hardly any doubt that the thigh pain which affects many of the patients treated with a cementless stem is connected to the type or quality of fixation of the prosthetic stem in the femur. According to Noble et al., 53 % of patients with a loose prosthetic stem had pain 1 year postoperatively, while this occurred in only 3 % of patients with a firmly anchored prosthesis [35]. On the other hand, however, firm bony integration of the femoral stem does not always guarantee freedom from pain [2]. Every division or resection of bone, which is necessary when an endoprosthesis is being inserted, disturbs the equilibrium of physiological biomechanics, which must be restored, among other things, by remodeling of the bone after insertion of the implant parts. For this reason the iatrogenic bone defect should be kept as small as possible. In the case of the femoral stem this means that as much of the femoral neck as possible should be preserved. The lower the resection through the femoral neck, the longer is the lever arm of forces attempting to lever the prosthesis from its intramedullary anchoring during varus-valgus movement and especially during rotation. Freeman rightly posed the question: "why resect the neck?" [15]. The forces acting in the direction of the femoral axis should also be transmitted as pressure by the endoprosthesis in the direction of the Adam's curve. We thus arrive at the requirement that the forces in cementless prosthetic systems should be transmitted as proximally as possible.

Transfer of forces in the proximal region is guaranteed only if the prosthetic stem is not inserted and fixed to bone distally. Distal stem fixation leads to relative movements and to stress protection in the proximal region. The latter leads to bone atrophy, which eventually encourages loosening of the stem.

Proximal force transmission (as occurs in the normal femur) should be achieved when cementless fixation of endoprostheses is carried out. This can be achieved by different types of proximal fixation such as use of a collar, structuring of the surface, press-fit etc. and also by deliberate prevention of distal stem fixation. The distal stem region should therefore have no surface structuring that could allow an ingrowth of bone tissue. This principle of deliberate prevention of distal fixation of the prosthetic stem is employed in the PCA, Harris-Galante and many other prosthetic systems.

Prevention of distal stem fixation and therefore of distal force transfer can be achieved by a prosthetic stem which can glide in a sleeve linked to the bony femoral shaft. This principle, which also shifts harmful shearing forces between the implant and bone into the interior of the prosthetic system, has been realized in the femoral stem which we have brought to the trial stage as a gliding prosthetic stem [25, 26].

Surface

With cementless fixation of an endoprosthesis, the composition, i. e., the structure of the implant surface and its material properties, is of crucial importance. We distinguish between structuring or macroporosity and microporosity. Moore can be considered to have carried out the first structuring with the perforation of his cephalic prosthesis, with which he was hoping to achieve greater bony stability for his implant [24]. By means of a microporous surface design the contact surface and thus the friction at the interface can be increased tenfold. The principle of microporosity derives from the experimental work of Galante et al. in Chicago who demonstrated the possibility of bony ingrowth with the fiber metal which they had developed [17, 18]. We know from the experimental investigations of Galante et al. [17], Pilliar and Bratina [37], Pilliar et al. [38], Bobyn and Engh [7], Engh et al. [9], Cameron [11], Ducheyne and Cuckler [13], Ducheyne et al. [14], and others that a surface structure must meet certain geometric requirements for bone to grow into it. Such a surface must have a pore size of at least 100 µm and a porosity volume of 30–70 %. We find porous surfaces in the form of small spheres sintered to the implant surface (PCA), such as the fiber metal mentioned above, as a plasma spray, or as a mesh coating.

Based on these findings, Sulzer Brothers in Winterthur, Switzerland, developed the Sulmesh mesh coating of pure titanium. This mesh consists of 4 metal meshes of precisely defined pore size and known pore volume sintered together and bound firmly together with polyethylene. Animal experiments in mountain sheep and histomorphological studies in cadavers have demonstrated the exceptionally good capacity for osseointegration of this implant coating [4, 28, 29, 39].

Material Properties of the Implant

The material properties of an implant are important for (a) biocompatibility with bone, (b) the gliding properties of the joint surfaces (tribology), and (c) for the mechanical properties, i. e., elasticity of the implant.

Biocompatibility of the Implant Surface

There has been great progress in the past two decades in the area of biomaterials. These are no longer regarded only as a substitute for living tissue which should have as benign a reaction as possible to it; an interactive function is now also expected of them. Beginning with simply biotolerant materials, the way led past bioinert substances such as titanium to bioactive hydroxyapatite (HA) which can form a true, i. e., chemical bond with bone tissue [21, 27].

Structuring the implant surface can increase it tenfold, which naturally increases the importance of biocompatibility. It is well known that metal surfaces corrode. Oxidation causes ions to go into solution and be excreted, cobalt and chromium especially in the urine [9, 23]. The larger the surface, the greater is the loss of ions. Chromium is a well-known allergen, and it has been possible to induce sarcomas in experimental animals with both chromium and cobalt [22]. However, the excretion of cobalt decreases with time, probably as a result of surface passivation. It is also reassuring to know that no proven malignant degeneration has been ascribed to implantation of a prosthesis. Malignant tumors have been described several times in the area of an implant as single case reports. In view of the great rarity of these observations and the frequency of foreign body implantation, this might very well be coincidental [36, 43]. The vanadium present in titanium alloys (Ti-6Al-4V) is highly toxic. In animal experiments it leads to a transient rise in lung tissue but does not obviously accumulate in any of the organs examined [45].

Hydroxyapatite. The most biocompatible material currently available in endoprosthetics is HA. It enables bilateral bone formation, i. e., bone is formed both by the host bed and by the implant surface, hastening osseointegration. In addition, larger gaps are bridged over by bone thanks to hydroxyapatite [5, 6, 16, 21, 41]. HA is thus not only highly bioinert but also has osteoconductive properties which directly stimulate osseointegration. There are also grounds for believing that a chemical bond exists between bone and HA, by which forces can be transmitted not only in the form of pressure but also as shearing and tensile forces. Although it has been demonstrated that the HA-bone bond is stronger than that between bone and titanium, the bond between HA and the implant is not beyond all doubt. Since HA is an extremely fragile material with a very high E modulus, there is a danger that it will separate when the implant deforms. In the course of time disintegration occurs, and the individual granules can be removed by macrophages. If any such extremely hard granules penetrate the joint (as is known to happen with bone cement), a very great degree of polyethylene wear can be expected [27]. This has already been reported [5, 6]. The clinical success of HA-coated implants depends on a series of factors, such as the thickness of the HA layer, the chemical purity of the HA, the quality of the bond between HA and implant, and the porosity of HA.

Rigidity of Implant Materials

The number of currently used implant materials is relatively large, although metallic materials have been used most frequently from the start. However, rigid implants, especially cementless femoral stems, run the risk of causing stress shielding with bone atrophy, which can compromise the fixation of the implant.

The observation in fracture management that rigid (metal) osteosynthetic plates can lead to atrophy of the osteosynthesized bone, led to the development in the early 1970s of so-called isoelastic prostheses [29, 30]. Such prosthetic stems should have the same deformability (isoelasticity) as the surrounding bone. Unfortunately, isoelasticity can never be achieved even from theoretical considerations, since bone tissue has anisotropic properties while artificial materials (especially the polyacetal resin used here) is isotropic. In addition, the bone constantly undergoes remodeling while plastic materials do not alter in their physical properties. There are also considerable differences between one bone and another. Corresponding adaptation of different prostheses to the individual variations is also not possible. In addition, not only the modulus of elasticity of its component material is decisive in the deformability, i. e., the elasticity of an implant. Its size is far more important, in fact to the fourth power. True isoelasticity is thus never achievable in practice because when a prosthetic stem is inserted into the femur, the rigidity of the implant is added to that of the femur. The degree of relative movement increases as a factor hindering osseointegration of the implant.

Stress shielding, on the one hand and relative movements between implant and bone, on the other, are influenced positively or negatively by the elasticity

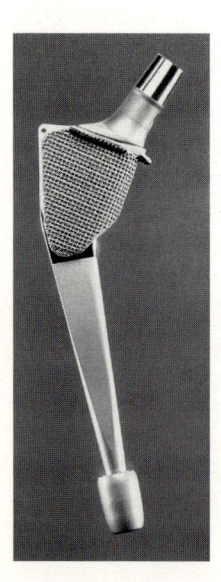

Fig. 1. Press-Fit Gliding Stem

or rigidity of the implant. The ideal elasticity of an implant does not exist, and the choice of material, i.e., titanium with relatively low E modulus or a cobalt-chromium alloy with an approximately doubled E modulus, as well as the size of the prosthesis, is always a compromise. The dilemma between preserving the original elasticity and thus the original bone substance and the avoidance of relative movements between bone and implant as a requirement for osseointegration can be solved neither by currently employed methods of stem fixation nor with an adaptation of the elasticity of the implant, whether this is achieved by the choice of a material of low E modulus or by adapting the implant's dimensions.

This realization led us to develop a fundamentally new modular cementless femoral stem prosthesis, the so-called press-fit gliding stem (Fig. 1), which is still being developed, but for which there are already 7 years of positive clinical observation.

Press-Fit Gliding Stem. One of the most fundamental features of this system lies in the fact that the leaflike prosthesis stem made of titanium is movably mounted in two sleeves. The sleeves themselves, in particular the proximal one through which forces are transmitted, are covered by the titanium mesh Sulmesh, already encountered in connection with the Press-Fit Cup and firmly bonded osseously with the cortex layer of the proximal femur end by the same. The prosthesis-bone bond is thus secured by bone ingrowth. By applying this gliding-bearing principle the micromovements occurring with every transmission of force can basically be transferred from the bone-implant interface into the interior of the prosthesis system thus to a "harmless" location.

Division of the sheath providing the bone-implant link into proximal and distal sleeves allows the transmission of force be controlled. On the one hand, forces are transmitted proximally from the pelvis to the femur in the natural hip joint, and proximal transmission of force is thus physiological; on the other hand, the distal transmission of force leads to proximal bone atrophy (stress shielding) with a possible subsequent loosening of the stem. Thus a cementless fixed stem prosthesis should basically be designed in such a manner that it guarantees proximal transmission of force. In view of the fact that the distal sheath virtually prevents a distal fixation of the prosthesis stem, the forces *must* be transmitted proximally.

The firm bone-implant bond in the proximal femur area, i.e., press-fit, is brought about by the fact that wedges of various thicknesses are inserted between the prosthesis stem and the laterally open U-shaped sleeve, which press the surface of the sleeve with the Sulmesh against the bone. The preload necessary to neutralize the harmful shearing forces is thus additionally created. The press-fit between the proximal sleeve and bone is further increased by the fact that the latter is shaped conically towards distal whereas the stem itself is designed plan-parallel. Since the forces have been introduced proximally, and the distal centering bush is relatively short, any stress shielding in the diaphysis area is rendered impossible (Fig. 2).

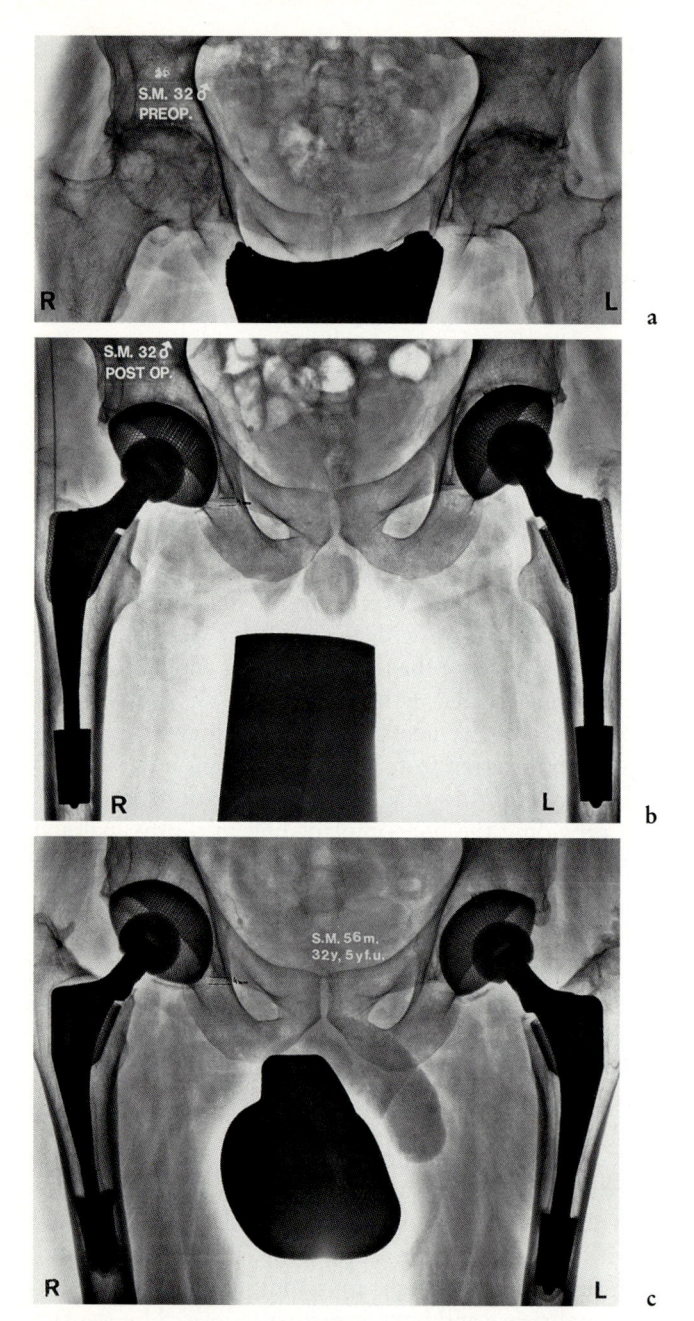

Fig. 2a. A 32-year-old man with rheumatoid arthritis of both hips. **b** One-stage hip arthroplasty simultaneously on both sides with press-fit cup and press-fit gliding stem. **c** Five-year result: pain-free, excellent movement and unlimited walking ability. Note: no stress shielding

The interior lining of the two sleeves is made of polyethylene, which not only allows shifts in position between the same and the prosthesis stem but also guarantees an elastic support of the prosthesis stem (shock absorption).

Admittedly, the deformation of the prosthesis stem under load causes more of a "rolling off" of the same on the medial plastic insert than an axial gliding, which for its part reduces the risk of shearing forces occurring between the proximal sleeve and bone. The transverse forces resulting from the rolling off as a consequence of the bending moments occurring are absorbed by the femur cortex layer through the distal shell.

Finite element studies have shown that the forces from the pelvis introduced through the prosthesis head and neck are passed on medially to the calcar femorale. This proximal transmission of force is possible of course only because the neck of the femur is resected high up, and the calcar femorale is retained.

Operating Technique

Uniform results can be achieved with cementless prostheses only if the system design and the instruments are so refined as to enable not only the developer but also the surgeon with average experience to use the prostheses with the precision necessary. In this respect, one can only confirm what Lunceford once observed: "A poorly performed cemented joint replacement often will function to the patient's satisfaction for a short time. A poorly performed non-cemented joint replacement will not have this grace!"

References

1. Albrektsson T, Brånemark PI, Hansson HA, Lindström J (1981) Osseointegrated titanium implants. Acta Orthop Scand 52: 155–170
2. Barrack RL, Jasty M, Bragdon C, Haire T, Horns WH (1992) Thigh pain despite bone ingrowth into uncemented femoral stems.
J Bone Joint Surg [Br] 507–510, 1994
3. Barrack RL, Mulroy RD, Jr, Harris WH (1992) Improved cementing techniques and femoral component loosening in young patients with hip arthroplasty. A 12-year radiographic review. J Bone Joint Surg [Br] 74: 385–389
4. Bereiter H, Bürgi M, Rahn BA (1992) Das zeitliche Verhalten der Verankerung einer zementfrei implantierten Hüftpfanne im Tierversuch. Orthopäde 21:63–70
5. Bloebaum RD, Dupont JA (1993) Osteolysis from a press-fit hydroxyapatite-coated-implant. J Arthroplasty 8:195–202
6. Bloebaum RD, Bachus KN, Rubman MH, Dorr LD (1993) Postmortem comparative analysis of titanium and hydroxyapatite porous-coated femoral implants retrieved from the same patient. J Arthroplasty 8:203–211
7. Bobyn JD, Engh CA (1984) Human histology of the bone-porous metal implant interface. Orthopaedics 7:1410–1421

8. Bobyn JD, Pilliar RM, Cameron HU, Weatherly GC (1980) The optimum pore size for the fixation of porous surface metal implants by the ingrowth of bone. Clin Orthop 150:263-268
9. Braun E, Schmitt D, Nabet F, Legras B, Coudane H, Molé D (1986) Concentration urinaire du cobalt et du chrome chez les patients porteurs d'une prothèse totale de hanche non cimentée. Int Orthop 10:277-282
10. Buchholz HW, Heinert K, Wargenau M (1985) Verlaufsbeobachtung von Hüftendoprothesen nach Abschluß realer Belastungsbedingungen von 10 Jahren. Z Orthop 123:815-820
11. Cameron HU (1982) The results of early clinical trials with a microporous coated metal hip prosthesis. Clin Orthop 165:188-190
12. Charnley J (1960) Anchorage of the femoral head prosthesis to the shaft of the femur. J Bone Joint Surg [Br] 42:28
13. Ducheyne P, Cuckler JM (1992) Bioactive ceramic prosthetic coatings. Clin Orthop 276:102
14. Ducheyne P, Martens M, De Meester P, Mulier JC (1984) Titanium and titanium alloy prostheses with porous fiber metal coatings. In: Morscher E (ed) The cementless fixation of hip endoprostheses. Springer, Berlin Heidelberg New York, pp 109-117
15. Freeman MAR: (1986). Why resect the neck? J Bone Joint Surg [Br] 68:346-349;
16. Furlong RJ, Osborn JF (1991) Fixation of hip prostheses by hydroxyapatite ceramic coatings. J Bone Joint Surg [Br] 73:741
17. Galante J, Rostoker W, Lueck R, Ray RD (1971) Sintered fiber metal composite as a basis for attachment of implants to bone. J Bone Joint Surg [Am] 53:101-114
18. Galante J, Summer DR, Gächter A (1987) Oberflächenstrukturen und Einwachsen von Knochen bei zementfrei fixierten Prothesen. Orthopäde 16:197-205
19. Gebauer D, Refior HJ, Haake M (1989) Micromotions in the primary fixation of cementless femoral stem prostheses. Arch Orthop Trauma Surg 108:300-307
20. Gebauer D, Refior HJ, Haake M (1990) Experimentelle Untersuchungen zur Primärstabilität von computergestützt-konstruierten (CAD) Individual-Hüftendoprothesen. Med Orthop Tech 3:138-144
21. Geesink R, De Groot K Klein C (1987) Chemical implant fixation using hydroxyl-apatite coatings. Clin Orthop 225:147-170
22. Heath JC, Freeman MAR, Swanson SAV (1971) Carcinogenic properties of wear particles from prostheses made in cobalt-chromium alloy. Lancet 1:564
23. Jorgenson TJ, Munro F, Mitchell TG, Hungerford D (1983) Urinary cobalt levels in patients with porous Austin-Moore prostheses. Clin Orthop 176:124-126
24. Moore AT (1952) Metal hip joint: new self-locking vitallium prosthesis. South Med J 45:1015-1019
25. Morscher E (1989) Endoprosthetic surgery in 1988. Ann Chir Gynaecol 78:242-253
26. Morscher E (1991) Experience with the press-fit cup and the press-fit gliding stem. In: Küsswetter W (ed). Noncemented total hip replacement, International Symposium, Tübingen 1990. Thieme, Stuttgart, pp 221-231
27. Morscher E (1991) Hydroxyapatite coating of prostheses. Editorial. J Bone Joint Surg [Br] 73:705
28. Morscher E (1992) Current status of acetabular fixation in primary total hip arthroplasty. Clin Orthop 274:172-193
29. Morscher E, Dick W (1983) Cementless fixation of „isoelastic" hip endoprostheses manufactured from plastic materials. Clin Orthop 176:77-87
30. Morscher E, Mathys R (1983) Erste Erfahrungen mit einer zementlosen isoelastischen Totalprothese der Hüfte. Z Orthop 113:745-749
31. Morscher E, Schmassmann A (1983) Failures of total hip arthroplasty and probable incidence of revision surgery in the future. Arch Orthop Trauma Surg 101:137-143

32. Morscher E, Bereiter H, Lampert C (1989) Cementless press-fit cup. Principles, experimental data and three year follow-up study. Clin Orthop 249:12-20
33. Mulroy RD, Harris WH: (1990). The effect of improved cementing technigues on component loosening in total hip replacement. J Bone Joint Surg [Br] 72:757-760
34. Nasser S, Campbell PA, Kiligus D, Kossovsky N, Amstutz HC: (1990). Cementless total joint arthroplasty prostheses with titanium-alloy articular surfaces. A human retrieval analysis. Clin Orthop 261:171-185
35. Noble PC, Alexander JW, Lindahl LJ, Yew DT, Granberry WM, Tullos HS (1988) The anatomic basis of femoral component design. Clin Orthop 235:148-165
36. Penmann H, Ring PA: (1984). Osteosarcoma in association with total hip replacement. J Bone Joint Surg [Br] 66:632-634
37. Pilliar RM, Bratina WJ (1980) Micromechanical bonding at a porous surface structured implant interface. The effect on implant stressing. J Biomed Eng 2:49-53
38. Pilliar RM, Cameron HU, Macnab I (1975) Porous surfaced layered prosthetic devices. J Biomed Eng 10:126-131
39. Schenk R, Morscher E (in press) Histomorphology of the implant/bone interface of the Press-fit-cup with the orderly orientated fiber mesh Sulmesh. 5th Biomaterial Symposium, Göttingen 1992
40. Stauffer RN (1982) Ten-year follow-up-study of total hip replacement. With particular reference to roentgenographic loosening of the components. J Bone Joint Surg [Am] 64:983-990
41. Stephenson PK, Freeman MAR, Revell PA, Germain J, Tuke M, Pirie CJ (1991) The effect of hydroxyapatite coating on ingrowth of bone into cavities in an implant. J Arthroplasty 6:51-58
42. Sutherland CJ, Wilde AH, Borden LS, Marks KE (1982) A ten-year follow-up of one hundred consecutive Müller-curved-stem total hip replacement arthroplasties. J Bone Joint Surg [Am] 64:970-982
43. Swann M (1984) Malignant soft-tissue tumour at the site of a total hip replacement. J Bone Joint Surg [Br] 66:629-631
44. Thomas BJ, Salvati EA, Small RD (1986) The CAD hip arthroplasty. Five- to ten-year follow-up. J Bone Joint Surg [Am] 68:640-646
45. Woodman JL, Jacobs JJ, Galante JO, Urban RM (1984) Metal ion release from titanium-based prosthetic segmental replacements of long bones in baboons: a long-term study. J Orthop Res 1:421-430

The Development of the Thrust Plate Prosthesis

A. H. Huggler, H. A. C. Jacob

The design of an artificial hip joint is not dictated primarily by purely mechanical requirements but rather by biological compatibility problems and surgical feasibility. Artificial hip joints are more or less always compromises [3]. The mechanical and biological requirements stand in close interactive relationship with the design and the materials used. To understand the behavior of an implant in the living bone it is necessary to investigate the reactions that occur due to the forces that act. One of the main problems in hip joint replacements is the unphysiological loading of bone. Wolff's law implies that the living bone, within certain physiological limits increases or decreases during turnover, thus adapting itself in form and architecture to the given loading situation [15]. A prosthesis should therefore transmit forces to the bone such that these lay within a physiological range. Kummer [7] compares living bone to a controller which regulates the bone turnover in such a way that the stress remains constant at a particular value.

By means of this postulated control mechanism, the bone alters its trabecular structure through apposition and resorption until this corresponds to the principle stresses (compressive and tensile stresses). An optimal orientation and dimensioning of these elements result so that a light construction issues [11].

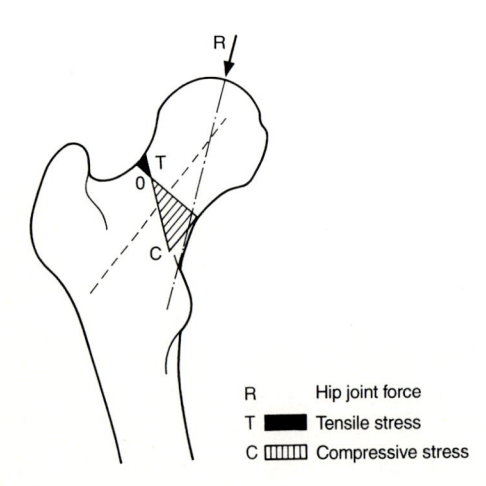

Fig. 1. Compressive and tensile stresses in the femoral neck

R — Hip joint force
T — Tensile stress
C — Compressive stress

Neither the physiological limits of stress to which bone might be exposed nor the exact mechanism by which this adaption takes place are known. As shown by Scholten et al. [12] in a finite element analysis, the dense cancellous bone of the femoral head is the main force-transmitting agent for the hip joint load, but further down, below the neck, especially in the diaphysis, it is the corticalis that takes over this function (Fig. 1).

The main problem of artificial implants is the mutilation of the bone during the implantation procedure, leaving the functionally adapted structure no longer in a position to readapt itself to the altered conditions. In spite of the practical clinical success now obtained with the majority of femoral prostheses of the intramedullarly anchored type, good long-term results of over 10 years are not the rule. Apart from the well-known problems associated with transversal forces (proximal-medial and distal-lateral), hoop stresses, change in the deformation behavior of the femur, etc., it must be pointed out that experimental stress analysis has shown that the proximal end of the femoral shaft with an intramedullarly anchored prosthesis stem suffers a stress reduction of as much as 60 % of the physiological level [5, 6]. The intramedullarly anchored stem therefore remains a biomechanically unsolved problem.

Experimental Investigations in the Development of the TPP

To maintain the physiological stress distribution with regard to both magnitude and direction the thrust plate prosthesis (TPP) was conceived by Huggler and Jacob in 1976. Since its first clinical application in 1978 several descriptions of this prosthesis have been published [2, 4].

The TPP differs in form from conventional prostheses. The principal element is the thrust plate which transmits the hip joint force directly to the medial cortical bone of the femoral neck stump, thereby largely maintaining the physiological stress distribution in the proximal femur. The thrust plate has a central hole which allows a mandrel to pass through and be seated upon this mandrel being fitted with a ball head. The mandrel, which is stiff in bending, is fixed to the bone by means of a single central bolt and a plate that is positioned on the lateral aspect of the femur, just under the innominate tubercle. The stiff mandrel and central bolt prevent the thrust plate from being lifted off the bone stump when under load. To accomodate different lengths of femoral necks, two 32 mm diameter heads with different neck lengths have been used. Presently heads of 28 mm diameter are available.

From 1976 to 1978 stress analysis on components, including material testing of the TPP, led to correct dimensioning. It was particularly important to determine the stress distribution within the bone just under the thrust plate. This was effected by means of a composite epoxy model furnished with strain gauges at its proximal end. The composite epoxy model was comprised of cancellous and cortical bone substitutes.

The model was loaded in one legged stance by means of beam that simulated the pelvis in which the abductors were replaced by cords attached to the great trochanter. Body weight was applied to the beam that simulated the pelvis. The TPP was also implanted in fresh human cadaver femora and loaded up to an equivalent of 150 kg body weight in one-legged stance. No movement at all was detected between the thrust plate and the bone. In a cyclic loading test the TPP was loaded between 30 and 780 kp for 5 million cycles.

Perren edt al. [9, 10] used a specially instrumented bone plate on intact, and on osteotomized sheep tibia to measure the compressive force acting within the bone. No steep drop in the compressive force was observed. Between the slow drop in compressive force and the haversian bone turnover that takes place over several weeks (months) a state of equilibrium is arrived at, in both intact and osteotomized bones. This slow drop in precompression is of relevance for the mechanical behavior of the TPP, especially just after implantation. The matter of torsional stability of the prosthesis within the host bone does not apply to the TPP.

Since the first implantation of a TPP in 1978 in Chur neither the concept nor the basic design of the TPP has changed. The TPP was initially built up of cobalt-chromium based alloys. While the central bolt is still made of a tough wrought CoCr alloy, the other main components are now made of titanium alloy. The initially circular thrust plate has been given an oval form already during the second generation. Experience with the second generation has shown that titanium is a suitable biocompatible material and therefore all parts that come to bear directly on bone (thrust plate, lateral plate for the central bolt) are made of titanium. The third, latest generation has a thrust plate integrated with the mandrel component and has a lateral plate for the central bolt, which fits snuggly under the greater trochanter (Fig. 2).

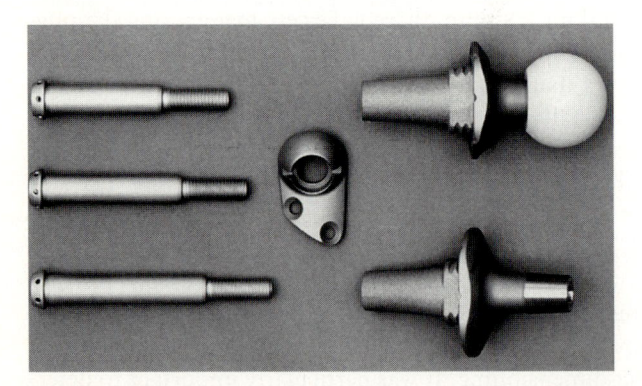

Fig. 2. The third generation with mandrel and thrust plate integrated into one piece

Indications

Generally speaking, if the life expectancy of the patient is such that a loosening of a conventional prosthesis might be expected, the TPP is considered indicated as the first implant. However, basic conditions such as size, form, structure and relationship of the main femoral access to each other must be also taken into consideration to ensure proper fit. If these basic requirements are fulfilled, practically all indications for a total hip prosthesis apply equally to the TPP. Contraindications are severe deviations of form (very short femoral neck or extreme varus, valgus or antetorsion of the neck) or pathological bone structure (osteopenia). Furthermore, acute trauma in the region of the femoral neck base is unsuitable.

If the indication for a successful intertrochanteric osteotomy in a young patient is questionable, implantation of a TPP should be considered. The TPP allows even young patients to continue their normal daily activities and theirs business occupations. There are no age limits; our oldest patient received a TPP at the age of 78 years. However, in the case of elderly patients when there is no reason to expect aseptic loosening of a conventional implant, there is no pressing reason to employ a TPP.

Surgical Technique

With a few special instruments and a proper preoperative planning (using radiographs), the surgical technique is quite simple. On exposure of the hip joint, a centering hole is drilled through the lateral cortex before the femoral neck is osteotomized. After the head is removed, a target plate is fixed to the resected end of the femoral neck and the drilling jig so attached that the hole is drilled right through the proximal femur, from the centering hole in the lateral cortex up to the target plate. This hole is now used as a guide for a milling device which planes the resected neck surface perfectly flat. Before fixing the thrust plate with the mandrel to the femoral neck it is advisable to first implant a cementless acetabular socket. After the mandrel with the thrust plate has been fitted to the neck or the femur, a central bolt that passes through a plate which lies on the lateral aspect of the femur is past through the guide hole to engage with the mandrel, thus holding the thrust plate firmly onto the bone. The lateral plate is furthermore attached to the bone by means of two cortical bone screws.

Virtually any of the usual surgical approaches to the hip joint may be used, and the postoperative treatment is the same as any which has proved suitable after hip surgery.

Clinical Results of the First and Second Generations

The first TPP was implanted in Chur in 1978. Since 1980 a field study together with the Orthopiedic Department Balgrist, University of Zurich, has been in progress [1, 2, 4, 13]. To evaluate the clinical relevance and indication of the TPP carefully a very limited number of patients received this implant: 115 at the Kantonsspital Chur and 47 at the University Hospital, Balgrist, Zurich (total 162). Since 1980 all patients have been regularly examined, clinically and radiologically. The average age was 53.2 years (19.9–78). Corresponding to the large number of male patients and the low average age, the most common indication for the TPP was idiopathic femoral head necrosis [1, 4, 13].

The majority of patients exhibited good to excellent range of motion and were able to walk freely more than 5 km. The postoperative walking distance progressively increased. Most of the patients improved by large in their daily activities and business occupations. They were usually painfree apart from a few of the first generation (see the description of the TPP) who complained of slight local pain in the area of the rather prominent lateral plate. The lateral plate was therefore decreased in size. The majority of patients were so satisfied with the results that they were willing to have the same operation performed again. The radiological examinations showed no signs of osteopenia or atrophy of the proximal end of the femur, especially in the region of the medial cortex of the neck. The clinical and radiological results were evaluated according to the Harris score (29–99 points) and reached 83 points on this scale. In six cases the TPP was implanted bilaterally. The longest follow-up period is now over 9 years. Four infections and four aseptic loosening occurred in the first series,

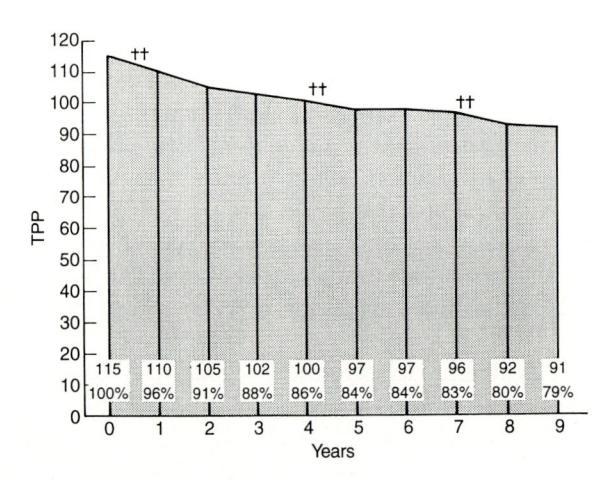

Fig. 3. The survivorship curve of the first and second generations ot the TPP. The results stabilize after 2 years. Six deaths are included. (From [4])

until 1986. Since then no such further complications have occurred. All eight loosened TPPs were easily replaced by conventional ones [3]. The survivorship curve, which also includes the patients who died, shows a leveling off after 2 years. The unsatisfactory cases usually appear during this initial period (Fig. 3). The majority of the aseptically loosened cases that required a revision, showed a loosened high-density polyethylene socket with considerable wear.

Case Histories

Case 1. A woman, born in 1903, with bilateral rheumatoid arthritis of the hips. Both hips were replaced by artificial joints. A TPP was implanted on the right, and 4 months later a conventional prosthesis with cement was implanted on the left side 1981. After 4 years some differences could be seen radiographically. On the right side dense cortical bone was seen in good contact with the thrust plate in the area of the calcar femorale which was in sharp contrast to the atrophied bone on the left side. A year earlier (1984) scintigraphy indicated higher activity in the left hip. The patient died in 1989, and both hips were subjected to histological examination. The histology (performed by R. Schenk) showed that the thrust plate, lateral plate and cortical bone screws, all made of cobalt-based alloys at that time, were fast embedded in newly formed bone. No intermediate layer of fibrous connective tissue was present (the crevice visible in the histological section is an artifact). The histology also clearly showed the strong, dense bone structure on the medial aspect of the proximal femur (Figs. 4, 5).

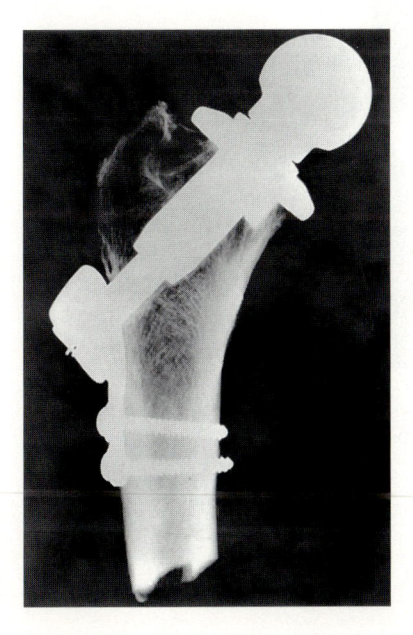

Fig. 4. Postmortem radiographs 8 years after implantation of a TPP shows a dense functional bone apposition in the area of the medial femoval neck

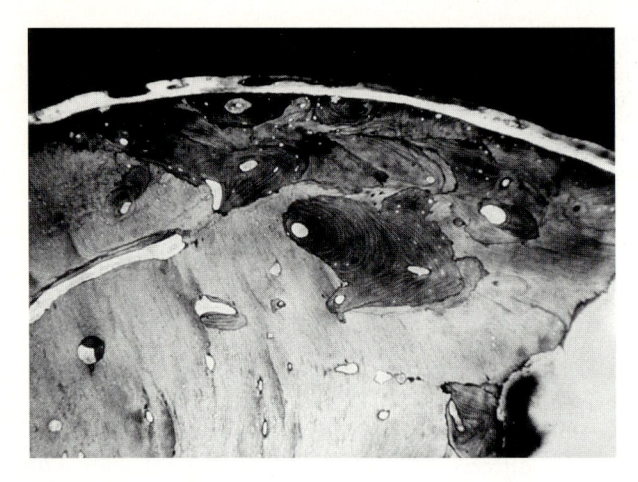

Fig. 5. *Case 1.* The histological findings confirm the formation of new bone (*dark*) at the medial aspect of the femoral neck. No connective tissue is visible; the gap is an artifact due to the fixation technique. (Provided by Prof. R. Schenk, Berne)

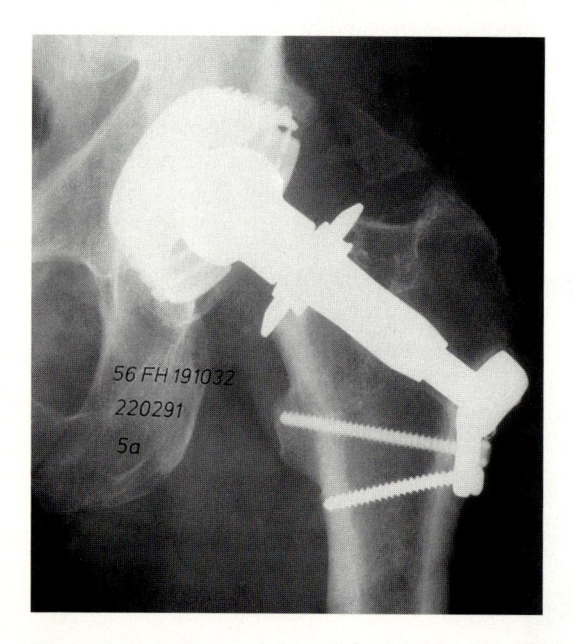

Fig. 6. *Case 2.* Osteoarthritis of the left hip. Excellent radiological result with thickened medial cortical bone of the femoral neck 5 years postoperatively

Case 2. A man, born in 1932. The patient had an invalidating coxarthrosis, left, which was treated by implanting a TPP of the second generation. Five years postoperatively the clinical and radiological results had remained good (Fig. 6).

Case 3. A man, born in 1928. A TPP was implanted in the right hip in 1981. Ten years later the socket loosened, and wore eccentrically. Replacement with a Stühmer stem prosthesis of size 5 and a Zweymüller socket (size 68) was easy and led to an absolutely trouble-free recovery because of the intact condition of the host bone.

Discussion

Based on stress analysis investigations, it seems most unlikely that the cancellous bone could ever be in a position to carry the loads imposed through the implantation of an intramedullarly anchored endoprosthesis. Moreover, the cortical bone too, in the proximal region tends to atrophy in the course of time, thereby leaving the prosthesis stem insufficiently supported. Therefore, a femoral prosthesis has been developed which transmits the hip joint forces directly to the medial cortical bone of the femoral neck. The TPP is particularly advantageous for use in young patients since revision surgery is easy with maximum availability of bone stock.

Wiles [14] and Mc Kee [8] described similiar prostheses, but the basic principles of the TPP are very different from those of these earlier designs. The TPP has resulted from more recent experimental investigations and clinical observations and is therefore an altogether new concept [2, 5, 6].

The axis of the TPP should coincide with that of the femoral neck. The thrust plate lies at a right angle to the axis of the mandrel, and therefore only with the prosthesis lying in the correct position relative to the femoral neck does the thrust plate come to bear on sufficiently thick cortical bone. In attempting to position the prosthesis more vertically, that is in valgus, the thrust plate no longer bears on sufficiently thick cortical bone and also probably interferes with the trochanter major in the region of the fossa. Also, with a more vertical position, the mechanical conditions begin to approach those of an intramedularly anchored prosthesis with collar [11]. The difference in axial stiffness between bone and implant would then lead to asliding motion between the central bolt and the lateral plate. The optimal position of the thrust plate would correspond to a neck angle of 125°/130°. A varus position is also unsuitable because the danger of slipping transversally off the neck increases. The specially structured surface of the thrust plate which seats on the bone resists the component of force by permitting interdigitation between bone and implant.

Summary

The TPP is employed as a routine procedure for corresponding indications. The surgical technique has been standardized. Cinical observations confirm that the TPP can withstand the hip joint forces and enables the medial cortical bone of the femoral neck to be loaded in a physiological manner. This has been shown in a histological examination of a specimen that had been implanted for 8 years. Taking Wolff's law into consideration, full integration of the TPP within the host bone might be expected and therefore better long-term results than presently obtained with conventional prosthesis.

References

1. Bereiter H, Jacob HAC, Huggler AH (1986) Die klinischen Erfahrungen mit der Druckscheibenprothese (DSP). Med Orthop Tech 1/86: 21–23
2. Huggler AH, Jacob HAC (1984) The uncemented thrust plate prosthesis. In: Morscher E (ed) The cementless fixation of hip endoprostheses. Springer, Berlin Heidelberg New York
3. Huggler AH, Weidmann E (1976) Design criteria of total hip replacements fixed with bone cement. In: Schaldach M (ed) Engineering in medicine, vol 2. Advances in artificial hip and knee joint technology. Springer, Berlin Heidelberg New York
4. Huggler AH, Jacob HAC, Bereiter H, Haferkorn M, Ryf C, Schenk R (1993) Long-term results with the uncemented thrust plate prosthesis (TPP). Acta Orthop Belg 59: 215–223
5. Jacob HAC, Huggler A (1978) Experimentelle Spannungsanalysen im menschlichen Oberschenkelknochen-Modell mit und ohne Prothese. Forschungsheft, Technische Rundschau, Sulzer, pp 73–83
6. Jacob HAC, Huggler AH (1980) An investigation into biomechanical causes of prosthesis stem loosening within the proximal end of the human femur. J Biomech 13: 159–173
7. Kummer B (1978) Mechanische Beanspruchung und funktionelle Anpassung des Knochens. Verh Anat Ges 72: 21–46
8. McKee GK (1966/1967) Developments in total hip joint replacement. Symposium on lubrication and wear in living and artificial human joints. Institution of Mechanical Engineers. London Proc 1971 4: 1–5
9. Perren SM, Huggler A, Russenberger M, Straumann F, Müller ME, Allgöwer M (1969) Kortikale Knochenheilung. I. Methode zur Messung von Druckänderungen an der lebenden Kortikalis. Acta Orthop Scand Suppl 125: 1–14
10. Perren SM, Huggler A, Russenberger M Allgöwer M, Mathys R, Schenk R, Willenegger H, Müller ME (1969) Kortikale Knochenheilung II: Reaktion der Kortikalis auf Kompression. Acta Orthop Scand Suppl 125: 1–14

11. Roux W (1895) Gesammelte Abhandlung über Entwicklungsmechanik der Organismen, vols 1, 2. Engelmann, Leipzig
12. Scholten R (1976) Über die Berechnung der mechanischen Beanspruchung in Knochenstrukturen mittels für den Flugzeugbau entwickeltes Rechenverfahren. Med Orthop Tech 6: 130–137
13. Schreiber A, Jacob HAC, Suezawa Y, Huggler AH (1984) First results with the thrust plate total hip prosthesis. In: Morscher E (ed) The cementless fixation of hip endoprotheses. Springer, Berlin Heidelberg New York
14. Wiles P (1958) The surgery of the osteoarthritic hip. Br J Surg 45: 488–497
15. Wolff J (1982) Das Gesetz über die Transformation der Knochen. Hirschwald, Berlin

Conical Stem Fixation for Cementless Hip Prostheses for Primary Implantation and Revisions

H. Wagner M. Wagner

Introduction

The conical fixation of femoral prostheses, where a conical prosthesis stem is pressed home in the conically reamed femoral medullary canal, ensures excellent primary stability in cementless implantation. The sharp longitudinal ribs along the prosthesis stem which cut into the bone provide strong rotational stability. The coarse-blasted surface of the titanium implant encourages osseointegration, gradually leading to permanent secondary stability. The conical design of the prosthesis fixation leads to smooth load transfer with more loading proximally, which accelerates the structural adaptation of the femur to the prosthesis.

Problems associated with the shape of the prosthesis stem

A decade of experimental and clinical experience permit the requirements for optimum prosthesis fixation to be clearly defined. The significance of a high degree of mechanical primary stability is no longer questioned. The fixation must be solid and reliable enough that the patient can be mobilized with partial loading of the leg immediately following implantation. The primary stability must also include significant rotation resistance. A high torque is placed on the prosthesis when standing up from the sitting position, and when climbing stairs, even under partial loading, and the fixation must be able to withstand this without relative motion. The initial, only mechanical primary stability from impacting can be maintained for only a limited time due to physiological bone restructuring. The design of the prosthesis stem must, however, be such that it is maintained until secondary stability from osseointegration gradually takes over.

According to the present state of the art for cementless prosthesis stems, a titanium alloy with a coarse-blasted surfaces is used which provides the best prerequisite for osseointegration [1, 2, 4]. Secondary stability is gradually achieved by the growth of new bone tissue directly onto the metal surface and gradual filling of the gap between the implant and the surrounding corticalis with bone. Osseointegration can proceed undisturbed only when relative motion between the implant and the bone interface is prevented by the high degree of primary stability. One can assume that the secondary fixation from osseointegration is gradually effective 3–4 months after implantation. Until that time the fixation strength must ensure the primary stability.

The original pressure between the implant and the bone is also lost after 3–4 months due to physiological bone restructuring at the bone/implant interface, so that there is a gradual transfer from primary to secondary fixation. The load transfer from the prosthesis stem into the bone should be smooth along the fixation area and should be greater proximally than distally, so that the femoral corticalis is uniformly loaded and is maintained during the physiological bone restructuring. Many varieties of stem design were developed in earlier decades with the objective of achieving smooth load transfer, particularly in the proximal area, and many of these designs where abandoned long ago. The most difficult problem with cementless stem fixation is evidently rotational instability, which shows itself quite early with pain in the thigh, long before structural change in the bone can be detected in radiographs.

For the improvement of rotational stability some designs have wing-like ribs at the lateral upper end of the stem which are pressed into the spongiosa of the trochanter major. These ribs are nearly useless because they are very close to the longitudinal axis of the femoral medullary canal and thus very close to the axis of rotation of the prosthesis stem. On the other hand there is the prosthesis head which transfers torque to the prosthesis stem, which is very far from this axis and thus has a long lever arm.

Prosthesis stems with a rectangular cross-section have a high degree of rotational stability but have the disadvantage that the individual shape of the medullary canal forces the implant to rotate and the operator cannot himself decide the anteversion angle. This is very important in the case of dysplastic hips, where the oval section of the femoral neck has pathological anteversion which turns the rectangular prosthesis stem to an undesired anteversion. A further disadvantage of the rectangular section prosthesis is evident where the proximal femoral segment is cylindrical. In such a case a solidly impacted cementless implant can lead to fracture of the bone. Prosthesis collars have not shown any value for cementless implantation. The collar concept is based on the idea that the collar sits on the medial corticalis of the femoral neck stump and ensures proximal load transfer. This load transfer, however, can only be effective when the stem is carrying little or no load. The collar then functions as a hypomochlion which, under load, forces the stem towards varus, which leads to relative motion and prevention of osseointegration. If the stem, on the other hand, is firmly anchored, elastic deformation of the femur under load causes oscillating relative motion between the collar and the medial corticalis of the femoral neck to occur, leading to osteolysis. The collar thus loses its effectiveness.

The most important question for the fixation of cementless femoral prostheses is that of the shape of the prosthesis stem, providing, on the one hand, the maximum primary stability and, on the other, following osseointegration, optimum load transfer into the proximal segment of the femur. Most cementless prostheses attempt a stem configuration which matches as closely as possible the anatomical shape of the femur, in order to thus produce the maximum surface contact between implant and bone. There is, however, one major reservation in this regard. The shape of the natural femur developed over the course of many years to adapt to the individual anatomical constitution and the corresponding loading situation. The morphology of the femur is therefore to a certain extent also a monument to previous function. For this reason, every femur is different because individuals exhibit considerable variations in biomechanical conditions. Standardized cementless implants therefore provide only a partial fit in the respective natural bone.

The biomechanical conditions in the proximal segment of the femur change decisively following implantation of a femoral prosthesis. Load transfer which was previously made mainly at the surface of the hollow bone now occurs via a pluglike implant onto the inner wall of the medullary canal. Furthermore the implant can only transfer compression and bending forces, and can scarcely absorb tension forces on the (lateral) tension side of the bone.

Given these loading conditions the question must be asked whether, following prosthesis implantation, the femur in fact needs the same morphological configuration as previously. This is certainly not the case, because the loading conditions have changed. This is evident not only theoretically from the change in the biomechanical configuration but also from long-term radiological follow-ups. Clinically and radiologically ideal prosthesis implantations *always* show an adaptation of the bone morphology to the implant over the years. Is therefore ideal cementless prosthesis implantation achieved by adapting the prosthesis to the given form of the bone, or is it better to choose an implant shape which provides the bone with optimum conditions for structural adaptation? There is a plausible answer: As the original morphological conditions in the bone cannot be maintained in any case, the shape of the implant should be such that optimum conditions are provided for the bone to proceed directly towards the permanent condition of structural adaptation.

How can these optimum conditions be defined? An cementless femoral prosthesis should meet the following requirements:
- Solid fixation with a high degree of primary stability.
- A high degree of rotational stability.
- A high degree of surface contact between implant and bone.
- Significantly proximal load transfer resulting from the shape of the prosthesis stem.
- Bone-friendly metal alloy for the implant, which encourages osseointegration.
- A good compromise between stiffness and elastic bending deformation of the prosthesis stem to reduce stress peaks during load transfer.
- Instruments for the gentle preparation of a well-fitting implant interface in the bone.

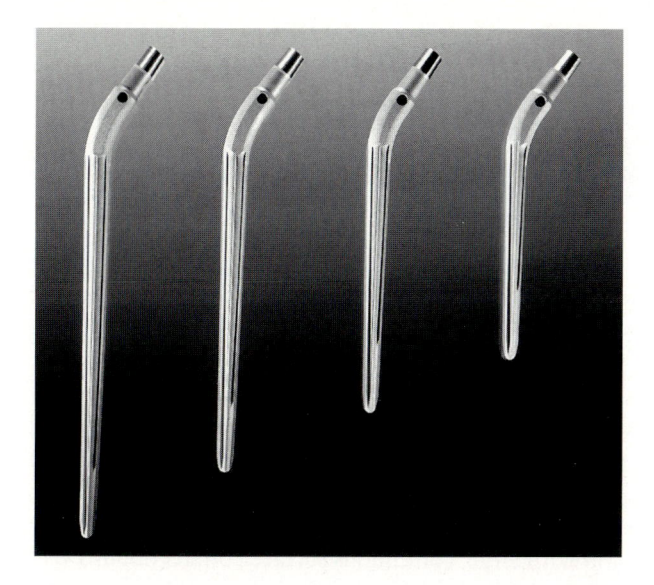

Fig. 1. Femoral revision prosthesis with a conical stem having a cone angle of 2° for prosthesis replacement. With millimeter diameter increments and four different stem lengths, a suitable prosthesis is available for the various anatomical canditions

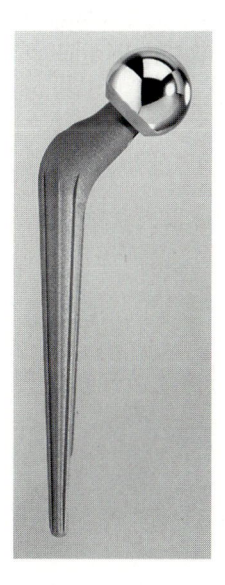

Fig. 2. Conical prosthesis with a conical stem having a cone angle of 5° for primary implantation

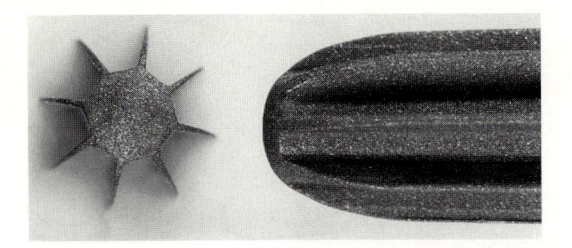

Fig. 3. Conical prosthesis stem with eight radial, longitudinal, sharp conical ribs around the circumference. The surface of the titanium implant is coarse-blasted

Conical stem fixation fulfills these conditions in a very impressive manner and has proven itself in the conical prosthesis for primary implantations and with the femoral revision prosthesis for prosthesis replacement (Fig. 1–3). Using this fixation principle, the conical prosthesis stem is impacted into the conically reamed medullary canal and with large, continuous surface contact obtains very firm fixation in a similar way to the well-known engineering solution using taper spigot connections. The osseous interface is prepared using sharp conical reamers in a simple and precise manner so that the conical prosthesis stem has full-fit contact with the bone [3]. The conical fixation provides high contact pressure between the implant and the osseous interface, which is available all over the full contact area (Fig. 4). This provides a high degree of primary stability with optimum use of the material strength of the bone.

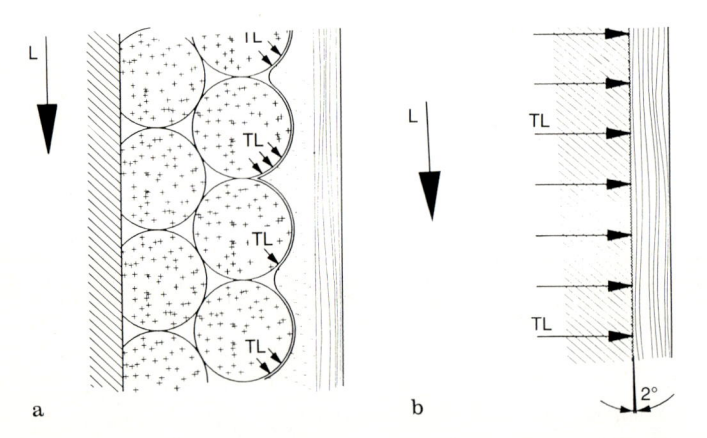

Fig. 4a, b. Load transfer *(TL)* between prosthesis stem and femur. **a** Discontinuous load transfer globular or coarse structured surface. **b** Continuous load transfer with conical fixation

Conical Stem Fixation for Cementless Hip Prostheses

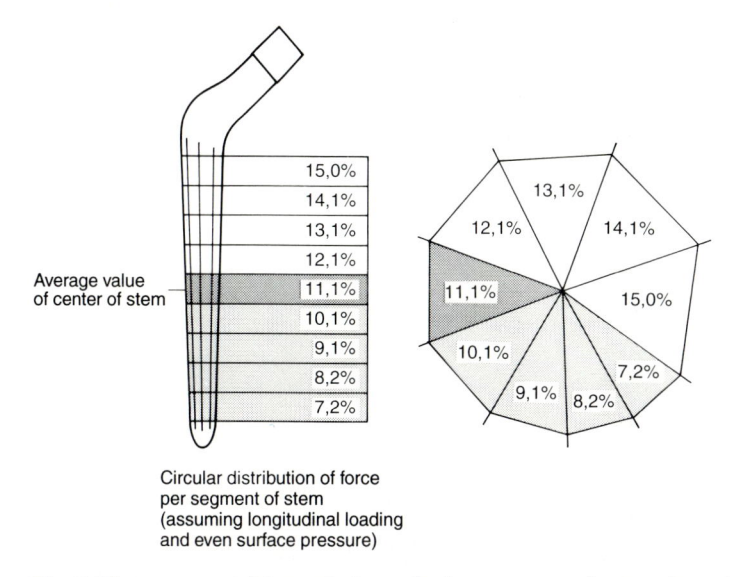

Fig. 5. The geometry of the conical prosthesis stem ensures increased proximal load transfer. In the proximal stem area the larger diameter ensures more load transfer surface per unit of length than in the distal stem region (given longitudinal force and continuos surface contact)

The cone angle of the prosthesis stems closely matches the natural morphology of the femur. The objective is that as little bone substance as possible must be reamed out during the preparation of the conical prosthesis interface. A cone angle of 5° has shown itself a good compromise for the conical prosthesis, which is used in the proximal segment of the femur. The associated reamer has a cone angle of 4°. This small difference in cone angles permits a somewhat tighter fit of the proximal prosthesis stem in softer bone than in the hard corticalis in the area of the tip of the stem. The conical prosthesis is not suitable for femora which open out trumpetlike proximally because the stem shape would permit sufficient fixation only in its distal half. For the femoral revision prosthesis, which is longer and is anchored predominantly in the more cylindrical diaphysial part of the femur, the cone angle is 2°.

With continuous surface contact between the conical prosthesis stem and the conical bone interface, a uniform load transfer per unit of area can be assumed. With the conical form of the prosthesis stem, the surface per unit of length increases with the diameter. The surface area per unit of length is thus greater in the proximal area than in the distal area of the stem. The conical prosthesis stem therefore has increased proximal loading from the stem geometry alone (Fig. 5). For this reason radiological follow-up observations of conical fixations dot not show the feared bone atrophy of the proximal end of the femur due to stress shielding, as has often been observed with coarse-structured cementless prosthe-

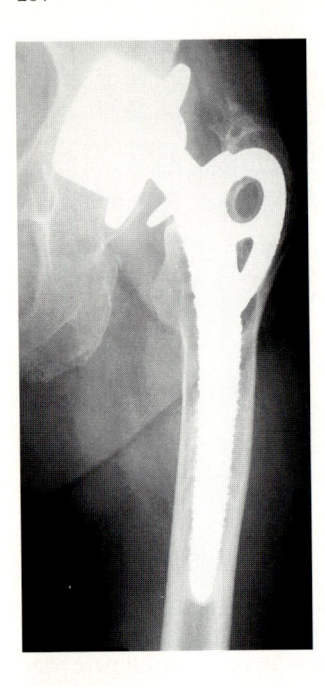

Fig. 6. Coarse-structured prosthesis stems with a mainly cylindrical shape dig into the surface of the bone, and this leads to a more rigid load transfer distally in the more solid corticalis than proximally in the elastic spongiosa. The resulting stress shielding in the proximal segment of the femur leads to bone atrophy

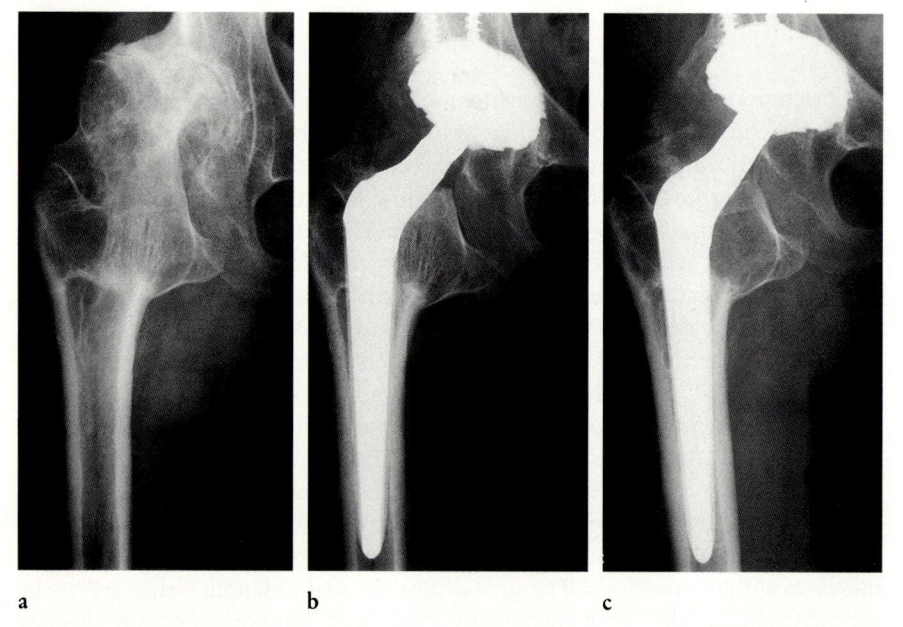

Fig. 7a–c. With conical stem fixation, increased proximal load transfer cause a deposition of bone mass in the proximal segment of the femur. Implantation of a conical prosthesis in a 43-year-old woman due to posttraumatic coxarthrosis *(right)* **a** Condition immediately before implantation. **b** Three weeks after implantation. **c** Two years after the operation, bone deposition in the proximal stem area, medial and lateral

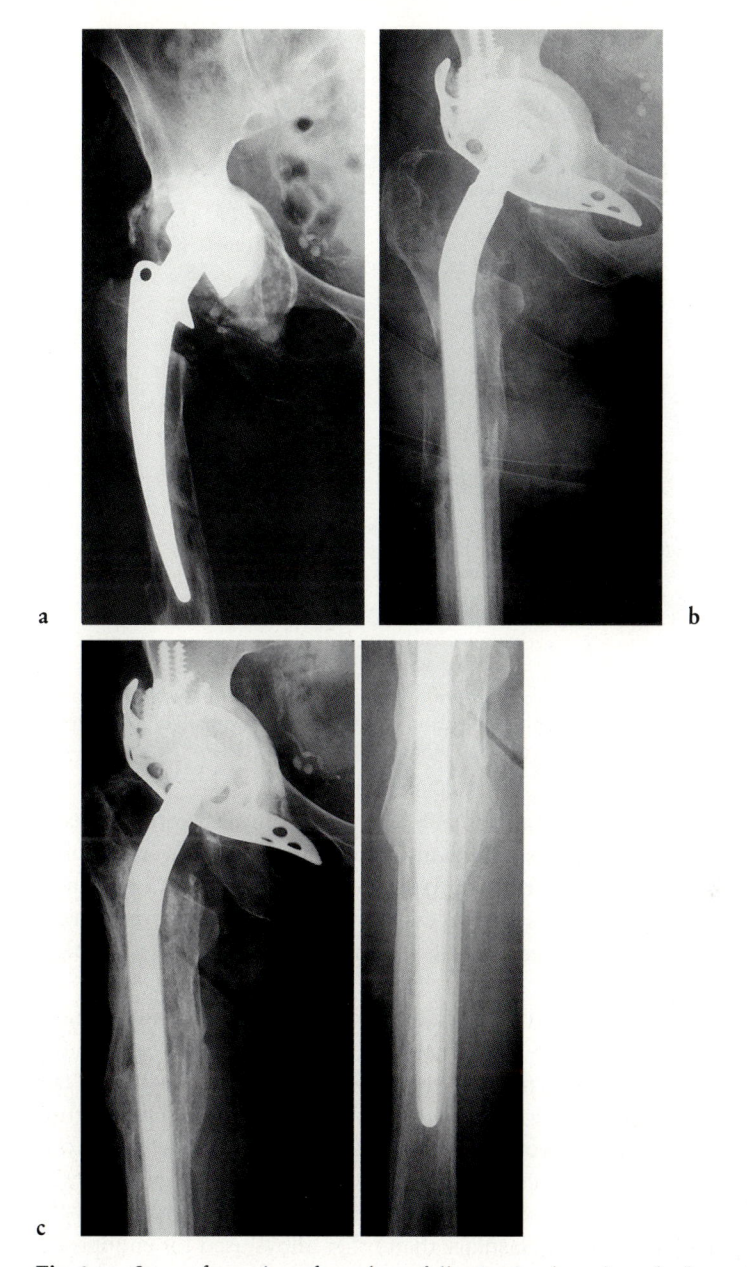

Fig. 8a–c. Strong formation of new bone following implantation of a femoral revision prostheses using transfemoral approach. **a** Preoperative condition of a 67-year-old woman with loosened prosthesis and severe bone resorption defects. **b** Three weeks after implantation of a revision prosthesis with bridging of the damaged femur segment. **c** Already 6 months after the operation there is extensive osseous filling of the defects with directional bone structures

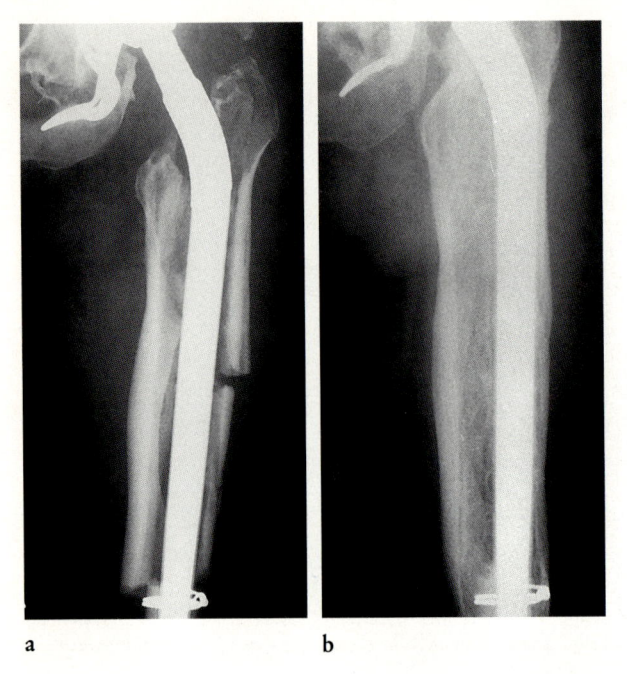

Fig. 9a, b. Bone regeneration after implantation of a femoral revision prostheses using transfemoral approach. **a** Condition 10 days after operation in a 40-year-old woman. **b** Voluminous, structurally aligned bone regeneration after 20 months

sis stems with other configurations (Fig. 6 and 7). The conical prosthesis stems have eight sharp longitudinal ribs uniformly around the circumference which cut slightly into the corticalis during implantation, thus leading to a very high rotationol stability (Fig. 3). This seems to explain why thigh pain is very rarely reported with the conical prosthesis and also with the femoral revision prosthesis.

The prostheses are manufactured from a tissue-friendly titanium-aluminium-niobium alloy and have a coarse-blasted surface, fulfilling the prerequisite for osseointegration, i. e., the formation of new bone substance directly on the metallic surface without an intermediate connective tissue layer. Histological investigations by Schenk and Wehrli [2] have shown additionally that the ongrowth of new bone occurs particularly at the raised areas of the implant. These phenomena encourage and accelerate the secondary fixation by bony ongrowth. The titanium alloy has a greater elasticity than other alloys used for endoprostheses. The resulting larger deformation under load applies especially to the longer revision stems and evidently plays a biomechanical role in the impressive regeneration of bone in the proximal segment of the femur following prosthesis revision with major bone loss [3] (Fig. 7–9).

An important point in conical stem fixation is achieving sufficient primary fixation by impacting the prosthesis into the medullary canal. The prosthesis is hammered into the femur using the impacting instrument. The penetration of the prosthesis must be carefully observed. The prosthesis penetrates further into the medullary canal with each hammer blow until the sound of the impact changes and further penetration does not occur with the same hammer force. It is essential that this condition be achieved during implantation, otherwise the prosthesis can subside postoperatively under load. While the subsidence provides subsequent fixation, albeit with leg shortening, this route to stability should be avoided. A subsided prosthesis is in fact insufficiently anchored and is thus unstable, and there is no assurance that subsequent stabiliziation meets the requirements for a high degree of primary stability. In fact, permanent instability may result, leading inevitably to prosthesis loosening. Subsidence has not been observed, even over longer periods of time, where there is adequate primary fixation, as evidenced by follow-up observations on a large number of hip joints.

References

1. Buser D, Schenk RK, Steinemann S, Fiorellini JP, Fox CH, Stich H (1991). Influence of surface characteristics on bone integration of titanium implants. A histomorphometric study in miniature pigs. J Biomed Mater Res 25: 889–902
2. Schenk RK, Wehrli U (1989). Zur Reaktion des Knochens auf eine zementfreie SL-Femurrevisionsprothese. Orthopäde 18: 454–462
3. Wagner H (1989). Revisionsprothese für das Hüftgelenk. Orthopäde 18: 438–453
4. Wong M, Witschger P, Eulenberger J, Schenk R, Hunziker E (1994). Effect of surface roughness and material composition on osseointegration of implant materials in trabecular bone. Orthop Res Soc 40: 598

Part VI
Noncemented Endoprosthesis Systems

The CLS Stem

L. Spotorno, G. Grappiolo, A. Mumenthaler

The CLS System

Conception and Evolution of an Idea

We have to face the fact that the prosthetic replacement of a hip joint using cement is still considered a standard procedure for the stem. Some authors even hold the opinion – whether right or wrong – that this system is still unsurpassable. The tendency for human beings to search for improvements and innovations has induced numerous researchers to investigate the so called biological anchorage. We were and still are protagonists of this idea. The search for a cementless anchorage began in 1976. Around 2000 stems of various manufacture were implanted before the CLS stem, which is still in clinical service, began to be used in December 1983. It is obvious that the stability of a cemented system is assured by the extensive bone cement surface and, in particular, because the cement with its very fine proturbances can claw into the cancellous bone structures. It is thus self-evident that with an uncemented prosthesis the reverse of this phenomenon was considered as the *primum movens*. Consequently, it is a question of trying to promote the growth of new bone formations of the trabecular structure onto the rough or macrostructured surfaces of the implant. From the very beginning, the idea of the porous coating was a popular solution and it is still widely supported today [8].

Our wide experience with the implantation of Lord prostheses [19] with a madreporous surface enabled us to adopt a critical stance with regards to the clinical and radiological findings, results which at least in some cases did not fulfil our expectations. Closer observation of the periprosthetic bone in a number of cases revealed an early cancellous transformation of the proximal cortical bone, combined with a spindle-shaped distal hypertrophy. This phenomenon reflects the bypass of forces in a distal direction, which is known as stress shielding. This phenomenon of the decompensated femur is manifested clinically by pain in the upper thigh.

This experience and the analysis of the good results achieved with cemented prostheses, which have a larger surface particularly in the proximal area, led to the development of the "Hedgehog" stem in 1980. This was a non-cemented prosthesis with a finger-shaped macrostructure limited to the proximal zone.

Nowadays, most authors agree that any form of macrostructurization and coating should be limited to the proximal zone.

The origin of the CLS prosthesis was the need to avoid the phenomenon of stress shielding. We interpret this frequently discussed occurrence as a lack of respect for the biotrophism of the femur. The biotrophism is preserved by giving the periprosthetic residual bone the chance to function according to its physiological model and to retain the quantity as well as the quality of the original bone. This concept, which basically conforms to morphofunctional criteria, can be applied to prosthetic replacements in general. In other words, preservation of biotrophism means facilitating longevity of the implant. In the full sense of the word, the changes in the periprosthetic bone are the result of iatrogenic influences.

We are now completely aware of the fact that the implantation of a prosthesis entails the decompensation of an osseous structure which has its own equilibrium, even if it is in a physiopathological state (thus justifying intervention). The prosthetic replacement must aim to restore the physiology of the joint and, at the same time, adapt the transmission of the forces to the physiology of the bone.

In actual fact we create a bone-prosthesis interface and, ideally a "discreet" intrusion, which accounts for a physiology-like transmission of the forces on the interface.

Our clinical experience has shown quite clearly that an implant which is too rigid prevents the bone from behaving in the same way as its physiological model (similar to when a prosthesis imprisons the bone from an inward direction). The bone also behaves unphysiologically when efforts are made to realise a distal anchorage according to the concept "fit, fill, and bone ingrowth".

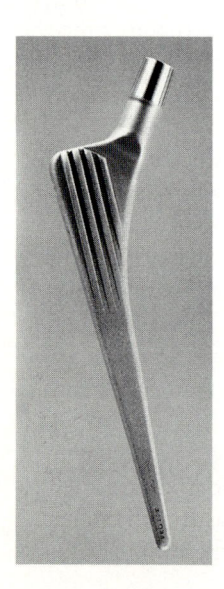

Fig. 1. The rough-blasted CLS stem with its three-dimensional wedge shape and proximal, pronounced axial ribs

The original idea from which the CLS prosthesis was derived, is based on this concept. Consequently, particular attention was given to the mechanical function of the proximal cancellous bone. The distal part was therefore kept small and the bone ingrowth concept abandoned in order to promote an anchorage in this region. In particular, preference was given to a shape (conical) and material (titanium) which, thanks to the calculation by means of the finite element method, proved to be favourable for the physiological transmission of the forces (Fig. 1).

Interplay Between Shape, Material and Surface

One of the most important aspects for the longevity of an implant is the effort made to match the transmission of forces as closely as possible to the physiological model. On the other hand, numerous other factors also play a role, e.g. primary stability and osseointegration, mechanical strength and the resistance to wear. The fact that we would like to emphasize here is that these factors depend on different variables (shape, material and surface quality) which also have a reciprocal influence [2]. If we consider a prosthesis as a system (stem and cup), it must embody a clearly defined basic concept.

Present-day knowledge – developed and refined through clinical experience, laboratory tests and theoretical studies – confirms the importance of the actual material properties, the surface treatment and the shape of the prosthesis for its respective integration.

The complexity of this problem is clearly apparent, inasmuch as the search for favourable materials, for example, can tend to make one factor dominant to the detriment of others. In other words, we must look for the necessary and satisfying conditions that will lead to the success of the implant, i. e. a favourable long-term result.

The ideal material must satisfy the following criteria:
– Appropriate mechanical characteristics,
– optimum biocompatibility,
– atoxicity,
– minimal tendency to abrade and become abraded,
– osteophilia,
– biocompatible modulus of elasticity [25].

Even though the mechanical strength can be tested quite easily in the laboratory, mechanical failures are still experienced in the clinical setting. They are usually associated with old prosthesis models. Nevertheless, the modularity can increase the mechanical risk. Strict laboratory testing and quality control of each piece are necessary to ensure that the material has the appropriate characteristics [24].

As far as biocompatibility is concerned, all the materials employed today fulfil the requirements, as least in vitro. This biocompatibility can be summarised in two specific properties:

- no toxicity (with metal, the release of ions must be reduced to a minimum),
- no activation of the immune system.

With regard to toxicity, the work performed by Semlitsch, for example, has shown that titanium alloys with niobium are superior to titanium with vanadium or pure titanium [31]. In addition, the problem of abrasion that arises with the sliding parts must be considered, something which is solved theoretically by means of in vitro testing. Using macrophage cultures, Haynes has shown that the abrased titanium is only slightly toxic, but releases a large amount of phlogogenic factors. On the other hand, chromium-cobalt particles have a direct toxic effect on macrophages, but result in a minor non-specific reaction [12].

The effective, induced immune reaction of the materials employed nowadays for the manufacture of implants is still not clear. However, the materials, through abrasion, do cause a non-spezcific reaction, i. e. simple macrophagic phagocytosis or even acute or chronic inflammation. In this sense, it appears that there are slight differences between the various materials. The non-specific reaction is definitely dependent on the quantity. Consequently, we must consider the materials with respect to their tendency to cause abrasion [15].

Laboratory investigations seem to confirm that bone cement is immunologically inert. However, they also reveal that there is a slight chemotactical effect on the mononuclear cells [27]. Hence in vivo, bone cement results in a foreignbody reaction with giant cells. The same thing occurs with polyethylene particles larger than 10 μm, the smallest polyethylene particles less than 3–5 μm in size are phagocytised, as in metallic abrasion. This maintains the non-specific inflammatory reaction [20]. On the other hand, ceramic can be incorporated by the macrophages and can accumulate there without causing any morphofunctional changes [6].

We know for certain, that hydroxyapatite does not act immunogenetically when an immune reaction takes place. On the other hand, we are also aware of the ability of osteosynthetic materials, such as hyaluronic acid and polyvinylpyrrolidate, to set off immune reactions of the thymus-dependent type. These products are not used in prosthetics but, as a theoretical example, they allow us to reflect on the way in which the chemical/physical denaturation of some materials might set off a similar reaction in vivo [7].

Osteophilia is dependent on the employed material, but is also influenced by the roughness of its surface [18]. The materials can therefore be biocompatible, bioinert or bioactive. Biocompatible materials do not permit direct contact with the bone: in other words, a layer of fibrous tissue, sometimes very thin, is interposed between bone and prosthesis. Bioinert materials permit osseous neoformations with direct contact. Their creation, however, is largely dependent on biomechanical conditions and the surface, which can be smooth, microstructured or macrostructured.

Buser and co-workers report the growth of bone onto all their investigated titanium surfaces [4]. Individually, bone growth of 20 % was observed on a smooth titanium surface and 40 % on corundum-blasted surfaces. Titanium plasma spray coating shows a growth of 60 % on the surface opposite the bone.

Macrostructurisation causes bone growth into the implant. In other words, it results in an ingrowth of bone irrespective of the material employed. We can obtain an anchorage between the prosthesis and bone without an on-growth. The macrostructured surfaces increase the mechanical risk and can lead to fragmentation. Moreover, with a similar quantity of material to match the larger surface they are subject to a greater release of ions. (For example, a simple macroporotic layer increases the surface area by about 200 %) [16]. The other disadvantages of macrostructurisation are undeniably the much more complicated removal of a prosthesis and the possibility of bone necrosis, set off by microtraumatic vascular crises.

Hydroxyapatite is the most interesting of the bioactive materials. According to Buser and Schenk, it facilitates extensive bonding, equivalent to 70 % of the surface area. As we know, it is completely histocompatible, but involves the danger of an interface crisis. The pull-out test indicates that forces with a magnitude of 18 MPa cause bone, hydroxyapatite and the prosthesis to become detached [5, 28] Calculation using the finite element method show that the bone prosthesis interface is subject to forces that fluctuate between 2 and 7 MPa, depending on the zone. These data would appear to be reassuring. Nevertheless, the effect of the cyclic repetition of submaximum loads in the long run are difficult to predict. The manner in which hydroxyapatite can cause abrasion is obviously indirect: fragments detached by the forces of pressure or abrasion of the surfaces that are subject to micromovements. Research is being carried out with the aim of minimising the risk in the interface.

The influence of biomechanical factors can never be completely ignored where bone growth is concerned. Schneider's classic investigations have shown that ample bone growth can be observed wherever a steel bolt or screw is subject to the forces of pressure, whereas on the opposite side there is a zone of microinstability which can still develop, i. e. which bone formation can occur, or which can allow the formation of a fibrous membrane.

In endoprosthetics, these biomechanical facts are obviously influenced by the shape and the employed material's modulus of elasticity. On the whole, the shape and modulus of elasticity enable us to define the concept of biocompatible elasticity. Other individual variables have to be considered as given facts, e. g. the shape of the femur as the recipient of the prosthesis, the lever arms of the muscular apparatus and the operative technique, all of which influence the biomechanical behaviour of the bone-prosthesis interface.

A rigid material, i.e. a material which is less elastic than cortical bone, tends to create a microinstability which is distally more pronounced, as animal experiments have confirmed. On the other hand, increased elasticity has the opposite effect: distal stability and proximal microinstability.

Proximal microinstability produces a fibrous membrane whose wealth of macrophages can activate an osteoclastic reaction through the production of prostaglandin. This phenomenon can be increased severalfold by the simultaneous presence of abrased products [38].

The significance of hydroxyapatite might be very important in this respect. Without doubt, hydroxyapatite promotes intimate and early bonding relatively independent of the material used. It might therefore favour proximal anchorage and reduce or even hinder the formation of fibrous membrane in this zone.

However, it would appear that purely biomechanical rules influence bone growth over the course of time, a fact that is confirmed by the recently introduced method of densitometrical measurement of bone. These measurements enable us to analyse the quantitative aspect of this phenomenon with great accuracy and to acquire a morphofunctional picture of the periprosthetic bone [9, 17, 21].

Bearing these points in mind, we want to show that, if a non-cemented implant is to be anchored in a favourable manner, we have to consider all the satisfying and necessary conditions when selecting the material, surface and shape of the prosthesis. In this respect we have also found that a number of factors interact and sometimes contradict each other, and it is very important to weigh up the interdependency of the various factors.

With the present state of knowledge, it appears that the compromise offered by the CLS titanium alloy stem with a corundum-blasted surface is a safe and applicable solution [1].

Stable secondary anchorage of the stem by means of osseointegration is absolutely dependent on the primary stability of the femoral component. This primary fixation is achieved by means of a three-dimensional wedge. It was our aim to include the adaptable trabecular structures with the primary anchorage. Anchorage in the proximal region means that the bulbus is at least partly responsible for the transmission and distribution of the load. The interpositioning of the trabecula reduces rigidity. The proximal, very pronounced axial ribs support this stabilising function by penetrating the cancellous bone thus achieving congruency. The likewise completely tapered, distal part of the stem is kept relatively slender, above all to avoid direct contact with the cortical bone. The CCD angle is relatively steep (145°), but it reduces the tilting moment considerably. The conical spigot connection 12/14 permits the choice of either ceramic or metal ball heads. The forged alloy PROTASUL-100 is used as material.

Indications

To reduce the risk for patients to a minimum, the indications for the CLS stem were rather limited to begin with. However, as a result of the increasing experience and the positive clinical results, they were progressively widened. The morphological classification shown here is considered a classical example:

The morphology of the proximal femur can be divided into three categories [6]:

The CLS System

- trumpet-shaped
- cylindrical
- dysplastic.

The latter can be allocated to one of the other two categories, depending on the individual case (Fig. 2).

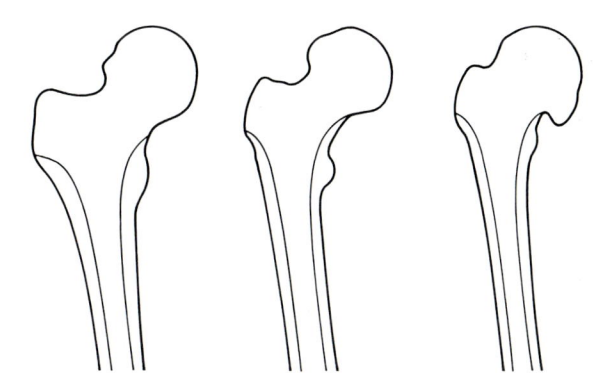

Fig. 2. Subdivision of the morphology of the proximal femur into three categories. *Left*, trumpet-shaped; *middle*, cylindrical; *right*, dysplastic

The diameter of the trumpet-shaped femur in the intertrochanteric region is about twice that of the diaphyseal isthmus with strong cortical bone. It is the ideal femur for the implantation of a non-cemented stem. Its morphology permits the proximal anchorage of a prosthesis of suitable design and results in optimal mechanical stability. This is a fundamental condition for secure biological stabilisation. A morphology such as this also enables us to provide a prosthesis with a relatively small quantity of metal, which takes the physiology of the bone better into account. In creating a prosthesis-bone interface, the elasticity should deviate as little as possible from that of the actual bone. Taking into account the elasticity of the interface, the proximal femur can change shape under physiological loads, something which preserves the trophism and thus contributes to a long functional life [39].

The diameter of the cylindrical-shaped femur in the intertrochanteric area is similar to that of the diaphyseal isthmus, i. e. the medullary cavity is cylindrical and in the case of osteoporotic development there is a thin layer of cortical bone. This is a problem in terms of mechanical stability and necessitates the use of larger implants, which increase the difference between the elasticity of stem and bone. It is a well-known fact that the creation of an interface system, whose characteristic features are greatly influenced by the prosthetic components, has a negative effect on the trophism of the bone.

The indication for the use of a cemented or a non-cemented stem is associated with a complex series of problems which are the subject of wide discussion [29].

Apart from the personal opinion of every surgeon, the reason for this may be found in the diverse factors that have to be considered in the case of each individual patient.

In order to develop the most objective and complete methodology possible, we elaborated a protocol for relative indications in 1985. It was based on the consideration of four clinical and radiological criteria. Each parameter is given a numerical value. The indication is formulated from the total aggregate of the various points [32]. The parameters assessed are age, sex, degree of osteoporosis and the morphology of the femur.

Age

Skeletal changes not only reflect the chronological age of the patient, they also have a real biological significance.

In general and for the purpose of simplicity, we assume that for patients aged 70 years or older a cemented stem – which facilitates rapid and painless rehabilitation – is indicated. The non-cemented stem is typically indicated for patients under 50 years of age.

Point ratings for age are as follows:
Under 50 years: 0 points,
50 – 60 years: 1 point,
60 – 70 years: 2 points,
more than 70 years: 4 points.

Sex

As far as bone quality is concerned, women (in whom there is a progressive incidence of osteoporosis, which is dependent on the hormonal changes that take place in the menopause) are certainly subject to a greater risk.

Point ratings for sex are as follows:
men: 0 points,
women: 1 point.

Osteoporosis

The presence of pronounced osteoporosis makes it more difficult to achieve primary mechanical stability; alternatively, it necessitates the implantation of an oversized stem with a diaphyseal anchorage, which impairs the preservation of the bone trophism. Points can be allocated according to the degree of osteoporosis using various radiological and instrumental methods (computed tomography, densitometry). The system we propose and use is simple in its application and is based on the evaluation of the trabecular adaption of the cancellous bone in the region of the neck of the femur, according to Singh.

We differentiate between four grades of osteoporosis:

The CLS System

physiological (Singh 7): 0 points,
slight (Singh 6–5): 1 point,
moderate (Singh 4–3): 2 points,
severe (Singh 2–1): 4 points.

Morphocortical Index

In our experience, the morphocortical index (MCI) is the most important parameter. The MCI is the ratio of the extracortical diameter, at the level of the middle of the lesser trochanter, to the intracortical diameter, which is measured 7 cm further distal (Fig. 3).

Point ratings for the MCI are as follows:
3.1 or higher: 0 points,
3.0–2.7: 1 point,
2.6–2.3: 2 points,
2.2 or lower: 4 points.

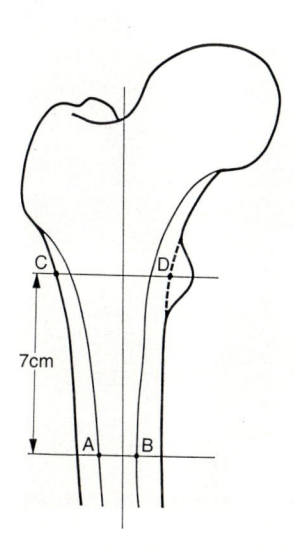

Fig. 3. Measurement to determine the morphocortical index (MCI), the ratio of *CD* to *AB*. See text for details

Final Assessment

On the basis of the points allocated with regard to the four factors that are assessed, the appropriate indication can be determined:
0–4 points, non-cemented stem,
5 points, indication with higher risk,
6 or more points, cemented stem.

Casuistics and Statistical Evaluation

In the following we report the mid- and long-term results obtained with a clinical series of CLS stems. More than 5000 of these stems were implanted in our clinic from 1983 to 1993.

The most interesting aspect of this evaluation is that it shows the results that have been obtained with a prosthetic model with proximal anchorage and a surface which does not offer any possibility for the ingrowth of bone (Fig. 4).

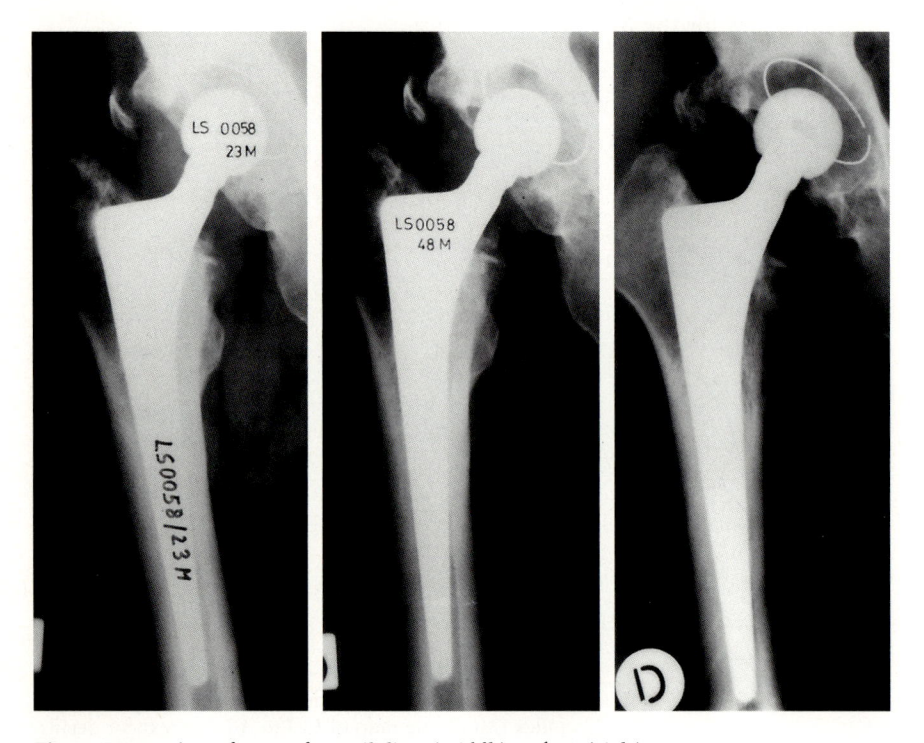

Fig. 4. Integration of stem after 2 (*left*), 4 (*middle*) and 10 (*right*) years

The evaluation of our clinical material was carried out in two periods: the first 300 patients with CLS stems combined with various cups, primarily non-cemented polyethylene and Lord screw-type cups [34] between December 1983 and April 1985, were requested to attend the clinic for a follow-up examination in November 1991. The CLS expansion cup was only combined with the CLS stem in the case of eight of these 300 patients.

The patients with a CLS expansion cup implanted in the period between December 1984 and December 1987 underwent a follow-up examination in

November 1992. This involved a total of 194 patients, in whom the expansion cup was mostly combined with the non-cemented CLS stem (n=171).

These statistics show that the clinical application of the CLS stem was more or less systematic from the very beginning (300 cases in 16 months). The use of the expansion cup was rather limited in the first phase (192 cases in 36 months), due to the minor technical improvement in the shape and the employed material. The average age of patients in the first two series was almost identical, namely 57.5 years for the first and 57.3 years for the second series. For the sake of simplification, the first series is referred to as the "stem series" and the second as the "cup series", even though in the second series the CLS stem was implanted in the majority of the cases.

In the stem series, the ratio of men to women was almost identical (154 women and 146 men), whereas in the cup series (106 women and 86 men) it corresponded to the general sex ratio of patients receiving a prosthesis.

The discrepancy between the two series is associated with the indication that applies for the implantation of the two components, namely that pronounced osteoporosis, which occurs more frequently in women, constitutes a relative contra-indication for the implantation of a cementless stem, but not for a cementless cup. Likewise, in the case of the preoperative diagnosis, some of the data in the two series do not correlate and have to be interpreted in terms of the indication. Rheumatoid arthritis, for example, which is frequently associated with deficient bone quality, was found in 6 % of the cup series and only in 2.5 % of the stem series. On the other hand, the effects of an acetabular fracture were observed in 6 % of the stem series and only in 2.5 % of the cup series. This shows that the expansion cup was implanted in less than half of these cases. As far as the stem series is concerned, 257 cases were followed up clinically and radiologically; 13 patients completed a questionnaire and them forwarded a recent X-ray, 20 patients had since died, seven had undergone a reoperation and three could not be found.

In the cup series, 172 of the 194 cases were followed up clinically and radiologically; six patients answered a questionnaire and sent an up-to-date X-ray, 11 had died, four had undergone a reoperation and one patient could not be contacted.

In short, a complete follow-up was possible with 257 implants in the stem series (average follow-up 82 months) and 172 implants in the cup series (average follow-up 70 months).

Reasons for Reoperation

Of the seven reoperations in the stem series, two were due to sepsis, three to loosening of the stem, one to loosening of the cup and one because of a defective prosthesis conical spigot following the attachment of a non-compatible ball head. Closer investigation of the aseptic loosening of the stem showed that the post-operative radiological follow-up had revealed the use of implants that were too small and were not in accordance with the basic concept. In the case of the third patient, it was established that a traumatic fracture of the femur with immediate subsidence of the prosthesis had taken place 8 months after the stem has been implanted. Four reoperations were performed in the stem series in 1992. One of these was due to sepsis, two to recurrent dislocation and one following rupture of the cup shell. It should be noted that, with the exception of the sepsis patient, no stems had to be changed in the second series.

Clinical Results

The rating scale according to Harris (HHS) was used for clinical evaluation [11]. Good and excellent results were established in 81 % of the stem series and 90 % of the cup series. It is evident that the HHS is influenced by factors that are not directly associated with the prosthetic replaced hip (condition of the other joints, general condition). In this respect, it is important to note that the average HHS rating for unaffected contralateral hips is 94 points, whereas in cases with arthritic hips or in any case with symptomatic opposite hips the score drops to 85.8. The most reliable clinical parameter for the rating of a hip with a prosthesis is related to pain. In the stem series, 84 % of the patients were without pain or only suffered slight, occasional pain (sensitive to weather changes).

In 13 % of the patients, the pain was slight, but constant during walking, and moderate in 2 %. There was no severe and invalidating pain in any of the patients. In 15 % of the patients with slight or moderate pain, the pain occurred in the groin and/or buttocks in 12.8 %, whereas pain was experienced in the upper thigh in only 2.2 %.

In the cup series, the pain-related data was even more favourable: 94.2 % had no or only slight, occassional pain (seven patients with slight pain and four with moderate pain). There were no patients with severe and invalidating pain in the second group either. Pain in the femur was experienced by seven patients, i. e. in 4.1 % of the cases. However, pain was extremely slight and only occurred occasionally in four patients, whereas pain was slight in two cases and moderate in one.

Radiological Results

Of the 272 femoral stems followed up, definite loosening was established in two cases (complete lucent line in one case, subsidence of 10 mm and migration in varus in the other). None of the 160 stems in the cup series showed radiological signs of loosening. Subsidence was established radiologically in four patients in the stem series and in six in the cup series. A significant subsidence (4–5 mm) was found in only one case in the first series and in one case in the second series. In the other cases, the displacement amounted to a maximum of 3 mm. Closer observation of the lucent lines revealed a complete absence in 57 % of the stem series and 85.6 % of the cup series. On the basis of the classifications according to Gruen [10], a high degree of demarcation (four to six zones) or a total demarcation (seven zones) was established in 4.3 % (eight patients) of the first series and in only 1.4 % (two patients) of the second series.

Discussion

The mid- and long-term results achieved with the CLS stem may be rated as excellent, not only clinically but also radiologically (Fig. 5). Of considerable importance is the fact that these results have been achieved with a femoral component whose characteristics are quite different from the other frequently employed designs [30].

It should be remembered that the CLS stem was designed to obtain a predominantly anchorage in the proximal region of the femur, without a macrostructure of its surface [33, 35].

We are convinced that the success of these femoral components is largely due to their three-dimensional wedge, a design which ensures an optimal press-fit in the proximal intertrochanteric region. In pursuing the concept of the press-fit

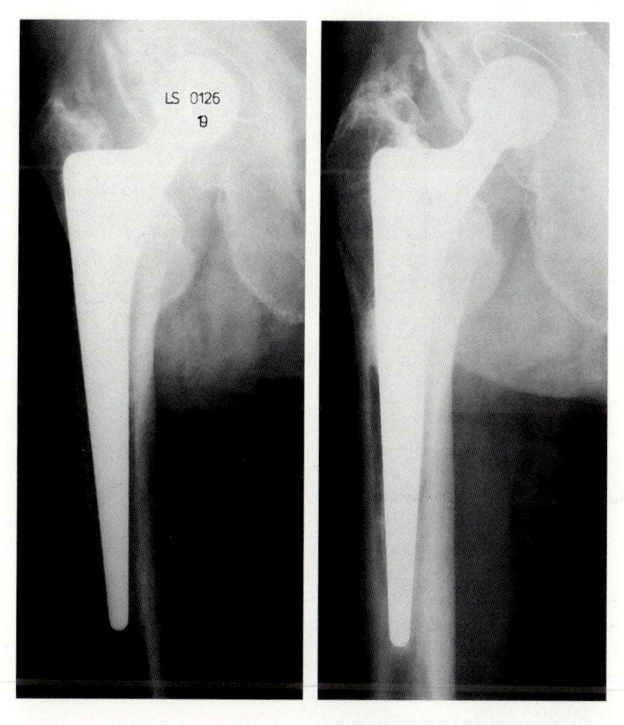

Fig. 5. Radiograph of the right hip 4 months (*left*) and 6 1/3 years (*right*) after the implantation of a CLS prosthesis with a polyethylene cup. Osseointegration with good trophism of the calcar and additional subtrochanteric blockage by new bone formations

and endeavouring to achieve stabilisation by means of viscoelastic deformation of the bony bed through the introduction of a slightly oversized implant of the same shape, we have found that the tapered shape is ideal for stability. The extremely rare occurrence of the stress shielding phenomenon indicates that with this system the proximal femur is somehow stimulated by the geometry of the implant and that the relative elasticity of the titanium alloy probably also plays a role (Fig. 6).

In comparing the two follow-up series, the following must be borne in mind. Apart from the different periods of observation, the better results of the second series can be explained by two factors. Firstly, we must make due allowance for the "learning curve", which may have influenced the indications and also the implantation technique. However, one decisive difference is that the stem in the stem series was combined with different cups (screw-type or non-cemented polyethylene cups), whereas it was always paired with the expansion cup in the cup series.

From the radiological standpoint, the results are excellent in both series, and there where only a few cases of subsidence, stress shielding and significant

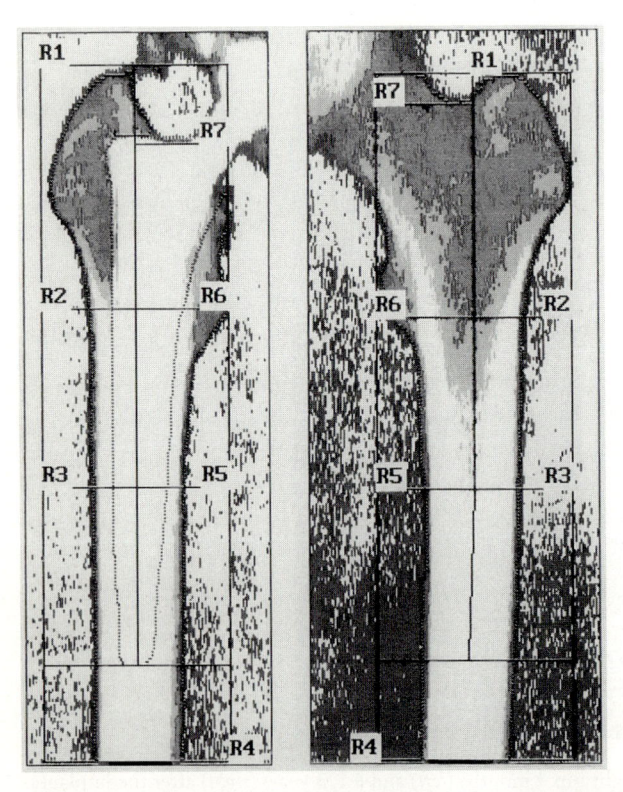

Fig. 6. Densiometry 10 years after the implantation of a CLS stem on the right side. Right panel healthy left hip. The density is comparable in the zone R7

osteolysis in the diaphysis. The only radiologically significant difference between the two series was the pronounced lucent line (always classified according to Gruen), with eight cases in the first series and only two in the second. This factor is now being analysed thoroughly so that the importance of this discrepancy can be explained. The difference might be dependent on the implantation technique, on the pairing of the stem with a different cup and, to a certain degree, on the mechanism of polyethylene wear.

Planning and Operative Technique

In order to create a bone-prosthesis interface which fulfils the prerequisites for primary stability in a patient, sacrifices only a minimum quantity of bone substance and takes the biomechanics of the joints into consideration to a sufficient degree. The operative technique is of primary importance. The preoperative planning and the operative technique are based on the experience that has been acquired with more than 5000 CLS prostheses.

As is confirmed by the studies of numerous orthopaedic surgeons, e. g. Pauwels, Bombelli, Charnley and M. E. Müller, preoperative planning is a generally accepted necessity in orthopaedic surgery.

The fundamental theoretical principles for careful preoperative planning are as follows:
- Preservation (or attempted restoration) of the physiological centre of rotation,
- preservation of a functionally correct relationship between the tip of the greater trochanter, the centre of rotation and the axes of the pelvis (correct tension of the M. gluteus medius),
- avoidance or correction of dysmetria.

On the other hand, the selection of the prosthesis size is part of the specific planning and depends on the concept behind each individual implant. In order to carry out the press-fit technique for the CLS stem and to obtain cancellous bone, thus preventing contact with the cortical bone, there must be an all-round clearance of about 1 mm between the outer limits of the prosthesis on the template and the inner limits of the medullary cavity.

During surgery, the measurements taken preoperatively enable us to determine the correct resection plane and help us to avoid dysmetria. It also makes it easy to establish the presence of a thin cancellous layer medial in a line with the resection plane, a layer that is planned preoperatively. The preservation of this cancellous layer is also proof of the correct positioning of the prosthesis. Nevertheless, to prevent the prosthesis from being implanted in a varus malposition, we should not forget how important it is to remove the cortical bone of the neck of the femur laterally with a small wedge of the greater trochanter. The following contributory factors for the correct centreing of the stem, which is vital for good biomechanical functioning of the prosthesis, still apply:

- The undersized distal end of the prosthesis (to prevent distal load transmission), but long enough to favour self-centreing.
- The resection level of the femoral neck, which is determined during the planning phase (e. g. with increased antetorsion, resection of the femoral neck must be performed nearer to the lesser trochanter).
- Preservation of the cortico-cancellous lamella, which is visible in the region of the calcar isthmus, also favours correct centreing in the sagittal plane. In addition, this cortico-cancellous lamella follows the straight lines and not the anatomical shape of the prosthesis. By preserving this structure, the proximal geometry of the femur matches the tapering shape of the prosthesis, whether right or left.

The geometric shape (taper) facilitates a more linear, easily foreseeable distribution of loads. The reduction of stress concentration is also advantageous from a biomechanical point of view. The CCD angle of 145° is a compromise to reduce the tilting moment. The object of the surgical procedure is to achieve perfect congruency between the prosthetic bed and the prosthesis itself, i.e. a cortico-cancellous "fit". However, the press-fit is not completely responsible for primary stability. We attach a great deal of importance to the pressure exerted during implantation. The surgeon's instinct of knowing just how powerful the blow with the hammer should be is also a constituent part and of fundamental importance for the operative technique. This load usually exceeds that to which the prosthesis will be subjected during the initial postoperative phase (muscle tension in the supine position, partial weight-bearing in the first month). On the other hand, the slight subsidence certainly enables the tapered shape of the prosthesis to attain a spontaneous press-fit.

The tapered shape is to some extent self-stabilising and represents the ideal geometry to maintain the press-fit. Sparing the transformable proximal cancellous bone simplifies the transition from primary mechanical stability to biological stabilisation through osseointegration.

The proximal rib structure constitutes an alternative possibility for the cancellous bone to give way during the impaction of the prosthesis. Moreover, these projections increase the osteophilic area and constitute a favourable geometry for the ongrowth of bone as bony neoformations prefer prominent parts. A further task for the rib structure is the enhancement of rotational stability.

In the latest generation of CLS stems, the ribs no longer form a stump in the proximal area, but are very sharp, in order to further reduce the possibility of fissures in the femur.

The CLS Expansion Cup

The projection of a cup component must take into consideration the physiological model of stress transmission, which is necessary for the biotrophism of bone.

Obviously, due allowance also has to be made for all the other factors, such as the extensive preservation of bone substance, primary stability, rough surface of the implant and the conditions that favour osseointegration [23, 36].

Physiopathology of the Acetabulum

In hip dysplasia the pathogenesis of secondary arthrosis can be explained by the significance of stress concentration in the region of the subchondral bone [37]. Due to the pathological architecture of the acetabulum, the alternating load generated through walking causes fatihue microfractures in the trabecular structure with consequential necrosis [26]. Radiologically, we first observe a subchrondral sclerosis, which gradually spreads to the bone of the ileum. The further development of this pathological process results in a resorption of the necrotic parts with the formation of cysts of a gelatinous character which are filled with connective tissue poor in cells. In turn, resorption leads to the complete disorientation of the subchondral bone with subsequent disintegration and loss of sphericity. Similar observations were made in the case of implanted non-cemented cups of the first generation. These cups were of a spherical shape and showed a very high degree of inherent rigidity, which explains the sclerotic reaction, cyst formation and loosening with migration of the acetabular components that result from stress concentration [13]. The reasons for the failure of the cemented cups are quite different [22]. This experience led to the search for a biocompatible cup system with a specific elasticity which would enable the system to transmit the forces acting on the three bones of the pelvis in a way comparable to the physiological model. Polyethylene, with its impact-damping effect, seemed to be an especially suitable material. However, its low osteophilic properties led us to seek other solutions with coatings. Rough-blasted titanium appeared to be the best coating or rather the ideal

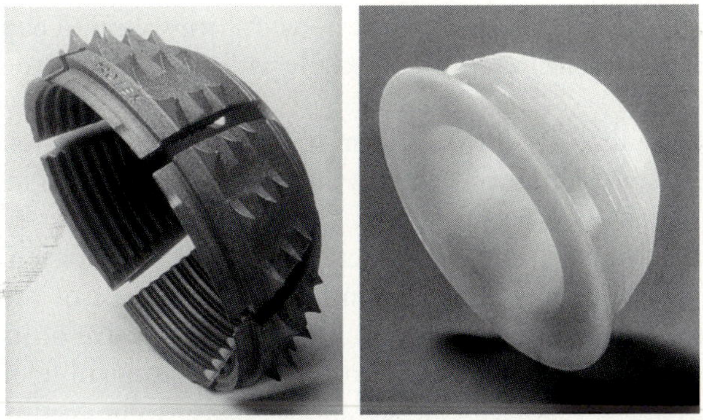

Fig. 7. The expansion cup consists of an elastic anchorage shell made of PROTASUL-100, with six lobes in a star-like arrangement with anchorage cusps and a polyethylene insert that can be screwed in

"metal-back". To avoid stiffening of the system, we subdivided the metal shell into six lobes, which are only joined in the pole area (Fig. 7). The basic shape of the shell is a slightly flattened hemisphere, which increases the equatorial distribution of forces; it is introduced into the acetabulum in a compressed state [14]. Since the outer diameter at the ends of the fixation cusps in the compressed state corresponds to the diameter of the acetabulum, the shell can be located in the desired position.

Release of the setting device causes the radially acting forces to press the fixation cusps of the titanium shell onto the bone. The insertion of the expansion cone expands the lobes radially, causing the full length of the fixation cusps to penetrate into the bone. Stable fixation and good tilting moment resitance are thus achieved. The implant is anchored primarily. The bearing insert corresponds exactly with the inner shape of the anchorage shell. The polyethylene insert has a flat rim, which, when inserted, covers the edge of the shell and thus prevents possible damage to the ball head.

Primary mechanical stability is achieved by real expansion, i. e. by means of an actual press-fit. Consequently, the manner in which the forces are transmitted to the pelvis is similar to that of the physiological kinetic model [14]. A test undertaken by the Biomechanical Institute of the M. E. Müller Foundation seems to confirm that the expansion cup is more suitable for the physiological transmission of forces than traditional hemispherical cups. With this test arrangement, three strain gauges were positioned around the acetabulum, each of them in the vicinity of one of the three pelvic bones, to measure the natural pelvis and a pelvis with the prosthesis. The relative micromovements were analysed by means of a simulated gait pattern. The natural pelvis showed a cranial displacement of 127 µm of the iliac strain gauge, whereas the strain gauges located on the ischiatic and pubic rami tended to come closer together. This corresponds to a jaw-like occlusion of these two bones and consequently a braking action on the head of the femur and thus a deviation of the forces with a decrease in the load at the level of the iliac bone. Apart from the absolute values of 125 µm the expansion cup exhibits a similar behaviour. A hemispherical cup with a high rigidity behaves quite differently, especially as far as the ischiatic and pubic rami are concerned.

The interpretation of these tests seems to confirm the phenomena observed with dysplastic hips. The lateral dislocation deprives the head of the femur of its normal loading characteristics. As a result, it does not allow the forces to be distributed to the ischium and pubis, and causes a cranial stress concentration. Likewise, the stiffening resulting from calcification and osteophytosis of the Lig. transversum is also a disturbing factor of joint kinetics. Irrespective of its shape, a cup prosthesis with excessive rigidity can reduce the functional life of the implant in various ways. The reported considerations seemed to be confirmed by the clinical, radiological and histological results obtained after more than 8 years' clinical application. Attention is drawn especially to the extremely low occurrence of lucent lines in zone III (according to Delee-Charnley).

Of particular importance is the phenomenon of the remodelling (functional adjustment) of the periprosthetic bone, which was observed during follow-up (Figs. 8, 9). It seems that the CLS expansion cup is not only capable of preserving the normal trophism of the periprosthetic bone, but also enables the cancellous structure to normalise itself once more with a reduction or disappearance of the subchondral sclerosis, as well as enabling the cysts to dissappear without having to use bone grafts during surgery. We even observed radiologi-

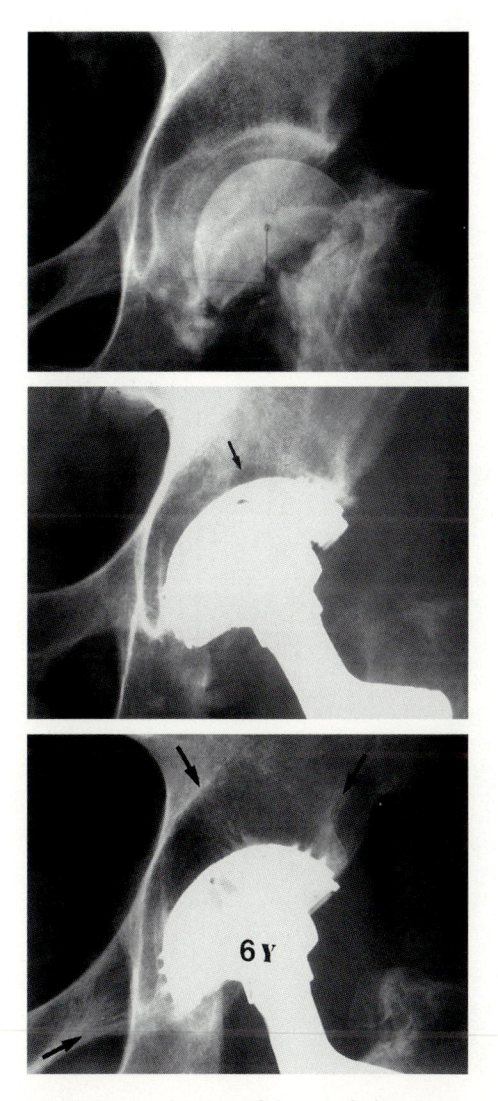

Fig. 8. Normalisation of the acetabular structure 6 years after the implantation of an expansion cup. *Top,* preoperative. *Middle,* postoperative. *Bottom,* after 6 years

cally an intensification of the trabecular structure in the presence of severe osteoporosis, whereby the trabeculae had oriented themselves to all three pelvic bones in accordance with the equatorial distribution of forces.

To sum up, we believe that the preservation of biotrophism is a fundamental prerequisite for the success of a prosthesis. It appears to be possible to attain

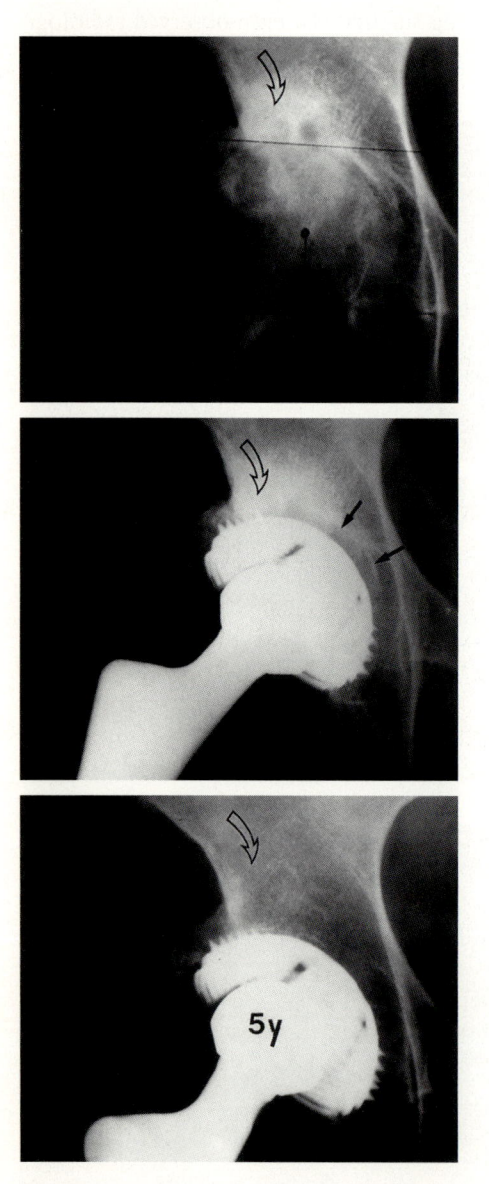

Fig. 9. Normalisation of the bone structure after the implantation of an expansion cup. *Top*, preoperative. *Middle*, postoperative. *Bottom*, after 5 years

and maintain this biotrophism, the basis of which is formed by various elements:
- A very high initial stability, which is attained through expansion, whereby the three rows of fixation cusps penetrate into bone over the circumference of the acetabulum to provide high rotational stability and tilting resistance.
- The press-fit produces a stable circumferential compression which, thanks to the microstructured titanium surface, quickly results in osseointegration and thus gives the implant a biological and lasting stability.
- The metal shell prevents direct contact between the polyethylene and the bone. The stability of the cup, i.e. the shell with the polyethylene insert, which is attained by means of screw insertion, is durable as long as the conditions for correct insertion are observed. Tests in the simulator with 5 million cycles have not revealed any polyethylene wear on the insert-shell interface.

However, it is obvious that the life expectancy of an implant is also influenced by other variables. The aspect most discussed at present is the search for a compromise, namely the combination of rigid materials with low degree of wear and polyethylene with a favourable modulus of elasticity, but with a high degree of wear. In this context, we investigated the current compromise Tribu-SUL, which resulted from tribological research and which provides for a pairing of polyethylene of a very high molecular weight with metal, a particularly favourable surface.

On the basis of experience gained so far, this approach appears to be feasible, because it is relatively rare that the radiological follow-ups performed after 8 years with normal methods reveal directly measurable wear of the polyethylene. On the other hand, we have learned to attach importance to other indirect indications, changes which occur especially on the femoral side and in our experience progress slowly. With the arising suspicion that polyethylene wear impairs the proximal anchorage of the stem, it would appear advisable to seak solutions or improvements in the tribological field and thus to develop an implant with sufficient residual elasticity so that the biotrophism of the periprosthetic bone is still influenced in a favourable manner. The technological progress made in the processing of materials now facilitate extremely interesting metal-metal pairings. Nevertheless, in view of the possible toxicity caused by metal abrasion, which has not been definitely dispoved so far, we shall have to view this solution with both confidence and caution. Only time will tell, although laboratory investigations have found the advantages of such metal-metal pairing to be quantitatively significant. Our development trends point to the manufacture of a cup whose metal insert retains a relatively residual mobility. One metal-metal cup is already available in this phase of development: it features a metal insert which is fixed to the outer shell of the cup by the interpositioning of polyethylene.

Indications

There is currently no cup prosthesis available which is suitable for every situation. However, the CLS expansion cup is suitable for a wide range of indications, even though a great deal depends on the operative technique as well as the acquired skill of the surgeon concerned. It is also possible to use the expansion cup for reoperations in the case of severe defects of the bottom of the acetabulum and, likewise, for primary implantations in patients suffering from severe osteoporosis or moderate hip dysplasia.

Consequently, it seems more expedient to emphasize the contraindications. Of particular importance is the need to obtain a peripheral anchorage and a stable press-fit. A relative contra-indication exists if a small segment of the circumference of the acetabulum is missing, and an absolute contra-indication if the defect accounts for one quarter or more of the circumference. However, if the defect is less than one sixth of the circumference, it is compensated for by the system and no special measures are necessary. It is also possible to implant the expansion cup if the defect is more than one sixth, but does not exceed one

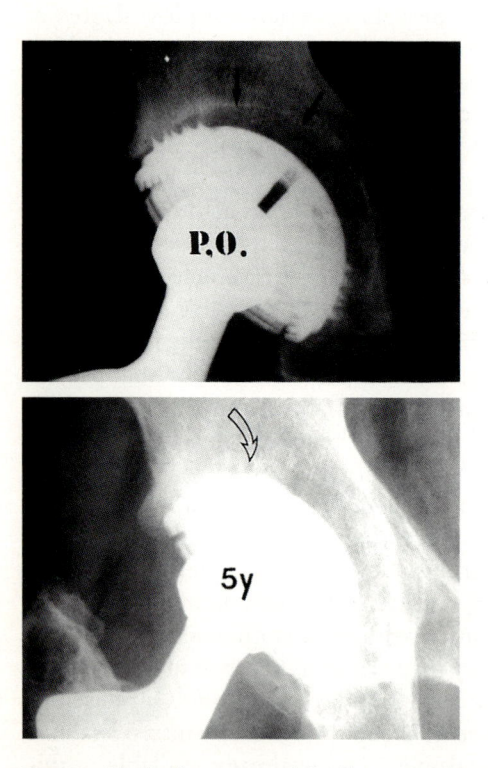

Fig. 10. The hollow space originally present between the bottom of the acetubulum and the pole of the expansion cup has been bridged by trabecular structure. *Top,* postoperatively. *Bottom,* after 5 years

quarter of the circumference. In such cases, the positioning of the lobes has to be performed with particular attention. None of the six lobes should remain without support in vital bone. From the biomechanics of the pelvis, we know that the greatest concentration of stress occurs in the posterocranial region of the acetabulum when a patient rises from the sitting position, for which due account must be made if there is a bone defect in this zone.

In summary, the expansion cup can be implanted with good results in all forms of idiopathic coxarthrosis, in femoral head necrosis and in rheumatoid arthritis. The expansion cup has also proven very successful in protrusions (Fig. 10), dysathrodeses and in conditions following acetabular fracture; the advantage is that the material of internal fixation can usually be retained. Restraint must be exercised, however, in cases of reoperation and dysplasia, where good results can still be obtained with correct planning and careful positioning.

Preoperative Planning and Operative Technique

As in the case of the stem, planning is done using the anteroposterior X-ray of the pelvis. The axial direction has to be accounted for in both cases. The objective of planning must be to preserve the physiological rotation centre or to restore it, with a minimum loss of bone substance. A compromise quite often has to be accepted in practice. The contact between the cup and acetabulum must be as large as possible, even if we have to put up with a slight medialisation of the rotation centre and possibly sacrifice part of the subchondral bone. From the functional aspect, the latter is "replaced" by the metal shell, because the shell is anchored peripherally and the press-fit acts antiprotrusively.

In the presence of a central osteophyte, it is possible to plan the reaming depth necessary to attain a physiological position of the acetabulum, i.e. to determine the quantity of bone to be removed. A piece of osteophytic bone, large enough to enable the reaming depth to be defined, can be removed with a hollow chisel or hollow reamer during surgery. Reaming is continued until the cavity made with the chisel or reamer is no longer visible.

It is advantageous to select a surgical approach (posterolateral or transgluteal) which facilitates a clear view of the acetabulum. In particular, the acetabular rim must be fully exposed. The soft parts have to be resected and any osteophytes removed. Complete exposure is necessary to enable the metal shell to be inserted correctly and then fully expanded. Likewise, the insertion of the polyethylene insert can then be carried out correctly without the interpositioning of any soft parts. A clear view of the cup edge facilitates the control of the equatorial anchorage and the penetration of the anchorage cusps.

With sclerotic bone, some of the cusps may not penetrate completely into the bone. In such cases, the maneuver using the expansion cone can be repeated. Experience has shown that any remaining gap is filled during the course of osseointegration.

With osteoporotic bone, however, it is advisable not to insert the expansion cone right up to its final position; complete expansion is then carried out using the polyethylene insert.

In summary, the most important operative steps are as follows:
- Clear view of the acetabulum
- Removal of an osseous cone above the incisura acetabuli (or at least in a central position) to serve as a basis for reaming and to determine the depth of reaming
- Initial reaming of the acetabulum with a reamer which is at least 4 mm smaller than the planned cup size
- Step-wise continuation of reaming, until the desired diameter is attained (e. g. 50-mm reamer for 50-mm cup)
- Checking of the acetabular rim (osteophytes) and the complete sphericity of the bony bed
- Exact positioning of the completely closed shell with the setting device (the shell must reach the bottom of the acetabulum)
- Checking of the coverage and the anteversion, whereafter the jaws of the setting device can be released
- Insertion of the expansion cone with moderate pressure
- Insertion of the polyethylene insert with strong axial pressure

The peripheral equatorial primary anchorage is decisive for secondary stability and lasting adhesion, as the structures are most powerful here and an anchorage in this zone also acts antiprotrusively.

References

1. Blaha JD, Spotorno L, Romagnoli S (1991) CLS press-fit total hip arthroplasty, Techn Orthop 6 3: 80–86
2. Bobyn JD, Mortimer ES, Glassman AH, Engh CA, Miller JE, Brooks CE (1992) Producing and avoiding stress shielding Clin Orthop 274: 79–96
3. Bombelli R, Santore R (1983) The morphology and classification of osteoarthritis: an anatomical and biomechanical perspective. J Rheumatol [supp] 9: 10
4. Buser D, Schenk RK, Steinemann S, Fiorellini JP, Fox CH, Stich H (1991) Influence of surface characteristics on bone integration of titanium implants. A histomorphometric study in miniature pigs. J Biomed Mater Res 25 (7). 889–902
5. Christel PS (1992) Biocompatibility of surgical-grade dense polycrystalline alumina. Clin Orthop 282: 10
6. Door LD, Faugere MC, Mackel AM, Gruen TA, Bognar B, Malluche HH (1993) Structural and cellular assessment of bone quality of proximal femur. Bone 14: 231–242
7. Eggli PS, Müller W, Schenk RK (1988) Porous hydroxyapatite and tricalcium phosphate cylinders with two different pore size ranges implanted in the cancellous bone of rabbits. A comparative histomorphometric and histologic study of bony ingrowth and implant substitution. Clin Orthop 232: 127–38
8. Engh CA, Bobyn JD, Glassmann AH (1987) Porous-coated hip replacement. J Bone Joint Surg [Br] 69: 45–55

9. Engh CA, McGovern TF, Bobyn JD, Harris WH (1992) Quantitative evaluation of periprosthetic bone – remodeling after cementless total hip arthroplasty. J Bone Joint Surg [Am] 74: 1009–1020
10. Gruen TA (1987) Radiographic criteria for the clinical performance of uncemented total joint replacements. In: Lemous JE (ed) Quantitative characterization and performance of porous implants for hard tissue application. ASTM STP 953. American Society for Testing and Materials, Philadelphia, pp 207–218
11. Harris HW (1969) Traumatic arthritis of the hip after dislocation and acetabular fractures: treatment by mold arthroplasty. J Bone Joint Surg [Am] 51: 737–755
12. Haynes DR, Rogers SD, Hay S, Pearcy MJ, Howie DW (1993) The difference in toxicity and release of bone resorbing mediators induced by titanium and cobalt-chromium-alloy wear particles. J Bone Joint Surg [Am] 6: 825–834
13. Hodge WA, Carlson KL, Rijan RS, Brugess RG, Riley PO, Harris WH, Mann RW (1989) Contact pressures from an instrumented hip endoprosthesis. J Bone Joint Surg [Am] 71 9: 1378–1386
14. Huggler AH, Schreiber A, Dietschi C, Jacob H (1974) Experimentelle Untersuchungen über das Deformationsverhalten des Hüftazetabulums unter Belastung. Z Orthop 112–144
15. Hunt JA, Remes A, Williams DF (1992) Stimulation of neutrophil movement by metal ions. J Biomed Mater Res 26 6: 819–828
16. Jacobs JJ, Skipor AK, Black J, Urban RM, Galante JO (1992) Release and excretion of metal in patients who have a total hip-replacement component made of titanium-base alloy. J Bone Joint Surg [Am] 73 10: 1431–1432
17. Kilgus DJ, Shimaoka EE, Tipton JS, Eberle RW (1993) Dual-energy X-ray absorptiometry measurement of bone mineral density around porous-coated cementless femoral implants. J Bone Joint Surg [Br] 75: 279–287
18. Linder L (1989) Osseointegration of metallic implants. I. Light microscopy in the rabbit. Acta Orthop Scand 60 2: 129–134
19. Lord G, Bancel P (1983) The madreporic cementless total hip arthroplasty Clin Orthop 176: 67–76
20. Marchant RE, Anderson JM, Dillingham EO (1986) In vivo biocompatibility studies. VII. Inflammatory response to polyethylene and to a cytotoxic polyvinylchloride. J Biomed Mater Res 20 1: 37–50
21. McCarthy CK, Steinberg GG, Agren M, Leahey D, Wyman E, Baran DT (1991) Quantifying bone loss from the proximal femur after total hip arthroplasty. J Bone Joint Surg [Br] 73: 774–778
22. Morscher EW (1992) Current status of acetabular fixation in primary total hip arthroplasty. Clin Orthop 274: 172–193
23. Pauwels F (1976) Biomechanics of the normal and diseased hip. Theoretical foundation, technique and results of treatment. Springer, Berlin Heidelberg New York
24. Ganz R, Perren SM, Rueter A (1975) Mechanische Induktion der Knochenresorption. Fortschr. Kiefer Gesichtschir 48–48
25. Poss R, Walker P, Spector M, Reilly DT, Robertson DD, Sledge CB (1988) Strategies for improving fixation of femoral components in total hip arthroplasty. Clin Orthop 235: 181–194
26. Johnston RC, Brand RA, Crowninshield RD (1979) Reconstruction of the hip. A mathematical approach to determine optimum geometric relationship. J Bone Joint Surg [Am] 61 5: 639–652
27. Santavirta S, Konttinen YT, Bergroth V, Gromblad M (1991) Lack of immune response to methyl methacrylate in lymphocyte cultures. Acta Orthop Scand 62 1: 29–32
28. Santavirta S, Nordstrom D, Ylinen P, Konttinen YT, Silvennoinen T, Rokkanen P (1991) Biocompatibility of hydroxyapatite-coated hip prostheses. Arch Orthop Trauma Surg 110 6: 288–292

29. Santavirta S, Gristina A, Konttinen YT (1992) Cemented versus cementless hip arthroplasty. A review of prosthetic biocompatibility. Acta Orthop Scand 63 2: 225–232
30. Sarmiento A, Gruen TA (1985) Roentgenographic analysis of 323 STH total hip prostheses (a low modulus titanium alloy femoral component). A two to six year follow up. J Bone Joint Surg [Am] 67 1: 48–56
31. Semlitsch M (1989) Twenty years of Sulzer experience with artificial hip joint materials. Proc Inst Mech Eng 203 3: 159–165
32. Spotorno L, Schenk RK, Dietschi C, Romagnoli S, Mumenthaler A (1987) Unsere Erfahrungen mit nicht-zementierten Prothesen. Orthopäde 16: 225–238
33. Spotorno L, Romagnoli S, Ivaldo N (1990) The Cementless CLS stem. In: Kusswetter W (ed) Noncemented total hip replacement. International Symposium Tübingen. 198–212
34. Spotorno L, Romagnoli S, Ivaldo N, Grappiolo G, Bibbiani E (1992) La crescita ossea nella protesi non cementata. Atti I Congresso Nazionale A.I.S.O., 79–82, Ott. 1992
35. Spotorno L, Morasso V, Romagnoli S, Ivaldo N, Grappiolo G, Bibiani E, Blaha DJ, Gruen TA (1993) The CLS system theoretical concept and results. Acta Orthop Belg 59 [Suppl]: 144–148
36. Van Syckle PB, Walker PS (1980) Parametric analysis of design for acetabular components of surface replacement hip devices. Trans Orthop Res Soc 5: 292
37. Vasu R, Carter DR, Harris WH (1982) Stress distributions in the acetabular region-i. before and the after total joint replacement. Joint Biomech 15: 155–164
38. Weinans H, Huiskes R, Grootenboer HJ (1990) Trends of mechanical consequences and modeling of a fibrous membrane around femoral hip prostheses. J Biomech 23 10: 991–1000
39. Zweymüller KA, Lintner FK, Semlitsch MF (1988) Biologic fixation of a press-fit titanium hip joint endoprosthesis. Clin Orthop 235: 195–206

The Cementless CLW System

D. Weill

CLW Threaded Cup

Together with the late Otto Frey we have been concerned with the development of our own, cementless self-tapping cup since 1982. We report our personal experience gathered over a period of 10 years. During this time the author has implanted more than 2100 of these CLW cups.

Philosophy and Description of the Implant

The tapered ring is made of pure titanium (PROTASUL-Ti). It has no bottom and is therefore less rigid. Consequently the acetabular bottom can be viewed through the ring throughout the implantation, and the volume of the implant is reduced accordingly (Fig. 1). Originally the surface of the ring was smooth and had a stairlike profile. In a second phase, however, since 1985, the profile has been given a truncated cone shape. The outer surface is roughblasted, the inner fine blasted. This truncated cone shaped ring has sharp, self-tapping laminar threads which penetrate into the subchondral bone of the acetabulum and thus ensure the primary anchorage of the implant. The work of Ungethüm and Blomer [5] indicates the particular suitability of the tapered shape not only for neutralizing the tilting moment but also for transmitting the load. The outer region of these slim lamina is elastic; therefore they can compensate to a certain degree for pelvic micromotion.

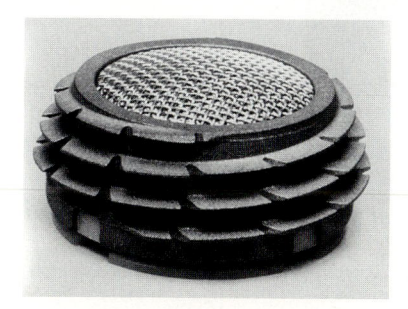

Fig. 1. CLW threaded cup. The convexity of the polyethylene insert is SULMESH coated

A polyethylene insert, also of truncated cone shape, is fitted in this metal ring with adhesive friction. The insert has a collar which lines up with the height of the joint. Furthermore, it covers the rim of the ring and prevents contact between the ball head and the titanium (e.g., in case of dislocation). The arch shaped dome is coated with a titanium net made of SULMESH. This prevents direct contact between polyethylene and bone and also reduces the deformation of the convex zone in weight bearing. It also improves the view of the bone/implant interface during radiological checks.

Only mechanical stability was assured with the first generation of rings, with their smooth surface. The change to a rough-blasted surface, which favors osseointegration, has influenced the long-term fixation and the results. Rough blasting of the surface in contact with bone facilitates osseointegration, i.e., direct bone contact, as well as an induction of load via a suitable bone structure.

Biomechanical Principle

Excellent primary stability is assured by the tapered shape and the pronounced threaded lamina, which facilitate an effective screw attachment. The structured surface also helps to neutralize the danger of loosening in the sense of unscrewing. Special conical reamers and the systematic grafting with autologous cancellous bone facilitates the optimal adaptation of the implant to the trimmed acetabulum. The primary stability achieved by means of the screw insertion is superceded by osseointegration. The large rough-blasted contact area between bone and implant, that is between the taper and the lamellar threads, favors the on-growth of bone, i.e., osseointegration. The large contact area also reduces the occurence of stress peaks between implant and bone. The marked protrusion of the lamellar threads is an important factor for osseointegration because expe-

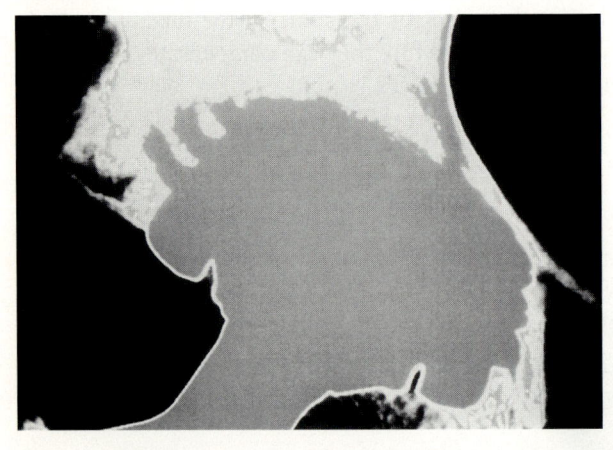

Fig. 2. Radiograph scan. Increased density of bone structure at the level of the lamellar thread

rience with various acetabular cups and femoral prostheses shows that osseointegration is usually favored on prominent parts of the implant (Fig. 2).

The experience gathered during the development of a threaded cup has enabled us to define various positive and negative factors. Negative elements include a hemispherical shape, insufficient height of the screw-thread pitch, excessive rigidity, and a smooth surface that does not allow any effective osseointegration. Positive factors include a tapered or truncated cone shape, effective lamellar threads, reduced rigidity (pure titanium, no bottom, relatively elastic lamellar threads), and a rough-blasted osteophilic surface. Confirmation of the actual occurence of osseointegration, which is important in achieving a cementless implantation, has been provided with a series of histological examinations by R.K. Schenk.

Range of Available Implants

Nine rings are available, with diameters of 44–66 mm in 2 mm steps. They are suitable for use with two inserts with outer diameters of different size. One of these fits rings of 44–48 mm and the other rings of 50–60 mm. Small inserts fit with the 28 mm prosthetic head and large inserts the 28 or 32 mm heads. We always use inserts with an inner diameter of 28 mm. Polyethylene inserts are also available, with an inner diameter of 22 mm. In addition, there are cup inserts with a radial, semilateral increased height of 10°. We also have paired inserts with METASUL inlays with METASUL heads for experimental purposes. The follow-up time for this metal/metal pairing is still too short to report results using it.

Instrumentation

Specific instruments are available for the implantation, including conical reamers, whose outer shape exactly matches the rings.

Operative Technique

The operation must be performed with care and precision. The size of the implant is determined preoperatively with the respective templates. The ultimate size of the implant is determined during surgery when the acetabulum is reamed. Transgluteal approach in supine position, resection of the femoral neck and head, and exposure of the acetabulum: The latter is to be prepared with particular care, the fossa acetabuli to be freed of soft parts and osteophytes. The acetabulum is reamed with hemispherical reamers until bleeding subchondral bone is reached. The exact shape is realized with the conical reamer, which is of the same diameter as the last employed hemispherical one. The acetabulum is reamed along the course of the future implant, improving penetration of the cup and precise implant/bone-fit (essential, from finite element analysis of the CLW cup by Huiskes [3]). The resection of additional bone material due to the use of a conical reamer is very limited.

Preparation with the conical reamer results in a circular ridge on the acetabular bottom. This can be removed normally during a final application of the hemispherical reamer of the same size. The prepared acetabulum is now checked with test rings. The diameter of the ultimate implant is usually 2 mm smaller than that of the last used reamer. In certain cases, when the bone is severely osteoporotic or relatively cancellous, a threaded cup of the same size may be implanted. The insertion is made with an inclination of 45° and an anteversion of 5 to 10°. An aiming device ensures the correct position. The attachment for this device is available in two versions, one for the supine and the other for the lateral position. The ring is easily inserted at the beginning, but the resistance increases quickly prior to complete blockage in the acetabulum. The ring must penetrate completely, a condition that can be checked through the inside of the bottomless ring. If the ring blocks before reaching the required depth of penetration, it must be removed, the acetabulum reprepared, or a smaller ring inserted.

When the final position is reached, the acetabular bottom is padded with bony pulp before introducing the insert. If a gap remains between the upper pole of the ring and the acetabular rim, it must be grafted.

During the preparation it is essential to preserve the anterior wall of the acetabulum. In dysplasia the anterior wall can be spared, namely by accentuating the reaming in dorsal direction. If this is not possible, the use of a threaded cup is contraindicated.

Indications

The studies by Amstutz [4] indicate the importance of bone quality for the use of threaded cups. We consider a more or less normal anatomy, good bone quality, and protrusions as a good indication for primary implantations. Rheumatoid arthritis and dysplasia are relative but justifiable indications; the operative technique must be carried out with particular care. Severe osteoporosis and serious dysplasia are contraindications [6, 11]. To ensure stable primary anchorage of the implant in revisions, this technique may be considered only for patients with bone of reasonable quality and quantity. In our clinical practice, the CLW cup is used for approximately 80 % of primary arthroplasties.

Peri- and Postoperative Complications

These complications were rare and do not depend on the peculiarities of the implant. Nevertheless, technical errors led to injury of the tabula interna in 23 cases in the early days, and postoperative luxations were experienced in 2 % of the patients. These were reduced without any recurrence.

Postoperative Care

Patients are allowed to get up on the third postoperative day and can – with the aid of two crutches – subject the operated leg immedialtely to partial load for a period of 3 weeks.

Results

Our series consists of more than 2100 implants; the maximum follow-up is more than 10 years. Of these, 648 were performed more than 7 years and 1109 more than 5 years ago [7–9 15]. Our report concerns the 556 oldest followed cases, which include 312 smooth and 244 rough-blasted threaded cups. The implantations were performed between 7 and 10 years ago. The difference between smooth and rough-blasted threaded cups is of decisive importance – their results differ substantially and probably explain the majority of failures experienced with other threaded cups.

We have been through two periods. The first phase was with smooth rings and only hemispherical reamers, excessive alignment of the implant with an inclination of 30°, and a liberal indication in cases requiring revision surgery (Fig. 3). In the second phase, since 1985, we have used rough-blasted rings and special

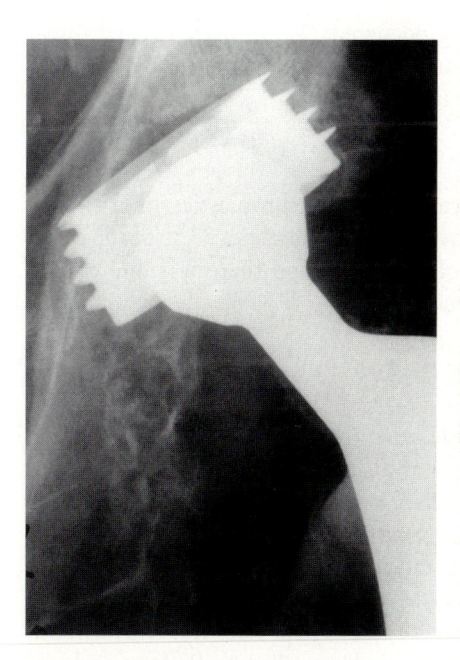

Fig. 3. A first-generation CLW treaded cup (smooth surface) at 10 years' follow-up

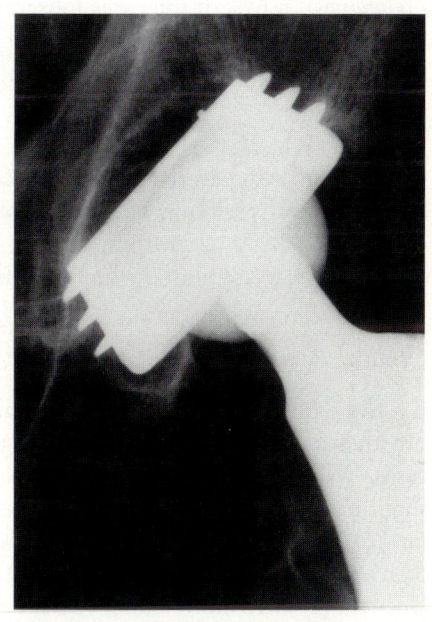

Fig. 4. A CLW threaded cup with rough-blasted surface and SULMESH-coated polyethylene insert at 7,5 years' follow-up

conical reamers, an inclination of 45°, and restricted revisions to patients with good bone quality of the residual acetabulum (Fig. 4). The results differ significantly.

In the radiological follow-up we attach great importance to identification and observation of lucent lines. A fine, non progressive lucency in zone III is without pathological significance, but a progressive lucency in zone I or II is pathological. We also pay special attention to possible migration and we rate the increasing normalization of the periprosthetic bone structures is a sign of good biomechanical acceptance of the implant and evidence of effective osseointegration with lasting stability.

Radiological Results

Radiolucent lines. In this series there were 79 cases of radiolucency among the 556 threaded cups. With the rough-blasted threaded cups this figure drops to 3 %, and almost all of these were non pathological radiolucent lines located in zone III.

Migrations. Migration occured in 8 % of the cases. With rough-blasted threaded cups this number sank to 0,5 %.

Loosenings. In 6 % of the cases loosening occurred. With rough-blasted threaded cups it was only 0,5 %. In addition, the percentage of loosenings with rough-blasted surface was 0,5 % compared with the 10 % of the series with smooth surface.

Ossifications. As in every series of non cemented hip arthroplasties, ossifications are by no means seldom. These were mostly asymptomatic in 33 % of the cases, severe in 6,5 % (2 % with impairment of function), and there was one case of extra- articular ankylosis, which required revision.

Clinical Results

On the whole the results are comparable with those obtained with cemented prostheses. Mobility: flexion over 90° and abduction more than 20° in 92 % of cases. Walking without crutches: 90 %. Pain: no pain in 82 % of the patients; slight pain occurring from time to time, but not necessitating the use of analgetics, 13,7 % (total 95,7 %); in 3,4 % comparatively severe pain, with 0,9 % severe pain – a sign of instability. It is interesting to compare our results with those of Decoulx [2] after more than 5 years. Perfect radiological stability: with smooth threaded cups 75 %; with rough-blasted threaded cups 99,5 %. Perfect implant/ bone interface: with smooth threaded cups 69,7 % with rough-blasted threaded cups 98,5 %. There is a significant difference between the results of smooth and rough-blasted threaded cups. Long-term results are excellent with rough-blasted cups if the indication and the operative technique are absolutely correct.

Conclusion

Experience over more than 10 years and the implantation of 2100 CLW cups shows the major differences in concept and operative technique as well as in the results obtained with the various threaded cups. With the elaboration and refinement of the operative technique, the introduction of special conical reamers, and the creation of a surface that promotes osseointegration the CLW cup shows excellent long-term results.

CLW Stem

Together with the engineer Otto Frey we developed a cementless femoral prosthesis made of forged titanium alloy in 1983. It has a proximal rotation-stabilizing wing and a pronounced distal slot. This slot reduces, the rigidity and thus enhances the transfer of load. The author has implanted some 700 of these CLW stems, whose maximum service life is more than 10 years. Of these, 261 prostheses were implanted 7 years and 442 more than 5 years ago.

Concept

This prosthesis is made of the forged titanium alloy PROTASUL-100. It is relatively long and slender and has no collar. The proximal wing ensures high rotational stability. Further characteristics are the distal slot, the pronounced longitudinally structured profile, and a rough-blasted surface, which favors the secondary stabilization by osseointegration [1].

A harmonious transfer of load prevents the proximal bypass and distal concentration of stresses. It is due to a rigidity which decreases continually from proximal to distal and particularly by a certain deformability in the distal part of the stem. This improves the transfer of stresses from the prosthesis to the femoral diaphysis. The stabilization is effected over a large area, and the primary anchorage is fundamentally proximal. The length of the rectangular stem facilitates automatic centering, which is almost always possible in the anteroposterior and the axial plane (Fig. 5).

The investigation of a generated model with the finite element method and also later radiological findings have confirmed the theoretical biomechanical concept. Distal anchorage of the stem must be avoided whatever the case. Its consequences are well known: pain, distal hypertrophy of the corticalis with proximal atrophy, and cancellization of the proximal femur.

Since the CLW stem is very slender and relatively long, it is appropriate for the continuous decrease in the rigidity of the bone/implant interface from

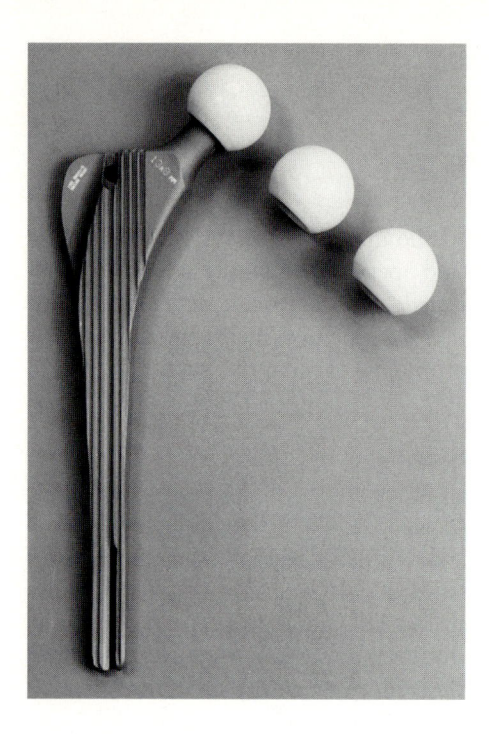

Fig. 5. CLW stem

proximal to distal. The amply dimensioned distal slot reduces the rigidity of this part. In the finite element model the greatest stresses occur in the middle and distal part of the femur, namely at a level of 220–99. The dark gray color of the corticalis can already be seen between the levels 113–99 and also further distally. This dark gray color signifies a stress of between 40 and 100 Nmm^{-2}. It also means that the transfer of the stresses to the corticalis is harmonious at a level with the prosthetic slot, a condition which has not been observed in any other rigid prosthesis. A light gray color (14–20 Nmm^{-2}) can not be seen over almost the whole corticalis. There are also stresses of 1–4 Nmm^{-2} in the prosthetic slot itself, a stress that enhances the formation of cancellous bone trabeculae, which is also visible in X-rays.

In our opinion the clearly reduced rigidity of the prosthetic tip is decisive. The need of a harmonious transition of the femur proximally stiffened by the prosthesis to the normal elasticity of the diaphysis is also met because the calculation with the finite element method of a femur without prosthesis produces almost the same picture of the distribution of stress at level 99. This slowly decreasing rigidity of the bone/implant compound from proximal to distal may also explain the absence of thigh pain and the fact that stress shielding with associated distal hypertrophy of the corticalis was not observed after correct implantation (Fig. 6).

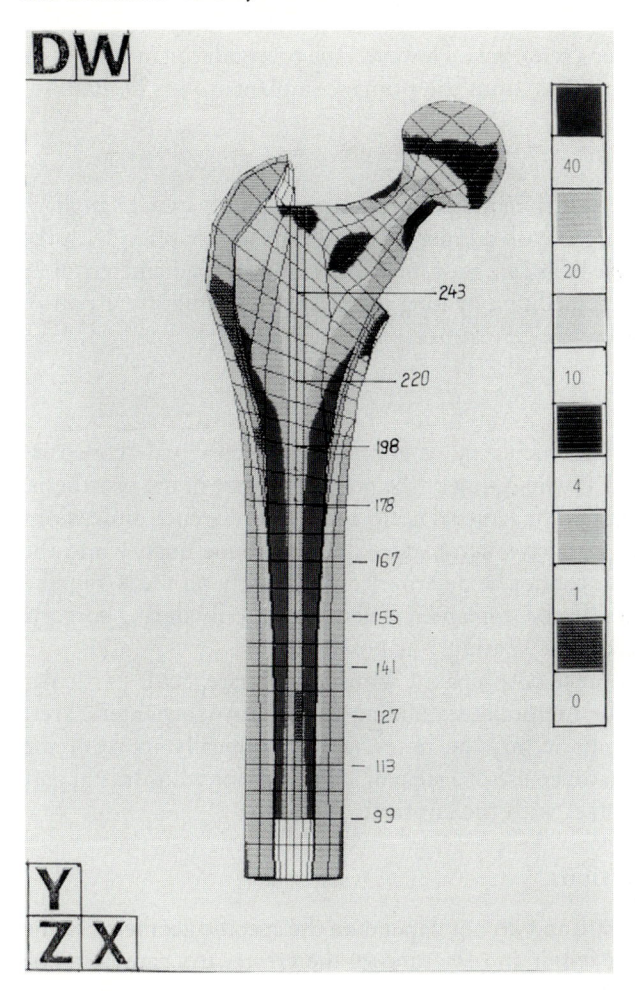

Fig. 6. Finite element analysis of a CLW shaft in a normal femur (1750 N)

Indications

We use this stem for approximately 35 % of primary total hip replacements. Shape, bone quality, age of the patient, severity of osteoporosis (according to Singh), and the morphocortical index must be considered. This stem is particularly suitable for cylindrical femora. With trumpet-shaped femora it is necessary to ream distally to avoid an undersized prosthesis and to prevent distal jamming in the dyaphisis. A particular shape of the femur (varus, antecurvatum) and insufficient bone quality (osteoporosis, rheumatoid arthritis) are contraindications. This stem gives good results in revisions because its specific shape facilitates the transfer of load over a wide area. However, the precondition in such cases is that the bone defect resulting from the primary implantation is limited.

Range of Available Stems

The stem is available in ten different sizes, from 6 to 15, with a CCD angle of 135°. The stems have a spigot with a taper of 12/14 mm for coupling with the ball head. Alternatively the balls can be of metal or ceramic with diameters of 28 or 32 mm, and with short, medium, or long neck. The most important part of the specific instruments are the ten rasps.

Operative Technique

The preoperative planning, which may be considered as the actual "construction drawing," is made on a plain X-ray of the pelvis. The size of the prosthesis, neck length, resection level of the femoral neck, and other reference dimensions are determined with the respective templates. Since the bone quality and the antecurvature of the femur cannot be determined sufficiently on the X-ray, the actual size of the prosthesis to be implanted is determined only during surgery. The femoral neck is resected as sparingly as possible.

The medullary cavity must be prepared with utmost care, with particular attention to the bed for the rotational stabilizing wing in the trochanteric area. In a trumpet-shaped femur it may be necessary economically to ream the medullary cavity to facilitate the use of a stem of sufficient size whose distal part does not make direct contact with the corticalis.

Perioperative Complications

These complications are rare and do not depend on the specific geometry of the prosthesis. Fissures of the femur and fractures of the greater trochanter can be avoided with a precise operative technique and proper preparation of the bony bed for the stabilisation wing.

Results

Our report concerns 277 cases of a series of 700 stems implanted in a period of between 7 and 10 years [12–14].

Radiological Results

- Pronounced periarticular ossifications in 6 %, but in general without any clinical effect (one patient with periarticular ankylosis had to be reoperated on).
- Hardly any change in the structure of the corticalis in 96 %, thickening in 2,5 % and partial cancellization in 1,5 %.
- Periprosthetic radiolucency with loosening: 1 %.

- Migration: none in 99,5 %, subsidence in 0,5 % (traumatic).
- Loosening: 2 %.

The very modest changes in the structure of the corticalis are remarkable. This fact confirms the good biomechanical acceptance of the implant by the femur (Fig. 7).

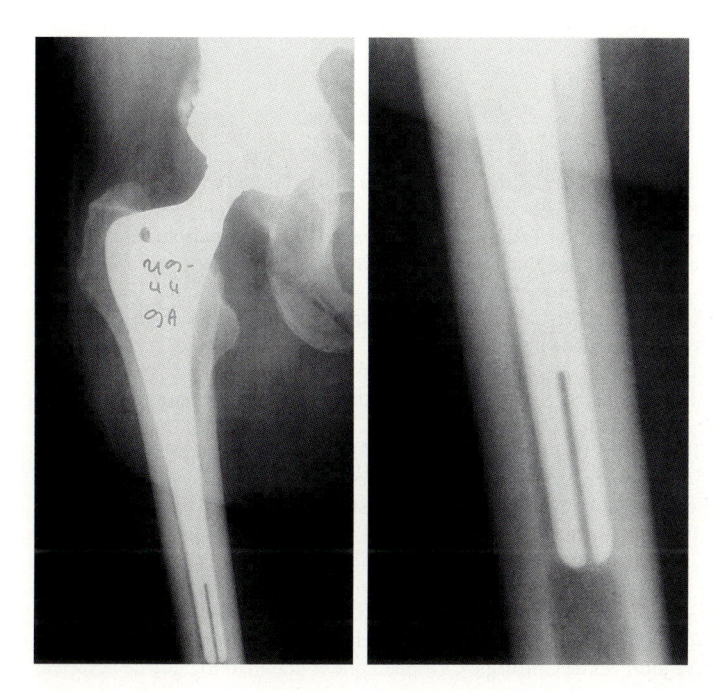

Fig. 7. At 9 years follow-up. **a)** Normal aspect of cortical bone and osseointegration. **b)** Detail of the distal region. Normal cortical bone, good osseointegration and newly built trabecular bone also in the slot of the prosthesis

Clinical Results

No pain: 85 %; slight pain from time to time: 10 %; stable hip: 85 %; no limping in connection with the prosthesis: 90 %; flexion equal or greater than 90 °: 90 %; pain in thigh, which usually disappears within 6 months: less than 5 %; subjective results good and very good: more than 90 %. The failures which led to revision (2 %), were usually associated with technical errors or with an incorrect indication (stem too small, insufficient bone quality). Overall, our results are therefore satisfactory. Under normal circumstances we attain absence of pain after a period of 3–4 months, and this condition is sustained.

Conclusion

The good results achieved with this stem can be attributed to its specific geometry, the decreasing rigidity from proximal to distal, and the rough-blasted titanium surface. The maintainance of femoral biotrophism with subsequent osseointegration leads to biomechanical acceptance of the implant and to its long-term stability.

References

1. Amstutz MC (1985) Arthroplasty of the hip. The search for durable component fixation. Clin Orthop 200: 343–361
2. Decoulx J, Laffargue P, Kapandji T, Thomas R, Chevance E (1993) Etude au dela de 5 ans des réactions osseuses autour des anneaux cotyloïdiens vissés en titane de type Weill dans une série de 810 prothèses totales hybrides de hanche. La Journée de Lille, 17 june
3. Huiskes R (1987) Finite element analysis of acetabular reconstruction. Non cemented threaded cups. Acta Orthop Scand 58: 620–625
4. Kody M, Kabo JM, Markolf KL, Dorey FJ, Delaunay C, Amstutz H (1990) Fixation mécanique initiale des anneaux vissés. Communication à la 64e réunion annuelle de la S.O.F.C.O.T. Rev Chir Orthop 76 [Suppl 1]: 83–84
5. Ungethüm M, Blomer W (1986) Biomechanische Aspekte zementfreier Hüftpfannen-Implantate mit Schraubverankerung. Med Orthop Tech 6: 194–197
6. Weill D (1986) Reconstruction du cotyle par greffe osseuse et anneau vissé autotaraudant non cimenté CLW. Acta Orthop Belg 52: 332–343
7. Weill D (1986) Cotyle vissé sans ciment CLW (et prothèse fémorale non cimentée expérimentale CLW) Etude préliminaire. Ann Orthop Traum 9: 65–77
8. Weill D (1986) Cotyle vissé sans ciment CLW. Ann Orthop 18: 126–131
9. Weill D (1987) Cotyle vissé sans ciment CLW et prothèse fémorale non cimentée expérimentale CLW. XVe Journées de Chirurgie Orthopédique et Traumatologique de l'Hôpital Bichat
10. Weill D (1991) Qualités et défauts des cotyles vissés. A propos d'une série homogène de 1400 implantations de cotyles CLW avec un recul maximum de 7 ans. 65e Réunion annuelle de la S.O.F.C.O.T. Rev Orthop 77 [Suppl 1]: 145
11. Weill D (1987) Reconstruction du cotyle par greffe osseuse et anneau vissé autotaraudant non cimenté CLW. In: Poitout D (ed) Greffes de l'Appareil Locomoteur. Masson, Paris, pp 160–169
12. Weill D (1991) Prothèse fémorale non cimentée CLW: à propos d'une série homogène de 600 implantations avec un recul maximum de 7 ans. Livre des Résumés – Congrès Européen de la S. O.T. Est, Troyes, 31 may, 2 june: p 17
13. Weill D (1992) Prothèse fémorale non cimentée CLW: à propos d'une série homogène de 600 implantations avec un recul maximum de 8 ans. Journées Communes de la S.O.F.-C.O.T. et de la S.P.L.O.T., 8–10 april
14. Weill D, Majidi-Ahi A, Auduy H, Bronner JF (1993) Prothèse fémorale non cimentée CLW: à propos d'une série homogène de plus de 650 implantations avec un recul maximum de 8 ans et 6 mois. Acta Orthop Belg 59 [Suppl 1]: 149–152
15. Weill D, Auduy H, Majidi-Ahi A, Bronner JF (1993) Le cotyle vissé CLW: Expérience personnelle de plus de 1900 implantations avec un recul maximum de 9 ans. Acta Orthop Belg 59 [Suppl 1]: 256–259

The Development of the Cementless Hip Endoprosthesis: 1979-1994

K. Zweymüller, F. Lintner, G. Böhm

Introduction

From the very beginning, the development of hip endoprostheses was governed by the wish for simple surgical technique, a minimum of implants, and maximum long-term stability of the artificial hip joint. The original route pioneered by Charnley and McKee is still valid today. The objective of every operation was optimum mechanical fixation, provided, according to the then state of the art, by the shape of the implant and the physical properties of the bone cement. It was only later that the term "biological fixation" was introduced, not least due to the work of Lintner [10] in the area of the histo-pathology of the cement interfaces and the clinical and experimental knowledge from dental implants provided by Albrektsson et al. [1]. This term was understood to mean the best long-term fixation of implants using own bone tissue through osseointegration. This biological acceptability could be achieved, however, only with the use of optimally biocompatible materials with a suitable surface structure and excellent primary fixation. Afterwards, the destiny of the implant depended upon the in- and ongrowth of own bone tissue, providing secondary fixation, the amount of loading due to patient behavior, and additionally upon wear and usage characteristics. Particularly the latter dictated the ultimate functional limit of hip endoprostheses.

First Generation of Stems

Our real experience in implants with cementless fixation began at the start of the 1970s. At that time the first step away from bone cement in the therapy of coxarthrosis was taken with the metal-ceramic prosthesis [22]. In this case a ceramic ball head was articulating in a conical cup with supporting "feet". The stem was cemented in the conventional manner. The logical further development with a view to doing without bone cement completely came in 1977 when, in cooperation with the Istituto Ortopedico Rizzoli in Bologna, a small series of ceramic-coated titanium stems were implanted without cement [5]. Here the stem cross-section was elliptical in the proximal area and round in the central and distal areas. The experience gained with the Rizzoli stem, particularly with regard to surgical technique, convinced us of the correctness of the selected methodology, but at the same time there were weak points regarding material and shape. The collaboration with Sulzer started in 1978 and made possible the interchange of our own experience with that of the experienced metallurgists and development engineers there. The first implantation of the new stem generation was made in the autumn of 1979.

The most important experience gained from the use of the Rizzoli stems was the fact that a round stem cross-section which almost completely fills the medullarary cavity is unsuitable. This is because it does not accomodate the anatomy of the proximal femur with its double curvature. In addition, the opening up of the femur with a rigid round drill often weakened the cortical bone in an uncontrollable way, causing an unacceptably high percentage of fractures. For this reason a wedge stem shape with rectangular cross-section was chosen from the start. Previous experimental investigations on cadavers in the spring of 1979 showed not only a negligible risk of fracture but also surprisingly good primary fixation of the implants, especially against torsional loads. An

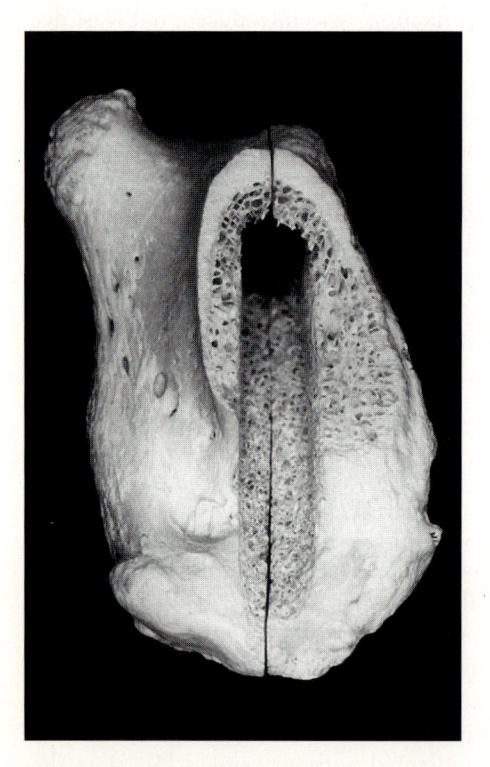

Fig. 1. Anatomical specimen after preparation of the proximal femur with the rectangular rasp. The major part of the dorsal neck cortical bone at the resection plane (*left*) ist retained. Following preparation, the bone was cut open exactly in the forntal plane

additional deciding factore, however was the study of the anatomy of the proximal third of the femur. The double curvature of the femur, the so-called anteversion-anteflexion and the ante curvature of the diaphysis, visible in every axial radiograph, permits the insertion of only a straight object without major destruction of the prexisting cortical bone when the diameter in the sagittal plane is small, i.e., when the cross section is rectangular.

There are a number of other advantages of rectangular wedge-shaped fixation as follows.

1. The dorsal femoral cortical bone can be retained in the area of the resection line of the femoral neck due to the relatively flat rectangular shape (Fig. 1). Fixation of the implant using a cortical structure is thus achieved directly upon entry of the prosthesis into the osseous cavity. This structure, which is important for the proximal fixation, is completely destroyed in the case of other prostheses intended to fill the medullary cavity or which represent cast models of the proximal femur, such as computer-generated custom prostheses.

2. A straight stem with a rectangular wedge-shaped cross section does not completely fill the medullary cavity of the femur. Because of this, portions of the endostal blood vessel supply are able to be maintained, which is very important for the formation of new bone structures. Avascular necrosis of inner sections of the cortical bone are thus not expected. The osseous cavity for the stem is prepared with sharp rectangular wedge-shaped rasps having the same shape as the prosthesis and inserted exactly along the longitudinal axis of the femur. This avoids the damage due to heat which can occur when using rotating medullary cavity drills. The use of sharp rasps also for the preparation of the cortical bone is to ensure that the fixation of the implant occurs using a larger area of direct bone contact. Fixation should thus not be at isolated points but across a larger surface.

3. The press-fit of a wedge-shaped straight stem ensures safe fixation under torsional loads. According to Plitz [21], the stability of a rectangular cross-section in torque is about nine times higher than that for a stem with a round cross-section. The relatively sharp edges of the implant play a central role here. Fears that bone resorption will occur in the area of the edges due to stress peaks have not materialized.

   The significance of the four edges of the implant becomes apparent in revision operations. In such cases, there remains practically no more cancellous bone but in most cases a thin eburnated cortical bone. Rasps are used in an attempt to cut a bony seat to receive the implant. In most cases the contact of the prosthesis edges in the cortical bone is sufficient to achieve a new stable primary fixation.

Originally the stem was wedge-shaped only in the frontal plane [27, 30]. In the sagittal plane the stem was thinner in its proximal third, with the intention of removing factors which might lead to splitting the bone (Fig. 2). This thinner

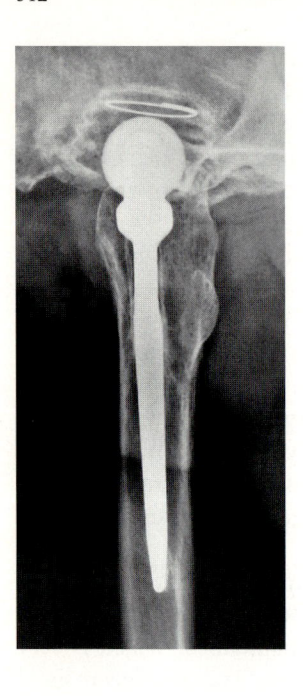

Fig. 2. Condition following implantation of the first generation titanium straigth stem. Axial view picture, 7 years postoperative. The stem is thinner proximally, showing a radialocent line, ventral and dorsal, down to the widening of the stem, with a double profile, ventral and dorsal, up to the widening of the stem

section was later gradually abandoned and with the introduction of the SL stem in 1986 replaced by a wedge form in the sagittal plane [31, 32]. The implant fixation thus occurs over large areas but even with the introduction of the second wedge form never fills the medullary cavity (Fig. 3). For a wedge-shaped straight stem with a rectangular cross-section it is evident that even a small surface is sufficient for absolutely stable primary fixation.

Experience with the first generation of wedge-shaped straight stems was good. Cementless fixation using the described principle proved biologically possible and could be maintained over a longer period of time [12, 15] (Fig. 4). Cementless fixation also differs in principle from cemented fixation inasmuch as implant integration increases with time after the operation. The comparison of ten each specimens with implantation times of up to 4 years and 5–7. 3 years showed significant differences in the bone-implant contact index, as described by Böhm et al. [2, 3](Tables 1, 2). It should be noted that in the majority of these cases the stem was used in combination with a polyethylene cup having direct cementless fixation in bone. The occasional missing or clearly lower coverage index in the most proximal segments can be explained by foreign body granulation tissue as a result of polyethylene wear between bone and cup.

Despite these inaccuracies due to polyethylene wear affecting the osseous tissue response in the most proximal stem areas, there appear to be differences in integration behavior between proximal and distal. The ability of the bone to bridge iatrogenic defects is considerably less in the cancellous bone area of the femoral neck and the trochanter than in the distal cortical bone area (Fig. 2).

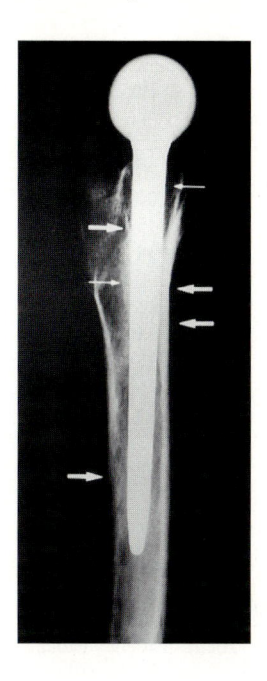

Fig. 3. Condition following implantation of an SL titanium straight stem. This has a continuous wedge shape in the sagittal direction. The proximal part of the stem thus has better fiaxation in the surrounding bone than in Fig. 2. *Large arrows*, implant contact with coritcal bone; *small arrows*, contact with cancellous bone. There is thus also direct proximal-dorsal contact with the femoral neck cortical bone (see also Fig. 1)

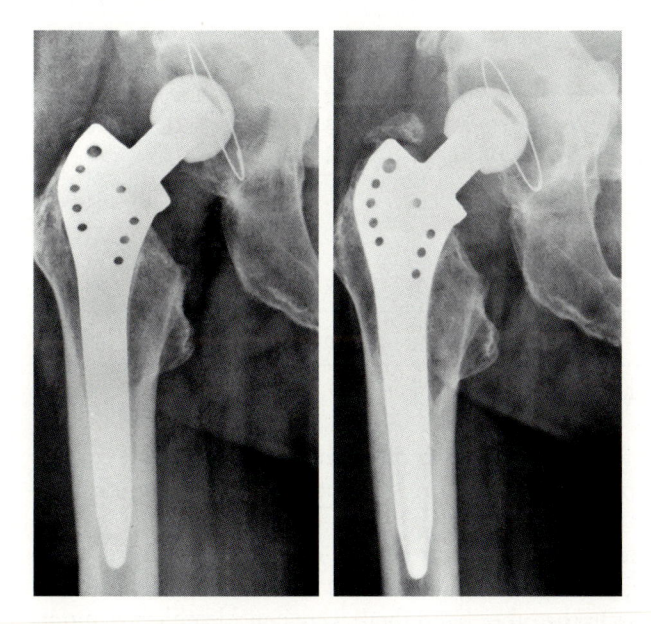

Fig. 4a, b. A 66-year-old man. **a** Condition following implantation of the first-generation wedge-shaped straight stem. One year postoperative. In this case the polyethylene cup was cemented. **b** Condition 13.5 years postoperative. Unchanged good implant fixation, no formation of radiolvcent lines, no indication of loosening

Table 1. Bone-Implant Contact Index – BiCi. Implantation period: 1,8–4,0 years.

Segment	Patient 1 (1.8 years)	Patient 2 (2.5 years)	Patient 3 (3.0 years)	Patient 4 (3.5 years)	Patient 5 (4.0 years)
1	40	00	00	00	00
2	49	77	11	28	00
3	39	48	34	33	45
4	49	56	62	31	38
5	50	77	65	35	50
6	49	72	77	38	45
7	58	68	65	46	44
8	73	76	73	47	48
9	72	68	65	61	76
10	63	79	60	54	81
Mean	54	62	51	37	49

Index mean, 49,5 %, bone coverage of the implant surface

Table 2. Bone Implant Contact Index – BiCi. Implantation period 5,0–7,3 years.

Segment	Patient 1 (5,0 years)	Patient 2 (5,0 years)	Patient 3 (5,3 years)	Patient 4 (5,5 years)	Patient 5 (5,5 years)	Patient 6 (5,8 years)	Patient 7 (6,0 years)	Patient 8 (7,1 years)	Patient 9 (7,3 years)	Patient 10 (7,3 years)
1	00	00	57	00	00	79	77	00	00	00
2	00	28	84	48	00	92	50	49	00	17
3	94	94	74	73	80	86	57	41	20	85
4	89	92	95	74	68	75	73	65	74	70
5	89	90	93	85	47	93	52	73	92	79
6	82	87	88	85	40	82	56	67	86	86
7	95	89	94	95	53	95	62	82	89	85
8	94	93	92	93	81	92	70	92	76	77
9	95	92	92	96	70	93	95	95	88	94
10	97	95	96	94	84	95	98	90	92	85
Mean	74	76	86	74	52	88	69	65	62	68

Index mean, 71 %, bone coverage of the implant surface.

The integration of the prosthesis tip, which often ends up far from the cortical bone, cannot, however, be explained by bridging of a large jumping distance [15].

The clinical and radiological follow-up studies of the first series of stem showed on the one hand, that not enough stem sizes were available to be able to offer a complete system. On the other hand there were considerable size jumps between short and long versions. Implanting the optimum model occasionally caused intraoperative problems. Further, the proximal thinning in the sagittal plane was seen to be counterproductive with regard to fixation in this area.

Combined with the threaded polyethylene cup, these factors led to postoperative thigh pain in a considerable number of cases. As a result of this the proximally thinner cross-section was gradually abandoned, without-being able to remove the other weaknesses.

The Stepless Stem

On the basis of the above experience the original form of the stem as used from 1979 on was developed further in 1986 into the so-called stepless (SL) stem. The SL stem was a wedge-shaped straight stem with a rectangular cross-section as before, and therefore nothing in the principle of fixation was changed. However, it had a continuous sagittal wedge shape. The size differences between the individual stems were no longer arithmetically determined but were based on so-called growth factors, where the differences were smaller in the smaller sizes and more pronounced in the larger sizes. Increasing stem sizes were not only longer and wider, but also thicker and thus also had increased stem surface [32].

Growth-based increases were also developed for neck lengths and trochanter areas. The problems of lateralization in the smaller sizes and medialization in the larger sizes were solved. The trochanter wing had shown itself over the years to be extremely useful on account of its proximal press-fit contribution to a considerably better proximal primary stability. The introduction of the SL stem coincided with a change in the alloy used. The Ti-6Al-4V alloy was replaced by Ti-6Al-7Nb, substituting the toxic vanadium with biocompatible niobium [23].

With the introduction of the SL stem, in combination with the cementless titanium threaded cup, the problem of thigh pain was a thing of the past. A review of our own midterm clinical and radiological stability results of a series of consecutive 96 cases after a follow-up period of at least 5 years showed no replacements and radiologically not a single case of loosening [9]. The first objective of the development of a prosthesis without cement fixation was therefore achieved, inasmuch as results were obtained which were well worthy of comparison with the short- and midterm results from cemented endoprostheses.

Surface Structure

The implant surface of the first generation stems was characterized by a macrostructure designed for secondary fixation due to the ongrowth of bony tissue, rather than for primary fixation. Together with the four edges of the implant, longitudinal grooves about 2 mm deep were provided. The pathological and histological results obtained from this macro structure showed that, although they were in fact filled up later with bone, there was no or little bone contact in the first postoperative weeks.

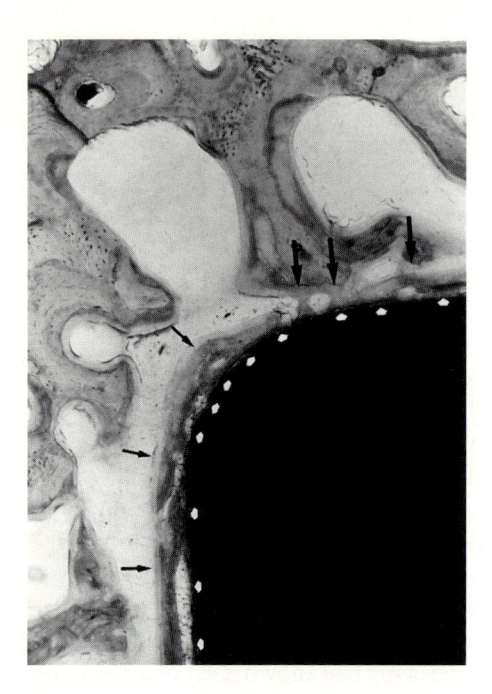

Fig. 5. A 79-year-old woman, 2.5 years postoperative. Cross-section in the metaphyseal region of a stable implanted SL stem. New formation of bone, initiating from preexisting interfacing bone, with bony ongrowth onto the implant surface (*large arrows*), and without the involvement of the interfacing bone surface (*small arrows*). The intimate contact of the ongrown bone with the rough implant surface can be seen (*small white arrows*)

Although fixation occurred at the implant edges and in those areas where there was a flat surface, the bone jumped over deep grooves in the surface. The longitudinal grooves therefore had no effect on the secondary osseous fixation starting immediately postoperatively. Rather, they reduced the primary contact area at the osseous interface and were thus counter-productive [11].

With the introduction of the SL stem and the pure titanium threaded cup shell, not only the macrostructure but also the microstructure was changed. Based on the above results, the grooves were abandoned. The new average micro-structure of 3–5 µm was the same as for the cup shells.

The growth of new osseous tissue begins immediately postoperatively, starting from the existing osseous interface and from bone particles, and this tissue adapts to the surface of the prosthesis and fills the unevenness (Fig. 5). Compared with the macrostructure, secondary fixation by the formation of new bone tissue leads to much earlier contact with the implant, which is osseointegrated by the coverage with new bone tissue in large areas after only a few wecks. It is thus very difficult to remove a well-implanted stem after about 2–3 months. The same applies for cups [12, 31].

Further Development of fhe SL Stem

The SL stem used since 1986 has proven itself in more than 50.000 cases. As a matter of principle has the senior author for years conducted every operation without patient selection. Without exception, therefore, every primary operation is carried out without the use of bone cement. This procedure also appears to be the only way to obtain reliable information on the value of the methodology.

The continuing search for ways further to improve the implant has led us recently to make changes to the stem, as for the cup. A modified SL stem has therefore been in use since the start of 1993, with the intention of improving the fixation in the proximal femoral section. A new form was developed for the calcar area, using the so-called calcar polynomial formula. The intention of this is to reduce the gap which sometimes remains between the implant and the medial-proximal femoral cortical bone. Together with the trochanter wing, this change thus represents an improvement of the proximal press-fit, provided by the increase in fixation surface in the proximal third of the femur (Fig. 6).

The use of the SL stem over the years has also shown that cementless fixation has good chances of success for revision operations, whether for loosened cemented or cementless prostheses. Following removal of toxic noxae in the form of foreign body granulation tissue and/or implant instability, the bone has the capability for regeneration. In cases of proximal destruction of the cortical

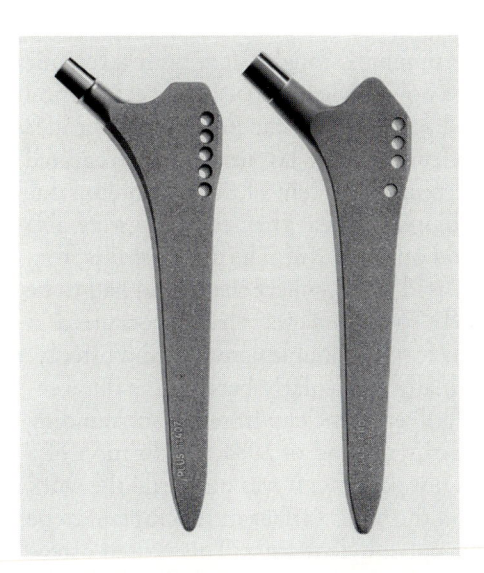

Fig. 6. Comparison of SL stems (*right*) and SL-plus (*left*). The SL-plus stem exhibits a changed proximal form, consisting essentially of an increase in volume in the calcar region. Using more surface of proximal press-fit, the implant thus has better fixation

bone due to loosening processes or previously implanted long-stem models, however, a long-stem model is desirable.

The SLR stem was specially designed for revision operations, based on the decision to transfer the fixation to a more distal region of the femoral diaphysis. It was therefore important that the fixation shape should not simply be a lengthened version of an existing SL or SL-plus stem. A new concept was therefore developed for the area of the prosthesis tip. The trochanter wing was also reduced, taking account of the frequently observed widening of the medullary cavity. In many cases having a trochanter wing as large as is necessary for primary implantations would necessitate cutting through the lateral-proximal cortical bone structures, leading to an additional weakening of the stem support area [34].

Nine sizes are available in the revision stem system, with lengths from 180 mm to 223 mm. This system is therefore suitable for the treatment of bone destruction up to 8 cm distal of the trochanter minor. The principle we have adopted, in contrast to that favored in the United States, is to include also the bone which surrounded the original implant in the fixation of the revision implant. This stem system can thus be used in the great majority of revision cases. The use of special systems or tumour prostheses is necessary for more distal bone destruction.

The Cup Implant

From October 1979 to March 1980 the titanium straight stem with a ceramic ball head was used in combination with a polyethylene cup using direct fixation in bone, and from March 1981 a threaded polyethylene cup [6, 7]. The basic idea behind the use of cementless polyethylene fixation lay in the then required relative isoelasticity, in particular concerning movement of the acetabulum due to load changes when walking. These biomechanical characteristics were also the basis of the Morscher cup concept and others [8, 18]. The initial results from the conical threaded polyethylene cups used by us, where the thread had to be precut in the bone, were good. Relatively soon, however, changes occurred in the surrounding osseous structure, in the form of double contours and osteolysis. We were unable to detect these originally particularly because the differentiation of the radiologically transparent polyethylene cup from the surrounding bone was difficult. However, it was clear by the end of 1984 that fixation of a polyethylene implant directly in bone is not possible. It was primarily the work of Lintner [13, 14] that the destruction on the outer surface of the implant to be caused mechanically, leading to massive polyethylene wear. This caused osteolysis of the surrounding osseous structure of the cup, and secondarily also of the stem [15]. The pathomechanism causing the loosening of polyethylene implants found by Lintner was also confirmed by others, but only much later.

From January 1985 a self-cutting pure titanium cup shell came into use [28]. The conical form of the implant was retained because this has clear advantages over hemispherical cups as regards resistance to tilting and the ability to apply prestressing during implantation. Additional fixation screws are therefore unnecessary. In recent 3 years the author has treated all primary patients but one operated by him with this implant. It was found in all cases that the primary stability was sufficient, so that additional cement fixation was not necessary. A further advantage of the conical cup form is that the polyethylene inlay can be controlled better than in a hemispherical cup [20]. Unoccupied screw holes carry with them the risk that polyethylene will penetrate into the recesses due to cold flow.

The prerequisite for achieving stable primary fixation is the exact preparation of the osseous interface in a conical form. In nearly all cases, with the exception of protrusion arthrosis, it is beneficial to carry out a medialization in the direction of the lamina interna. Implantation of the metal shell in the area of the cup osteophytes, with the selection of too big an implant, is thus avoided. In dysplasia arthrosis with a frequently occurring double acetabular floor it is essential to carry out an optimum medialization extending right up to the lamina interna, which thus helps to avoid having to use the resected femoral head as an extension of the cup roof.

The microstructure of the cup shell surface, which is 3–5 μm, as is the stem, has shown itself to be very good. With ongrowth processes analogous to those on the stem, microstructure ingrowth processes on the cups start immediately postoperatively, leading to secondary implant fixation by means of osseointegration.

The thread blades forming the macrostructure achieve the intended primary stability with prestressing. They also serve as starting points for the secondary osseous fixation (Fig. 7). The frequently expressed fears that bone resorption would occur in the area of the thread blades due to stress peaks have not materialized. The results after 5 years from our own material can be considered positive [9]. Müller was able to show in an ambitious follow-up investigation that the failure rate is extremely low, adding that his clinic is a training clinic with implantations carried out by up to 30 surgeons.

The osseointegration of cups was not only of interest for primary operations. It was obvious to consider this implant also for revision operations to replace loosened cemented or cementless cups. The observed formation of new bony substance as with stems occurs only with firmly implanted cups. The achievement of primary stability is therefore also a sine qua non for revisions. This stability must be sufficient, even in a hip immobilization cast, to prevent subsidence or tilting of the implant.

Further Development of the Conical Threaded Cup

The titanium threaded cup shell first used in 1985 has been implanted in Europe in several 10 000 cases. Despite the prevalent opinion in the United States that a conical cup is not the solution, there is very valid evidence that this fixation principle is very significant.

The repeated criticism of the strictly conical cup form compared with hemispherical cups was that more medial bone resection was necessary. Another problem was faced in several cases where, due to very hard subchondral bone, it was not possible to screw the cup shell in far enough that it was in contact with the reamed cup floor. It was felt necessary that all thread blades should cut fully into the bone, which was often impossible where the bone was very hard. However, as primary stability is also achieved in these cases, and the formation of new bone structure begins at the tips of the thread blades, this represented no disadvantage in particular with regard to the permanent fixation [16].

Both the unnecessary bone resection at the base of the cup and the occasional difficulty in screwing the cup down the reamed depth caused us to consider modifications. These changes affected firstly the base of the implant, which is now provided with a conical bevel. With the main conical form being maintained for the rest of the circumference, the outside of the new cup has a double conical form. The advantage of this is reduced bone resection while maintaining the basic conical cup form. Additionally, the cutting ability of the thread blades was increased, so that in almost all cases direct contact of the base of the implant with the bone can be achieved (Fig. 7)

There are now also two different forms of thread flank, one for hard, sclerotic bone and the other for softer, osteoporotic bone. The locking mechanism of the polyethylene insert was also modified, so that micromovement in relation to the metal cup shell is no longer possible. Both cup types, the Bicon "standard" cup and the Bicon "porosis" cup, have not only proven themselves for over two year in primary operations in several hundred cases. It also appears that the double conical form is significantly better for revision operations. In any case, the use of Burch-Schneider cages has declined significantly since the introduction of the Bicon cups. The Bicon cup has been further improved with a newly designed antiluxation insert, providing a better "roof" for the ball head, and so designed that there is no limitation of mobility. The dysplasia insert can thus be implan-

Fig. 7a–d. A 79-year-old woman, a Extensive coxarthrosis (*right*). Head collapse with subsequent destruction of the acetebulum. b, c Radiograph and microradiograph of the Bicon cup. Good implant contact with the prepared osseous interface. The medial part of the cone is in direct contact with the lamina interna. All thread blades have cut well into the bone. d Enlargement of the region of the second thread blade (*right*, c). The blade has cut deeply into the original cortical bone (*K*). Extensive formation of new bone at the tip of the thread (*asterisk*). Progression of growth of new bone tissue from the thread tip to the flanks (*arrows*). 2.5 months Postoperative.

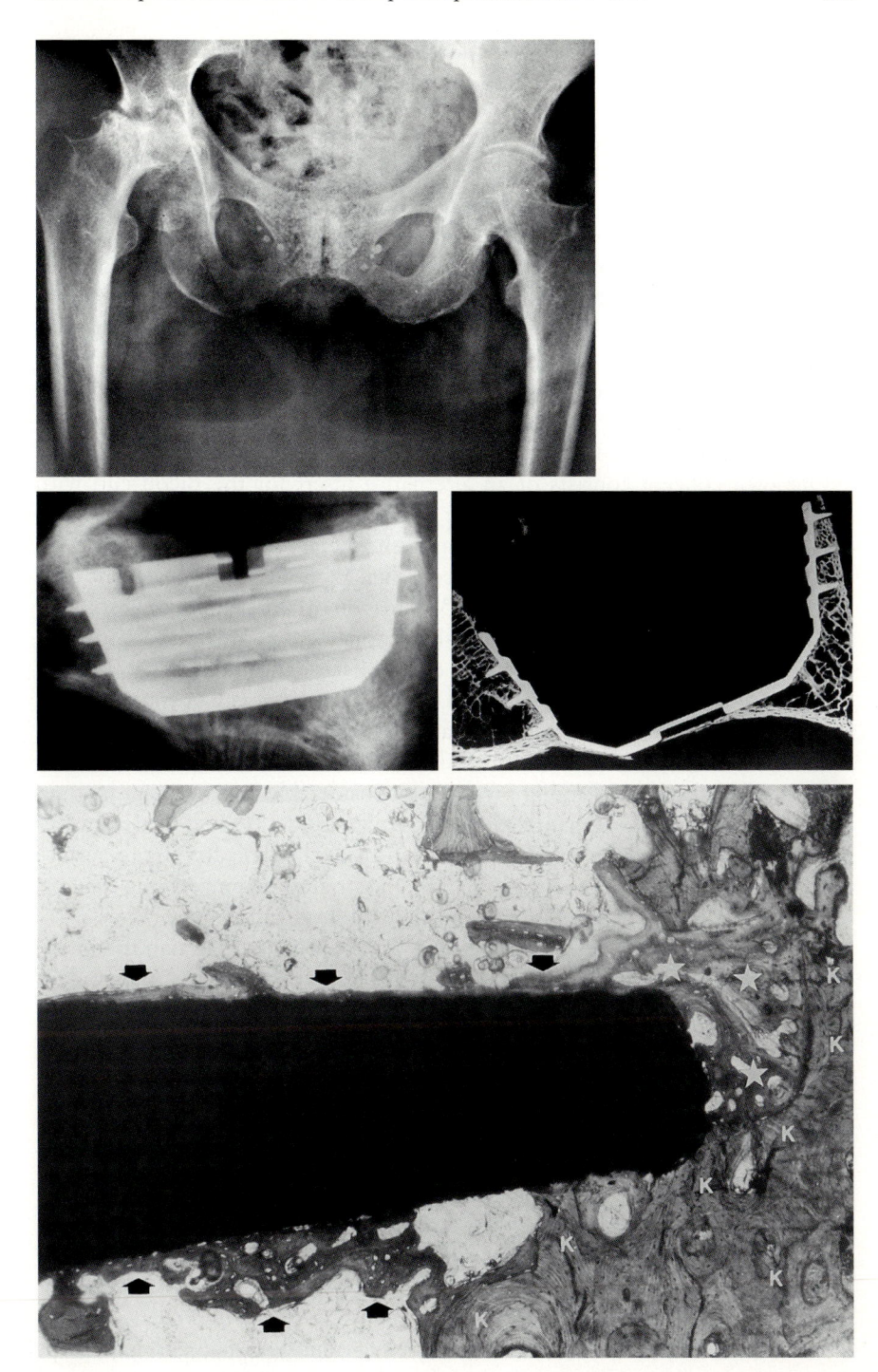

The Development of the Cementless Hip Endoprosthesis: 1979–1994

ted for luxation tendency due to various causes without any limitation of mobility, compared to the standard insert cup.

Metal-Metal Articulation

The ceramic-polyethylene material combination has been used by us since 1979 [24]. This achieved a clear reduction in the amount of polyethylene wear compared with metal-polyethylene articulation, but in no way eliminated it [4, 23]. We just met Charnley's requirement for low friction with the combination of a ceramic ball head with a polyethylene inlay. This requirement must however be supplemented with the requirement for low wear. Weber, in collaboration with Semlitsch, addressed the problem of low wear with the introduction of a modern articulation technology with a metal ball head and metal inlay [25, 26].

Our own concept consists of an alternative insert for the Bicon cup with metal-metal articulation. From the very beginning we placed much importance on a solid multi stepped conical fixation of the metal inlay in the polyethylene support, which is itself held in the Bicon shell without micromovement by a multistepped conical fixation design [33]. This important element of absolutely no relative motion at the polyethylene shell connection permits the elimination of polyethylene wear due to the cup design itself. The metal inlay and the articulating ball head are manufactured from a chromium-cobalt-molybdenum alloy which has been implanted for many years. The vacuum melting method achieves a purity ten times better than the ESU (Elektro-Schlacke-Umschmelz) process, and subsequent forging produces a considerable improvement in grain refinement and a uniform distribution of the fine carbides. This in turn improves the mechanical and chemical properties and forms the basis for a high surface finish. Using a special polishing procedure, the strictest manufacturing tolerance requirements for the metal inlay and the ball head can be met.

Long-term simulator tests indicate that, using optimum material, the intended sphericity and manufacturing tolerances, the wear rate falls after only a short running-in period to 1 μm per million cycles and component [33]. The reduction in the running-in period contributes significantly to minimizing the amount of wear from the very beginning. Organic loading due to wear products is not expected, due to the fact that their level is that of trace elements and can thus be ignored. Thanks to new technologies metal wear has been reduced sufficiently that we have reached a satisfactory safety margin for the concept. We thus routinely implant metal-metal components in younger patients.

Discussion

Surveying the 15 years of experience with the system described above, perhaps the most interesting is the on-going product development, not only of the stem but also of the cup. This did not happen suddenly, but instead gradually, using the gradual experience gained. We were frequently criticized, particularly as regards the stem, for "changing models" and this was considered disadvantageous or inconsistent. In fact, however, the principle of rectangular fixation of a wedge-shaped straight stem was maintained from the very beginning until today. Only the form of the implant changed. Coarse structures were deleted, a wedge shape also introduced in the axial plane and the fixation moved further proximally away from distal. With the recent widening of the proximal prosthesis portion in the calcar region, there is a further step towards balanced fixation distally and proximally. At the same time, the rotational stability of the stem was increased. Together with the trochanter wing, this stem is now able to guarantee a proximal press-fit. Many cadaveric implantations have confirmed to us that the trochanter wing is well able to offer proximal support of the implant.

A similar situation applies for the cup. The starting position was different, however, in that a polyethylene threaded cup was implanted in direct contact with bone until the end of 1984. As soon as it became clear from ongoing follow-up investigations of patients with these cups that this isoelastic suspension was impossible for cup implants, an immediate change was made to the pure titanium cup shell. This change eliminated the problem of massive polyethylene wear. It has also been shown that the opinion held in the United States, that a conical threaded cup does not function, is false. It is in fact correct that good prestressing and the tilting stability of a conical implant plays a significant role in achieving permanent secondary fixation. However, even here changes were necessary, such as using single-pitch thread instead of double-pitch [29] and making the thread blades sharper. Remaining was the problem that many surgeons felt there to be a unnecessary amount of bone resection at the floor of the implant. The recent change to a double conical form is now being implemented. The further improvement of the cutting ability and the improved fixation of the polyethylene insert in the cup shell may be regarded as small steps, but both were considered as an absolute necessity. We are also convinced that Weber's "back to the future" principle of lowering the volume of wear particles represents a further step in the right direction. It appears that McKee's brilliant idea [17] of "low friction and low wear" has now, with a delay of several decades, gained the upper hand over Charnley's "low friction" principle.

Low friction and low wear ensure the promotion and maintenance of permanent implant fixation. The prerequisite is primary stability, biocompatibility and the surface structure of the prosthesis. The replacement of toxic vanadium by biocompatible niobium and the use of a implant surface microstructure are changes directed to not only primary but also permanent fixation.

References

1. Albrektsson T, Brånemark PJ, Hansson HA, Lindström J (1981) Osseointegrated titanium implants. Requirements for ensuring a lomg-lasting, direct bone-to-implant anchorage in man. Acta Orthop Scand 52: 155
2. Böhm G, Lintner F, Brand G, Obenaus C, Klimann S (1990) Morphometrische Befunde an einzelnen Titaniumschäften. In: Zweymüller K (eds) 10 Jahre Zweymüller-Hüftendoprothese. Huber, Bern pp 61–65
3. Böhm G, Lintner F, Tuppy H, Brand G (1994) Bone-implant-contact-index, a method for the biological rating of implants. In: Willert HG (ed) 5. Biomaterial Symposium Göttingen. Hogrefe-Huber, Toronto (to be published)
4. Bos I, Meeuwssen E, Henßge EJ, Löhrs U (1991) Unterschiede des Polyethylenabriebes bei Hüftgelenkendoprothesen mit Keramik- und Metall-Polyethylenpaarung der Gleitflächen. Eine Untersuchung an Operations- und Autopsiematerial. Z Orthop 129: 507–515
5. Chiari K, Zweymüller K, Paltrinieri M, Trentani C, Stärk N (1977) Eine keramische Hüfttotalendoprothese zur zementfreien Implantation. Arch Orthop Unfallchir 89: 305
6. Endler M, Endler F (1982) Theoretisch-experimentelle Grundlagen und erste klinische Erfahrungen mit einer neuen zementfreien Polyethylenschraubpfanne bei Hüftgelenkersatz. Acta Chir Aust (Suppl) 45: 1
7. Endler M, Endler F, Plenk H (1983) Experimentelle Aspekte und klinische Früherfahrungen einer zementlosen Hüftgelenkpfanne aus UHMW-Polyethylen. In: Morscher E (eds) Die zementlose Fixation von Hüftendoprothesen. Springer, Berlin Heidelberg New York
8. Knahr K, Salzer M, Frank P (1983) Erfahrungen mit zementfrei implantierten Polyethylenpfannen. In: Morscher E (eds) Die zementlose Fixation von Hüftendoprothesen. Springer, Berlin Heidelberg New York
9. Kutschera HP, Eyb R, Schartelmüller T, Toma C, Zweymüller K (1993) Das zementfreie Zweymüller-Hüftsystem. Ergebnisse einer 5Jahresnachuntersuchung. Z Orthop 131: 513–517
10. Lintner F: (1983) Ossifikationsstörung an der Zement-Knochen-Grenze. Histologische und klinische Untersuchungen – Experiment und Klinik. Acta Chir Austr (Suppl) 48
11. Lintner F, Zweymüller K, Brand G (1985) Die knöcherne Reaktion auf zementfrei implantierte Titanium-Schäfte. In: Maaz B, Menge M, (eds) Aktueller Stand der zementfreien Hüftendoprothetik. Symposium Düsseldorf 1985. Thieme, Stuttgart, New York
12. Lintner F, Zweymüller K, Brand G (1986) Tissue reactions to titanium endoprostheses. Autopsy studies in four cases. J Arthroplasty 1: 183–195
13. Lintert F, Böhm G, Brand G, Endler M, Zweymüller K (1988) Ist hochdichtes Polyethylen als Implantatmaterial zur zementfreien Verankerung von Hüftendoprothesen geeignet? Eine histomorphologische Untersuchung an explantierten Polyethylenschraubpfannen. Z Orthop 126: 688–692
14. Lintner F, Böhm G, Bösch P, Brand G, Endler M, Zweymüller K (1990) Results of histological and mikroradiographic examination of cementless implanted polyethylene threaded hip sockets. In: Willert HG, Buchhorn GH, Eyerer D (eds) Ultra-High Molecular Weight Polyethylene as Biomaterial in Orthopedic Surgery. Hogrefe-Huber, Toronto
15. Lintner F, Böhm G, Brand G, Obenaus C, Klimann S (1990) Gewebliche Reaktionsformen des Titaniumschaftes. In: Zweymüller K (ed) 10 Jahre Zweymüller-Hüftendoprothese. Huber, Bern pp 47–60
16. Lintner F, Böhm G, Huber M (1994) Zementfreie Schraubpfannen. Morphologische, Mikroradiographische und Morphometrische Untersuchungen zum Einbauverhalten. Med Orthop Tech 114: 233–237

17. McKee GK (1970) Development of total prosthetic replacement of the hip. Clin Orthop 72: 85-103
18. Morscher E, Dick W (1983) Zementlose Verankerung einer Hüftgelenkpfanne aus Polyethylen. In: Morscher E (ed) Die zementlose Fixation von Hüftendoprothesen. Springer, Berlin Heidelberg New York
19. Müller, W, Lindenfeld, T, Egloff, TP Baumgartner, R, Friedrich, NF (1995, in press) Erfahrungen 1982-1994 mit dem zementlosen Hüfttotalprothesensystem Zweymüller 1979-1992. In: Zweymüller, K (Hrsg) 15 Jahre Zweymüller-Hüftendoprothese. 3. Wiener Symposium. Huber, Bern
20. Önnerfält R, Franzén H (1991) Separation of plastic and metal in an acetabular cup. Acta Orth Scand 62/5: 489-490
21. Plitz W (1992) Biomechanik zementfreier Endoprothetik. Vortrag DGOT-Kongreß, Mannheim
22. Salzer, M, Zweymüller, K, Locke, H, Zeibig, A, Stärk, N, Plenk, H, Punzet, G (1976) Further experimental and clinical experience with aluminium oxide endoprostheses. J. Biomed. Mater. Res. 10: 847-856
23. Semlitsch M (1990) Stand der Werkstofftechnik des Zweymüller-Hüftprothesensystems nach 10 Jahren klinischer Praxis. In: Zweymüller K (ed) 10 Jahre Zweymüller-Hüftendoprothese. Huber, Bern
24. Semlitsch M, Lehmann M, Weber H, Dörre E, Willert HG (1977) New prospects for a prolonged functional life-span of artificial hip joints by using the material combination polyethylene/aluminium oxide ceramic/metal. J Biomed Mater Res 11: 537-552
25. Semlitsch M, Streicher RM, Weber H (1989) Verschleißverhalten von Pfannen und Kugeln aus CoCrMo-Gußlegierung bei langzeitig implantierten Ganzmetallhüftprothesen. Orthopäde 18: 377-381
26. Weber BG (1992) Metall-Metall-Totalprothese des Hüftgelenkes: Zurück in die Zukunft. Z Orthop 130: 306-309
27. Zweymüller W (1986) A cementless titanium hip endoprosthesis system. Basic research and clinical results. In: Anderson LD (ed) The A.A.O.S. Instructional Course Lectures XXXV. Mosby, St. Louis
28. Zweymüller K, Samek V (1990) Radiologische Erkenntnisse der Titaniumpfanne. In: Zweymüller K (ed) 10 Jahre Zweymüller-Hüftendoprothese. Huber, Bern
29. Zweymüller K, Semlitsch M (1986) Weiterentwicklung des zementfreien Hüftendoprothesensystems aufgrund spezieller Indikationen. Med Orthop Tech 106: 11-14
30. Zweymüller K, Semlitsch M (1982) Concept and material properties of a cementless hip prosthesis system with Al_2O_3 ceramic ball heads and wrought Ti-6Al-4V stems. Arch Ortho Trauma Surg 100: 229
31. Zweymüller K, Lintner F, Semlitsch M (1988) Biologic fixation of a press-fit titanium hip joint endoprosthesis. Clin Orthop 235: 195-206
32. Zweymüller K, Deckner A, Lintner F, Semlitsch M (1988) Die Weiterentwicklung des zementfreien Systems durch das SL-Schaftprogramm. Med Orthop Tech 108: 10-15
33. Zweymüller K, Deckner A, Kupferschmidt W, Steindl M (1994) Weiterentwicklung der konischen Schraubpfanne. Med Orthop Tech 114: 223-228
34. Zweymüller K, Deckner A, Steindl, M (1995 in press) Der SL-Plus- und SLR-Plus-Schaft. Konzept und erste Ergebnisse. In: Zweymüller, K (Hrsg) 15 Jahre Zweymüller-Hüftendprothese. 3. Wiener Symposium. Huber, Bern

Part VII

Knee Joint Arthroplasty

The Gschwend-Scheier-Bähler Knee Prosthesis

N. Gschwend, H. Siegrist, H. G. Scheier, A. Bähler

Knee arthroplasty can be considered a routine operation in orthopedics today. Its numbers are increasing almost yearly in specialized clinics. Our own statistics also confirm this trend (1990, 221 knee and 477 hip arthroplasties; 1993, 326 knee and 512 hip arthroplasties). The fact that knee arthroplasty lags behind hip arthroplasty in number may be attributed to the following:
- the arthritic knee joint is more amenable to conservative measures (physiotherapy, injections) than the arthritic hip joint;
- osteotomy in the area of the knee joint has a high success rate (83 % outstanding and good results, improvement in 90 % of cases) [5, 11];
- due to complicated joint kinematic knee arthroplasty reached its success rates 10–15 years later than hip arthroplasty, so that both physican and patient are now more actively involved in this procedure.

A glance at the latest world literature shows optimism specially among the specialists who perform knee arthroplasty on an almost daily basis. Their success rate of almost 95 % justifies them in thinking that the results of knee arthroplasty are superior even to those of hip arthroplasty [4, 10, 12].

At least two limitations must be considered:
- We do not yet have very long term experience with the newer knee arthroplasty system (which is been considered here), to compare with the Charnley school with the original method of hip arthroplasty.
- Knee arthroplasty is, in comparison with hip arthroplasty, technically more demanding; faulty surgical technic at implantation, especially of the condylar prosthesis, can easily lead to bad results.

The question: "Wich knee prosthesis is the best and recommended for surgery?" cannot be answered satisfactorily without the added question "For which patient?" and "Who is the surgeon?" To abtain a definitive answer there is a need for multicenter studies which compare repeatable evaluation criteria among a homogeneous group of patients. The publication by Tew and Waugh [13], based on the survival curves comparing various prostheses implanted in the same clinic, should be assessed with caution [13, 14, 17]. Based on the 10-year survival rates of different knee prostheses implanted in the same clinic, the authors compare the results. From the study it would appear that the newer prostheses are better. However, this conclusion is not justified. It is clear that results of condylar prostheses depend, among other factors, on whether the postoperative tibiofermoral angle is between 4° and 10° valgus. In other words, the postoperative tolerance range of axis deviation can only be 3° [3]. Insall [10] narrowed this range even further.

For lasting and objective follow-up our patients are always assessed by the same person, a qualified orthopedic surgeon and rheumatologist. She sees the patients at regular intervals and completes the Eular Knee Assessment Chart or Eurpean Rheumatoid Arthritis Surgical Society (ERASS) knee form. Both data and those from many other clinics are evaluated at the Documentation Center in Edinburgh. Our data are also saved in our clinic computer system. This allows us to meaning fully compare our data with that of others.

The concept of the GSB Knee Prosthesis

The GSB knee prosthesis was developed in 1972, because the inflexible metal-metal hinge prosthesis was, with respect to joint dynamics, unphysiological. Because of excessive stresses on the bone, these prostheses frequently did not last long. Moreover, there was a need to sacrifice a relatively large amount of bone for implantation, so that when complications arose, there was no bone reserve. The then available unconstrained condylar system (Gunston, St. Georg sledge prosthesis, and somewhat later among others the Geomedic prosthesis), required a functional ligament apparatus preoperatively. In cases with severe deformity or poor bone quality, as in many of our patients with rheumatoid arthritis, implantation was contraindicated.

The GSB I prosthesis (Fig. 1a) was characterized by careful adaptation to the femoral und tibial condyles yet with minimal bone resection and following the low-friction principle. The femoral component lacked a patella gliding surface, due to this, the posterior surface of the patella was not replaced.

The GSB II prosthesis (Fig. 1b, c) was a further development based on the analysis of the pitfalls of the GSB I prosthesis, namely (a) pain in the femoropatellar region and (b) abnormal kinematics in the sagittal plane from 80° flexion onwards (the femur was too ventral in relation to the tibia). Moreover, the recurrently observed tendency to metallosis was of concern, and it was possibly correct to presume that the higher rate of late infection could be related to this phenomenon. A flattened femoropatellar flange was introduced, and the posterior patella surface was replaced by a cement-free fixed polyethylene prosthesis. The metallic axis was eliminated and replaced by a central stud. This formed a stabilizing element, on the one hand, and, on the other, a virtual axis gliding on

Fig. 1a–f. Gschwend-Scheier-Bähler (GSB) prostheses. **a** GSB I. **b, c** GSB II: Flat. patellar shield and high-desity polyethylene patellar prosthesis. **d** GSB III, with total polyethylene covering for the tibia. **e** GSB revision prosthesis. **f** GSB III, with raised lateral portion

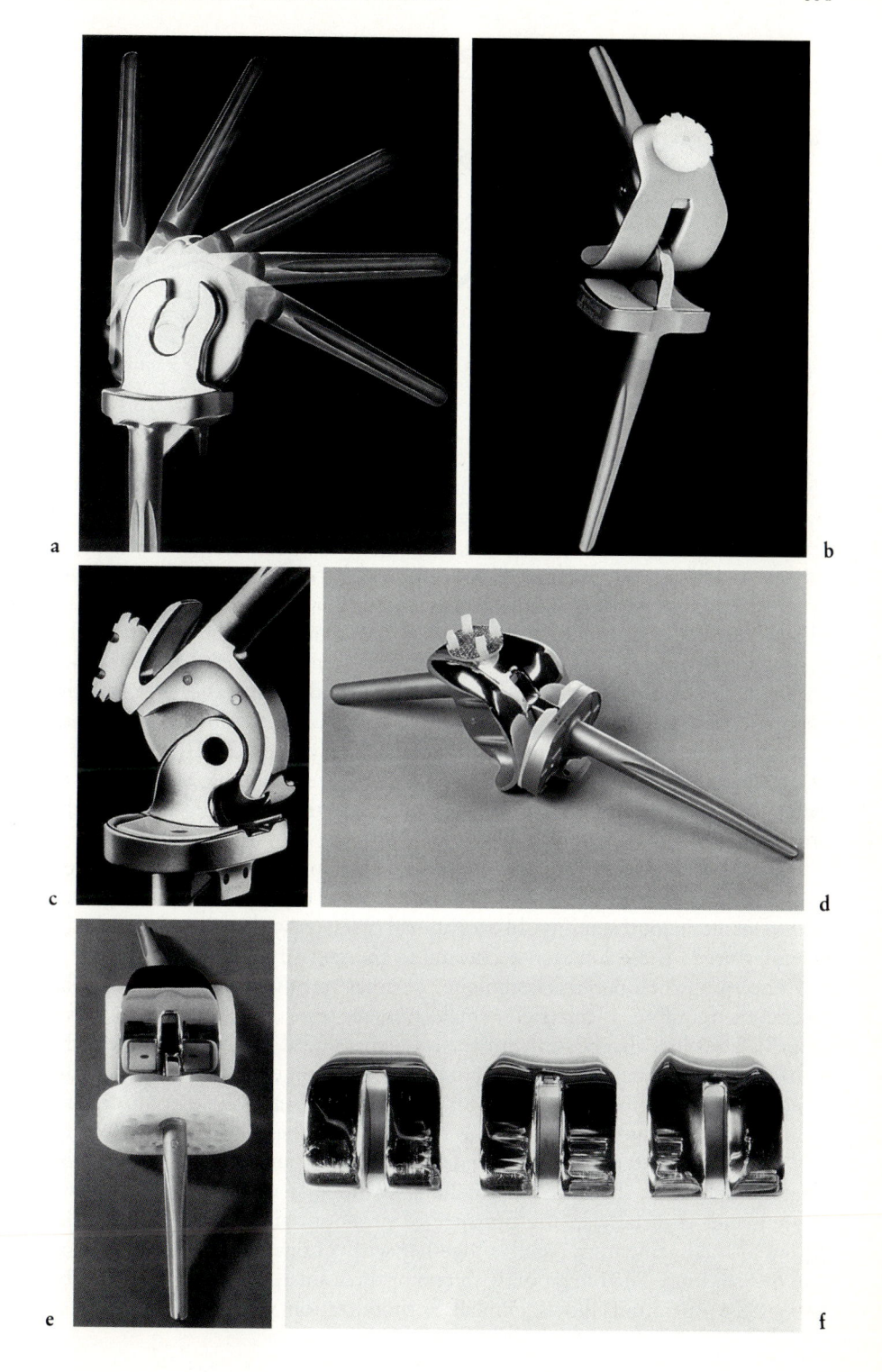

The Gschwend-Scheier-Bähler Knee Prosthesis

a

b

c

d

e

f

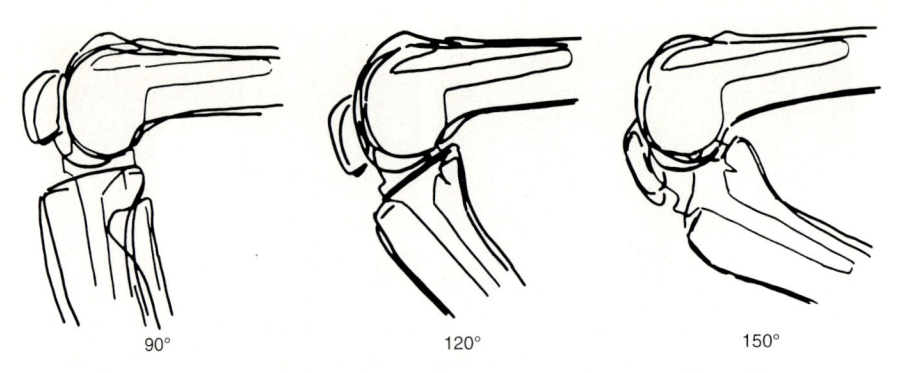

Fig. 2. Kinematics of GSB III prosthesis in comparison with a normal knee joint

a polyethylene base. The kinematics corresponded to those of a normal joint in the sagittal plane. The normal femorotibial relationship was still maintained even at flexion greater than 100° (Fig. 2).

In the GSB III prosthesis (Fig. 1d), metal contact at the condylar surfaces of fermur and tibia was eliminated, and replaced by a thick polyethylene layer completely covering the oval tibial plateau. By this means, we attempted to more closely reproduce the anatomy of the patellar-femoral articulating surface. By raising the lateral portion, we prevented the recurrently observed patellar dislocation or subluxation (Fig. 1f). Another fundamental modification involved the shape of the patella and its cement-free fixation, using a Sulmesh – network made from titanium for the posterior surface. Today, the GSB III prosthesis is available in three sizes. The medium or standard size is suitable for 80–85 % of patients, 10–15 % require the large prosthesis, and the remaining 5 % need the small size.

For revision surgery or patients with greater bone loss (e. g., tumors), a revision prosthesis (Fig. 1e) with additional parts is available, to replace the missing bone and to maintain joint stability. In exceptional cases, individual prostheses can be manufactured. These function according to the same dynamic principle.

Concerning the operative technique, we refer to other publications [6]. The operation requires a relatively small number easy-to-handle instruments (Fig. 3). Thus it is also possible for the less experienced surgeon to implant the GSB prosthesis correctly. Another point of note is that even considerable faults concering axial alignment of the GSB prosthesis at operation do not necessarily imply failure (as opposed to the condylar prostheses). There is also the advantage of the lateral approach under routine step-cut lengthening on of the lateral retinaculum. Because the patella is less mobile with this approach, we recommend, especially in the presence of pronounced valgus deformity, the lifting of the ligamentum patellae together with a bone lamella 2–3 mm thick and 6–7 cm long. The refixation with two or three small fragment screws at the end of the operation allows immediate mobilization without the danger of

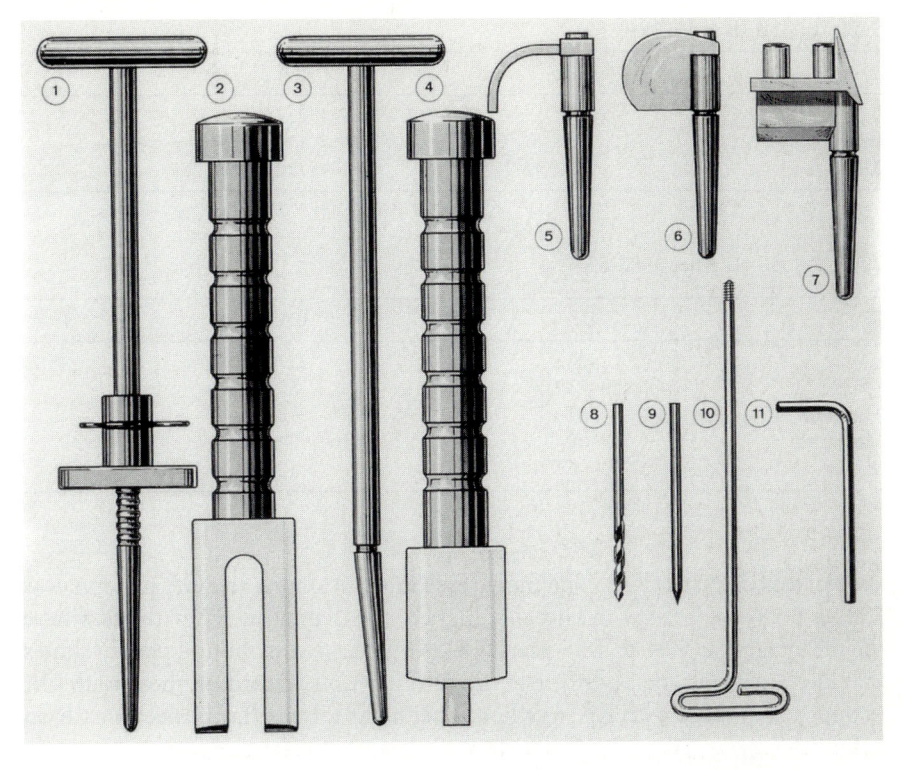

Fig. 3. Instruments for implantation of the GSB III prosthesis

loosening of the ligament and consequent weakening of the extensor apparatus.

The postoperative treatment is relatively simple. On day 1 postoperatively the patients is allowed to stand up with a splint and walk a few steps. After removal of the Redon drains, the knee is laid on a Kinetec splint at least twice daily, and the patient is instructed to walk on two crutches in three point mode. We expect achieving flexion of at least 90° and full extension in the first 3 weeks. If the joint mobility is substantially below these values, we mobilize the knee joint under general anesthesia. Walking without support is only allowed after 2–3 months.

Case Reports and Results

During 1980–1993 we implanted 712 GSB III knee prostheses at the Schulthess Clinic. During 1980–1989 638 patients received a GSB III knee prosthesis (Table 1). Of these patients 421 (66%) had osteoarthritis (OA) and 217 (34%) had

Table 1. GSB III Knee 1980–89

	OA		RA	
n	421		217	
Female	352	84 %	175	81 %
Male	69	16 %	42	19 %

Table 2. GSB III Knee 1980–89

	OA	RA
n	421	217
⌀ age	73,6 y	59,4 y
Minimun	51	18
Maximum	88	84
± s	6.9	12.5

rheumatoid arthritis (RA). The mean age (Table 2) among the OA patients was 73.6 ± 6.9 years (51–88) and notably higher than that of the RA patients, where the mean age was 59.4 ± 12.5 years (18–84). The age distribution clearly shows that knee arthroplasty is performed only from age 50 onwards in those with OA as opposed to those with RA, in whom knee arthroplasty may be necessary even before the age of 20 years, to ensure the patient's walking capacity.

The Role of Pain

Pain is the major indication for all knee arthroplasties. It is the major determinant of the patient's ability to walk and also plays a major role in general mobility. This is the reason why, in most evaluation of results, the relief of pain is given the highest rating.

Of all the criteria (mobility, stability, axial alignment, gait, and X-ray findings), pain is the most subjective and thus can be evaluated with only limited precision. In addition, pain depends on the amount of stress and the condition of the neighboring joints. A separate consideration of basic disease, age, and specific individual needs is necessary. It is important to determine exactly the localization of the pain, if it is associated with changes in the femoral or tibial components, and whether its source is patellofemoral, which is most common, or in the soft tissues. The aim of any operation in which pain is the major indication, must be to alleviate the pain completely, if possible. Any amount of pain reduction is considered successful. Expressed as a percentage, 95 % experienced very significant pain reduction, and only 4.2 % experienced the same or worse pain.

Pain recurrence postoperatively is also of interest as it gives us some information with regard to duration of success. The recurrence of pain postoperatively

Table 3. Pain n = 120

preoperative		postoperative
0	None	74
2	Mild	26
27	Moderate	15
91	Severe	5

was determined by data collected by one examiner at 1, 3, and 5 years after the GSB arthroplasty for RA and OA. Members of the ERASS enter their results in to the ERASS computer this guarantees a most reliable comparison between various parameters because we have follow-up studies from other authors (using different knee arthroplasty systems) utilizing the same form.

The total condylar system interests us especially, being a minimal constraint and nonlinked system. After 5 years 73 % of patients with rheumatoid arthritis had no pain and 18 % had mild pain. Thus, for 91 % of patients the operation was highly successful. On the other hand, only 52 % of OA patients had no pain and 26 % had mild pain. Thus this rate of 79 % is obviously less successful than in the RA group. Retropatellar pain plays a large role in OA patients.

Comparison of pain at 1, 3, and 5 years after operation for GSB III and total condylar knee shows, that patients with the total condylar knee had markedly less pain. This difference becomes less noticeable when one compares the mild, occasional pain and the lack of pain in a group. It is noteworthy that patients with the GSB prosthesis have less pain as the years progress, at least in the RA patients.

A separate consideration of anterior knee pain in the GSB and total condylar knee prosthesis, shows that the main reason for knee pain in the GSB prosthesis is the less physiological patellar articular surface. In the total condylar knee the limited rotation appears to be the cause. The rather extensive flexion-capacity with the GSB knee increases the patellofemoral stresses compared with the total condylar knee. As a result pain is elicited more easily in the more physically active OA patients then in RA patients.

Mobility

The good average mobility of the GSB knee prosthesis postoperatively is an undoubted advantage of the system. in RA patients a marked improvement in mobility was noted: 90 % achieved flexion of 100–120° and > 120° 1 year postoperatively and 8 % flexion of 80–100°. Among OA patients 85 % had 100–120° and > 120° flexion and 14 % 80–100° flexion. In the comparative study of GSB III knee patients determined by the ERASS score with other knee systems, evaluated separately for OA and RA, the GSB III prosthesis confirmed its advantage. The improvement in extension is noteworthy. The ability fo flex over 100°, especially on standing up from a sitting position, is of great importance for the patient's independence. Considering mobility, over 80 % achieved 100° and approximately 1/4 exceeded the 120° limit 5 years postoperatively. there was no notable difference between OA and RA patients. Also, extension deficit of the knee was rare. In approximately 85 % of both RA and OA patients full extension was possible 5 years after operation. In 15 % there was a relative limitation of the extension (range inbetween −1° and −11°). These values are obviously less favorable with the total condylar knee, with which only approximately 30 % of OA patients could reach the 100 degree limit and only 5 % greater than 120°. In RA patients the values were similar to ours. Inability to extend the knee postoperatively was demonstrable in 50 % of the patients with the total condylar knee.

Instability

The instability of the GSB knee due to the linkage of the two components is not a major problem. When a patient experiences an episode of instability, it may be due to instability in the region of the patella.

Walking capacity

The improvement in gait is the main goal of knee arthroplasty in other words to prevent the inability to walk. In the majority of cases the gait before and after operation shows a definite improvement; 84.6 % showed a marked improvement. Approximately 60 % were able to walk more than 1 km postoperatively and a further 25 % achieved a distance of 1 km. Approximately 90 % (89.74 %) were satisfied with the gait they had achieved. The difference between OA and RA patients is seen in our second cormputerized study in which we compared the behavior of gait 1, 3, and 5 years postoperatively. The RA patients did less well over time due to the other extensive joint involvement. This was also the case among OA patients, for the following reasons: a) the average age at operation was 73.5 years, b) at 5 years follw-up the patients were already approaching 80 years of age, and c) many of these patients also had progressive degenerative changes in the opposite knee or in the hip or ankle joints. Despite these disadvantages the goal of the operation was achieved in the majority of patients. The same can be said for the RA patients with GSB knee prosthesis and additional joint disease. Due to the small numbers of cases with total condylar knee the comparison with the GSB knee joint was not possible.

The great majority of patients do not need a regular walking aid, for example, a walking stick. This is particularly true in RA due to the RA patient's difficulty in using stick because of pathological changes in the upper extremity.

Comparison of Two Knee Prosthetic Systems in the Same Patient

With increasing specialization newer condylar type knee prosthetic systems, cemented and uncemented, are being used, initially for less advanced joint destruction and deformity and now even for more advanced knee joint destruction. The porous-coated anatomic knee prosthesis was the first condylar prosthesis used at our institution; after some disappointments the low contact stress (LCS) prosthesis was used. The LCS system is convincing not only from the kinematic point of view but especially with respect to the longterm results showing minimal polyethylene wear. We compared two different knee systems in the same patient. This comparison is particularly significant because all patient data (age, sex, weight, etc.) and physical requirements were constant. We evaluated 18 patients with a LCS system on one knee and a GSB prosthesis on the other. The results were as follows: a) postoperative flexion of 110° was the same in all 18, and with 2 exceptions all reached full extension; b) in both groups 3 patients had anterior knee pain and 15 were pain free; c) in 15 of the LCS prostheses no patellar replacement was necessary, but in 14 patients with the GSB prothesis the patella was replaced, and d) with respect to subjective patient's satisfaction, no difference was noted. It should be noted that the dual cruciate retaining model of the LCS system was most commonly used initially, and this later turned out to be the most problematic model.

Complications of the GSB III Prosthesis

Careful analysis of all complications is a deciding factor in the evaluation of a method. In follow-up of 5 or more years (1980–1989) the following complications were most common:

Infection. Especially late infection (appearing as a acute or low grade infection after years (1–12 years) was the most common complication. This affected 30 patients with 32 knee prostheses (22 = 3.4 %) of OA patients and 8 (1.3 %) of RA patients. A total of 34 operative procedures were undertaken: 15 revisions, 14 primary or secondary arthrodeses, 4 above-knee amputations, and 1 synovectomy. A further development (in the last 4–5 years) in the presence of infection has been revision in one or more commonly two stages (mainly to a cement-free system). Only when this fails is a secondary arthrodesis performed. Due to this the number of arthrodesis has decreased remarkably.

Aseptic loosening or fracture of the Prosthesis. This has presented no problem with the GSB knee prostheses. Among the total of 638 GSB prostheses there were only two fractures and one loosening. In both cases revision was performed successfully. In two cases there was dislocation of the prosthesis: one following a patellar dislocation and one following trauma, whereby the patient suffered a fracture of the lateral femoral condyle and a quadriceps tendon rupture. Postoperative reconstruction of the extensor apparatus was successful.

Despite improvement of the femoral patellar articulating surfaces, and the use of a newer patellar prosthesis, relatively many operations were performed on the extensor apparatus up to 1988 (total 49 = 7.7 %): 12 repositionings of the extensor apparatus by repositioning of the tibial tuberosity (8 had a lateral release), 15 patellectomies or hemipatellectomies (9), 12 revisions of the patellar prosthesis, 8 removals of the patellar prosthesis, 2 removals of the tibial tuberosity, and 1 simultaneous cranialization.

Initially, the polyethylene covering was thin, and the surface attached to bone was covered only by a Sulmesh (titanium) net, and positioned cement free. Because of this the polyethylene wore through, and the Sulmesh net disintegrated; in four cases removal of the patella was necessary. In some cases which required a patellar revision a simultaneous synovectomy or partial synovectomy was performed. The results of these revisions were disappointing because only 50 % of patients were pain free or had less pain than preoperatively. Despite these operations fracture of the patella or lateralisation of the patella was common (one-third of patients).

In the past 5 years the number of these types of procedures has markedly decreased. The improvement in the laterally raised articulating surfaces at the femoral component and the use of the reinforced Sulmesh patella has had a positive effect. Concerning patella fractures the management has become more conservative because in the majority of these cases the continuity of the extensor apparatus is maintained and therefore an operative procedure is not absolutely necessary.

The *survival curves of the GSB III knee prosthesis* after 10 years shows an obvious improvement in comparison with the older GSB I system. As expected, the percentage of removed GSB III prosthesis is higher in the OA than RA patients, presumably related to the differing demands among these patients (Fig. 4).

The relatively high *infection rate* in the GSB III prosthesis has been associated with the following two factors:
1. the lessened resistance of the bone to circulating infections agents and
2. the higher wear of polyethylene in the small contact surface between the metal and the polyethylene.

Considering the former point. The use of cement in the medullary cavity and on the condyles influences negatively the blood circulation in the bone and thus the resistance to infection. The majority of late infections are hematogenous. *Concerning point 2:* The excessive thickening of the capsule in the reoperated infected knee joints showed extensive necrotic areas due to the increased wear (especially high-density polyethylene, but partly also metal). Due to this,

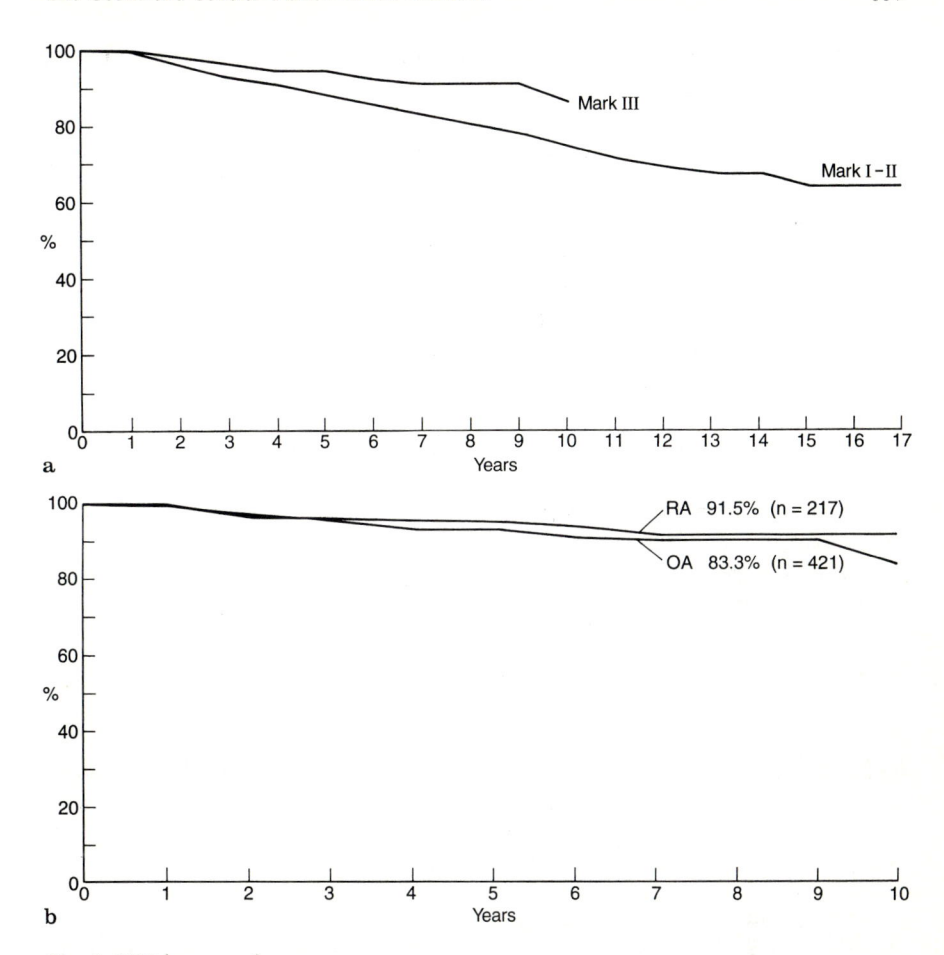

Fig. 4. GSB knee survivor curve

the resistance to infection in the joint was decreased. this was the main reason why we chose the LCS joint for all our cases of OA and RA that did not have extremely severe varus, valgus, or flexion deformities. In the LCS prosthesis the lowe contact stress and the meniscuslike articulating surface of polyethylene leads to minimal friction. The kinematic of this prostheses are more physiological. This has reduced the need for cement fixation and for an artificial replacement of the patella in the majority of cases.

Survival curves of prosthetic system supply us with information regarding the longterm results of a system. The number of necessary revisions is reflected by a downward trend in the curve. A requirement is that the survey within a specific time period encompasses all prostheses of patients who died or were referred for treatment elsewhere. Naturally the percentage shown in the curve at a specific time is not identical with the success rate in that it includes patients with prosthetic loosening or significant pain. A survival curve cannot enable one to make binding predictions. Still, it is a good method of comparing different knee prosthetic systems and the same system in different patients (e. g. RA and OA). We have seen that RA patients with fewer demands regarding ability to walk, and despite their nonideal bone conditions (e. g. steroid osteoporosis) and younger age, need fewer revisions.

Because of the long-term experience and obviously lesser risk of complications in the LCS system we use this system for the majority of RA and OA patients. We reserve the GSB III system for severe deformities in older patients (> 75 years old). We also believe that in wheelchair patients with marked flexion deformities, the GSB knee has a much better chance of achieving flexion greater than 90° than other condylar systems. This is because in the GSB system ligaments and bone-sparing soft-tissue surgery can be avoided in the interests of a greater range of motion.

In summary, the GSB III prosthesis plays an important role, even today, in the treatment of severe knee deformities. It promises as highly dependable success rates as the surgeon could expect with technically more demanding joint systems.

References

1. Abraham W (1988) Long-term results of patellar replacement. Clin Orthop 236: 128–134
2. Bayley JC, Scott RD (1988) Failure of the metal-backed patellar component after total knee replacement. Clin Ortop 235: 82–87
3. Denham RA, Bishop RED (1978) Mechanics of the knee and problems in reconstructive surgery. J Bone Joint Surg [Br] 60: 345–352
4. Ewald FC (1984) Kinematic total knee replacement. J Bone Joint Surg [Am] 66: 1032–1040
5. Gschwend N (1990) Vortrag anläßlich des Golden Jubilee Symposiums, Karolinska Hospital Stockholm
6. Gschwend N, Löhr J (1981) Der Gschwend-Scheier-Bähler (GSB)-Ersatz des rheumatischen Kniegelenks. Reconstr Surg Traumatol 18: 174–194
7. Gschwend N, Ivosevic-Radovanovic D (1988) Proven and non-proven facts in knee arthroplasty, results with the semiconstrained GSB-Prosthesis. Arch Orthop Trauma Surg 107: 140–147
8. Insall J (1983) Principles and techniques of knee replacement. Zimmer, Warsaw, Indiana
9. Insall JN (1984) Total knee replacement. In: Insall JN (ed) Surgery of the knee. Churchill Livingstone, New York, pp 587–696
10. Insall JN, Hood RW, Flawn LB, Sullivan DJ (1984) The total condylar knee prosthesis in gonarthrosis: a five to nine-year follow-up of the first one hundred consecutive replacement. J Bone Joint Surg [Am] 65: 619–628
11. Kleinert B, Scheier H, Munzinger U, Steiger U (1985) Ergebnisse der Tibiakopfosteotomie. Orthopäde 14: 154–160

12. Ranawat CS (1985) Total condylar knee arthroplasty: technique, results and complications. Spriger, Berlin Heidelberg New York T.ky.
13. Tew M, Waugh W (1982) Estimating the survival time of knee replacements. J Bone Joint Surg [Br] 64: 579–582
14. Tew W, Waugh W, Forster IW (1985) Comparing the results of different types of knee replacements: a method proven and applied. J Bone Joint Surg [Br] 67: 775–779
15. Walker PS (1973) Trends in knee prosthesis development. Engl Med 2: 76
16. Waugh W (1983) Knee replacements. In: McKibbin B (ed) Recent advances in orthopaedics, vol 4. Churchill Livingstone, Edinburgh, pp 45–64
17. Waugh W, Tew M, Johnson F (1981) Methods of evaluating results of operations for chronic arthritis of the knee. JR Soc Med 74: 343–347

Total Knee Replacement at the Royal London Hospital: 25 Years' Experience (1968–1993)

M. A. R. Freeman, K. M. Samuelson

Introduction

This contribution describes the evolution of a series of prostheses, each a modification of its predecessor. The first of these was entitled the Freeman-Swanson prosthesis; the second the ICLH (Imperial College/London Hospital) prosthesis, and the third the Freeman-Samuelson prosthesis. As this contribution is being written, the third version of the prosthesis has been modified in certain respects and is known as the Freeman-Samuelson modular prosthesis.

Work began on the design of this prosthesis in 1968 in the Biomechanics Unit at the Department of Mechanical Engineering at Imperial College, then directed by Prof. S. A. V. Swanson and the present authors. We sought a device which would resurface the whole of the tibiofemoral joint with a polyethylene component articulating with a metallic femoral component. Both components were to be attached to the bone with the aid of polymethylmethacrylate cement.

It was intended that this device should be used for the severely damaged knee. To realign such knees, it was anticipated that the cruciate ligaments would have to be resected. A further reason for resecting the cruciate ligaments was to abolish the roll back/forward that was then believed to occur between the femur and tibia during flexion and extension. By abolishing this movement it was planned to provide an area of contact between the femoral and tibial components by making both surfaces curved with the same radius. Only by doing this did it seem possible, by calculation, to provide acceptably low stresses on the polyethylene surface.

The resultant prosthesis (Fig. 1) was first implanted at the London Hospital in 1969. So far as the author is aware, this represented the first implantation of a total knee replacement prosthesis of the condylar kind.

The tibial component was initially attached to the tibia with the aid of two staples, whose function was simply to steady the prosthesis while the cement set. This proved an unsatisfactory method of fixation. The femoral component did not replace the whole of the patellofemoral joint and was of only one size, so that in a large knee the short anterior flange was buried within the femur. The result was to produce an irregular surface over which the patella travelled. This potential problem was addressed initially by carrying out a patellectomy. Wound healing following patellectomy proved difficult in the first ten knees,

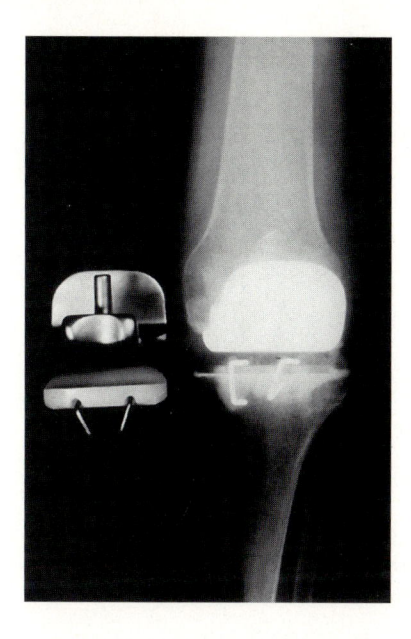

Fig. 1. The Freeman-Swanson prosthesis inserted at the London Hospital in 1969

and thereafter the patella was left in place. The posterior flange of the femoral component was not divided at the intercondylar notch, in order to increase the contact area with the polyethylene tibial component. As a consequence, it was difficult to extract cement from the posterior aspect of the knee.

Over the first 10 years of clinical experience at the London Hospital, a number of problems and complications were encountered which were enumerated in the *Journal of Bone and Joint Surgery* in 1978 [15]. In that paper the authors concluded that the operation of condylar knee replacement was clearly possible, and that the short-term results were encouraging. However, attention was drawn to four major problems: an unacceptably high incidence of tibial component migration and loosening; an unacceptable incidence of patellar pain; wear of the polyethylene component; and an inability reliably to align and stabilize the knee in extension. In the following years these problems were addressed, and in doing so both the prosthesis and the operative technique were modified.

Tibial Component Loosening and Migration

The initial tibial component was made in only one size and therefore was smaller than the top of the tibia in most knees. A radiograph illustrating a typical consequence is shown in Fig. 2.

In 1978 Bargren et al. [4] proposed, on the basis of cadaver studies in the laboratory, that larger tibial components should be available which would cover

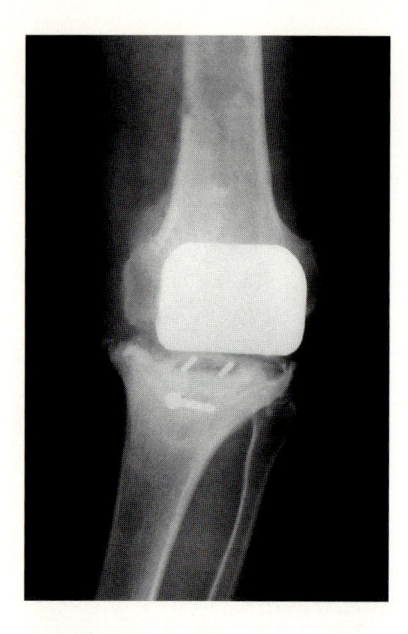

Fig. 2. Tibial component loosening with downward medial migration: a common complication in the early series of prostheses

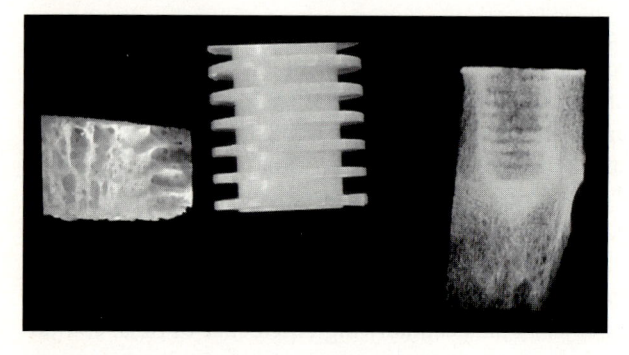

Fig. 3. Macerated postmortem specimen (*left*) and radiograph (*right*) to show interlock between a flanged polyethylene peg (*centre*) and the tibia

the whole of the top of the transsected bone, and that the tibia should be resected as proximally as possible since the bone was point-for-point stronger proximally than distally. Clinical studies with the modified device showed that the loosening rate was indeed reduced but that it was still not acceptable.

Because of wear produced by cement debris (a subject discussed below), the method of tibial fixation was then modified to permit fixation without cement. The resultant prosthesis was attached to the tibia by medial and lateral flanged pegs which could be expected to interlock with the cancellous bone of the tibia (Fig. 3). Early experience with this device, fixed both with and without cement [6] showed an acceptable early loosening rate.

By the early 1970s the need to develop a technique for revision arthroplasty had become evident. In many knees requiring this procedure the bone of the proximal tibia was significantly damaged. Accordingly, in 1978 an additional component was designed consisting of a horizontal metal element upon which the polyethylene tibial component was placed. The metal back had a stem on its undersurface. Because of the fear of infection following revision arthroplasty it was decided not to cement the stem but instead to use cement simply to fill defects in the bone under the horizontal component. The early results of this revision technique were reported by Bertin et al. [5] who drew attention to the fact that at a maximum follow-up of 5 years there had been no case of aseptic tibial loosening.

Thus, by 1983 four techniques of tibial fixation were available: the purely polyethylene component fixed with cement, the polyethylene component fixed without cement, and the polyethylene component placed on a metal-back and stem, the latter having cement under its horizontal surface or being entirely without cement. In the short term it proved difficult to distinguish between the rival merits of these four possibilities, in particular because Blaha et al. [6] had demonstrated that conventional radiography is an insensitive method of measuring component migration (migration of less than 2 mm and of less than 3° could not be detected).

Fortunately, in the late 1980s the technique of roentgen stereophotogrammetric analysis (RSA), introduced initially by Selvik, was reported in its application to the early measurement of tibial migration by Ryd [22]. We were fortunate at the Royal London Hospital in being able to work in cooperation with Ryd in Lund and in so doing were able to compare the quality of early fixation achieved by the alternatives then in clinical use. In 1990 Albrektsson et al. [1] reported that without cement the purely polyethylene component was statistically significantly less stable both at 1 and at 2 years than was the same component placed upon a metal back and stem. These workers not only reported that the metal back and stem was more stable but also that the reduction in migration concerned particularly the tendency of the component to tilt into varus/valgus and antero/posteriorly. This finding was of particular interest because a short experience of an uncemented, metal-backed device without a stem had produced an obvious increase in early loosening as compared with the purely polyethylene device [1]. It thus appeared that rigidity made fixation worse, but that this disadvantage could be more than offset by the addition of a stem.

In clinical practice it was found that the use of the stem in primary arthroplasty carried with it a difficulty: if such a stem was too long, there was a danger that it might contact the inner cortex in short or unusually curved tibiae. If the tip of the stem contacts the inner cortex, it tends to displace the upper horizontal portion of the prosthesis and thus makes fixation worse. Clinical experience suggested that most tibiae could be accommodated by an 80-mm stem, but that some tibiae required a 50-mm stem. Two investigations were therefore carried out. Firstly, the 80-mm stem fixed without cement was evaluated by RSA and compared with the same device having cement under the horizontal surface [2]. This study demonstrated that the 80-mm stem was on average slightly more stable than the earlier 110-mm stem used by Albrektsson et al. but not to a statistically significant degree. On the other hand, the addition of cement produced a statistically significant improvement in early migration, mean total point motion (MTPM) now falling to 0,5 mm at the end of the first postoperative year. This figure represented the lowest value for early tibial MTPM delete recorded in the literature.

Secondly, a modular version of the tibial component (the prosthesis being known as the Freeman-Samuelson modular prosthesis) was introduced to enable the surgeon to adjust the length of the stem to suit the particular tibia under operation.

Although demonstrating that certain configurations are more stable in the first year or two postoperatively, RSA is open to the criticism that it may have no relevance to the long-term failure rate. It is therefore interesting to note that studies at the Royal London Hospital of the long-term failure rate of the various configurations studied by RSA produce a ranking order identical to that of their stability at 1 year (Table 1) [3].

Table 1. Tibial component fixation, early migration measured by RSA versus late revision rate

Prosthesis and fixation	MTPM (mm) at 1 year	Revision rate
Polyethylene press-fit	2.0	17 % at 10 years
Metal back 110 mm plus stem	1.5	10 % at 8 years
Press-fit 80 mm	1.3	
Metal back plus stem proximal cement	0.5	0 % at 10 years

In summary, it would appear that a tibial component placed as proximally as possible, covering the whole of the tibia and having a metal back, a medial and lateral peg and a central stem 50–80 mm in length can be securely fixed to the proximal tibia with the aid of cement placed only under the horizontal surface. Cement used in this way produces no significant invasion of the bone and appears to have no obvious disadvantages.Having said this, the author is at present evaluating a cementless device having exactly the same configuration but with hydroxyapatite on the undersurface of the metal back in the hope that this may provide even lower early migration rates.

Patellar Pain and the Evolution of the Femoral Component

Anterior pain was a major problem in the early years and was attributed to the fact that the unreplaced patella had to make its way across an uneven, bony and metallic surface. In 1973 the posterior surface of the patella was replaced, and the anterior flange of the femoral component was lengthened. The latter step necessitated the introduction of femoral components of varying anteroposterior size.

Initially it was feared that patellar component loosening might represent a major hazard, and therefore an attempt was made to design a relatively unconstrained patellofemoral joint to reduce the shear stresses that might otherwise have been generated at the patellar bone/prosthesis interface. The resultant prosthesis had a flat anterior flange in the mediolateral direction and was known as the "ICLH". Unfortunately, lack of constraint at the patellofemoral joint, although it was indeed associated with a low incidence of component loosening, was also associated with an unacceptable incidence of lateral patellar subluxation [17]. However, in patellae in which tracking was satisfactory anterior knee pain almost disappeared [18].

In view of these findings it was decided to provide the anterior part of the femoral surface with a deep groove having a single radius as viewed from the side. The patellar component was made of polyethylene and was saddle-shaped to provide, firstly, an area contact (and thus low stresses) when articulating with the femoral component and, secondly, a significant area laterally to resist lateral patellar dislocation. The design of this part of the prosthesis was particularly attributable to the work of Dr. K.N. Samuelson. The patellar component could be fixed with or without cement.

A review of the results of this mode of reconstruction was reported by Elias et a. [9]. A summary of their findings is contained in Table 2, from which it can be seen, that the incidence of patellofemoral complications has now fallen to an acceptable level. We have measured, in a small unpublished series, the rate of forward migration of the patellar component through the patella when fixed without cement over the course of 7 years. The average migration rate was found to be 0,1 mm per year.

Table 2. Patellar complications after patellar replacement: 122 and 18 cemented prostheses[a]

Anterior pain requiring analgesia	1
Fracture Intraoperative	2
Fracture Postoperative	2
Subluxation	2
Dislocation	0
Aseptic loosening	0

Inserted 1980–1987; average follow-up 5 years

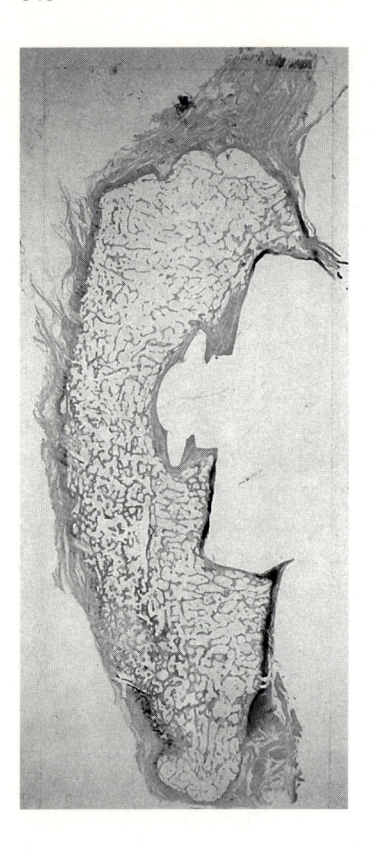

Fig. 4. The histological appearances of the patella beneath a press-fit polyethylene component. Note the presence of chondroid metaplasia where the interface is loaded in compression

Histological studies of well-functioning knees retrieved at postmortem have shown that the patellar component is contained in a fibrous tissue bed which undergoes chondroid metaplasia where it is loaded in compression (Fig. 4). Since the patellar component is recessed into the patella rather than being placed on its transsected surface, the peripheral portion of the original articular surface of the patella also carries load. This surface also becomes covered with soft tissue which, as in the bed of the prosthesis itself, undergoes chondroid metaplasia.

Certain features of the patellofemoral reconstruction are of importance. Firstly, it has been reported [16] that in the natural knee exhibiting recurrent patellar subluxation, the anatomical defect is in the proximal extremity of the lateral prominence of the femoral condyle so that patellar maltracking starts between 0° and 10°. In view of this it seems appropriate to provide the femoral component with an anterior flange of sufficient height to engage the patella throughout its range of extension.

Secondly, the natural femoral surface around which the patella tracks is circular as viewed from the side (Fig. 5). In a similar way the patellar articular surface of the femoral prosthesis should be circular to provide smooth tracking

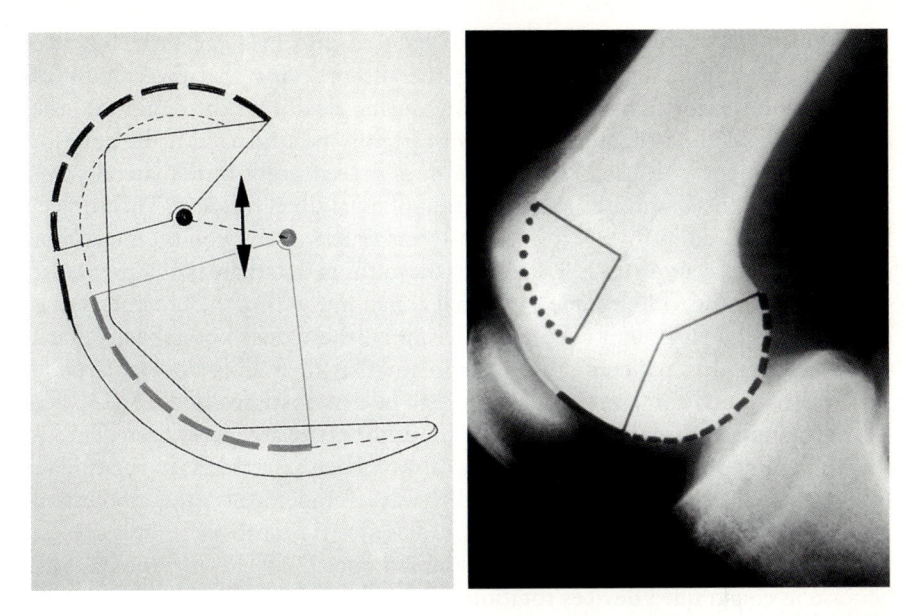

Fig. 5a. A lateral radiograph of the knee, and **b** a diagram of the prosthesis to show the circular patella and tibial surfaces of the femur

for the patella throughout the range of flexion (Fig. 5) [9]. It is important that the patellar component should be adequately recessed into the bone, and that the patellar articular surface of the femur should be anatomically placed anterodistally. If the femoral component is displaced forwards, or the patella is made too thick by replacement, the extensor mechanism is rendered unduly tense as the knee flexes. This may contribute to "pull-off" lateral patellar fractures, to limitation of flexion, and perhaps to anterior pain.

With regard to its tibial surface, the essential feature of the femoral component is that it has a single radius articulating with a tibial trough of the same radius. Two things follow from this geometry: firstly, all the femoral components may be interchanged with all the tibial components; secondly, the stresses on the polyethylene may be reduced to acceptable levels. Rostoker and Galante [21] have argued on the basis of experimental data that polyethylene stresses should not rise appreciably above 1 000 lb/in^2. For the medium size of Freeman-Samuelson prosthesis this stress is produced by the application of three times the bodyweight using the existing conforming geometry. Thus, for relatively flat tibial components (having a larger radius of curvature than their matching femur), the operating stresses must be above the levels recommended by Rostokker and Galante.

A consequence of a fully conforming tibiofemoral joint which is not at the same time meniscal is that anteroposterior translation of the femur on the tibia during flexion and extension cannot occur. Neither can axial tibial rotation.

Space does not allow these topics to be entered into in detail here, but two observations may be made. Firstly, it is the authors' view that the amount of obligatory posterior translation occurring during flexion of the femur (at least on the medial side) is negligible and can certainly be neglected if the anterior cruciate ligament is divided. Translation does indeed occur in the lateral compartment, but this is simply a manifestation of axial tibial rotation. This subject has been discussed in the context of posterior cruciate resection by the author elsewhere [11]. Secondly, it is not clear to the authors that there is any particular disadvantage in providing some rotational constraint within the prosthesis as is done by a roller-in-trough geometry. Certainly, there does not appear to be a functional penalty: patients do not complain that their tibia does not rotate axially. Rotational component migration can be demonstrated by RSA [13], but actual rotational loosening has, so far as the author is aware, never been demonstrated for any prosthesis, although it has always been asserted that a rotationally constrained bearing would fail in this way. Paradoxically, the amount of rotational migration occurring in Ryd's studies of various prostheses was greater in unconstrained implants than in constrained ones [22]. This may perhaps be because in constrained devices rotation is actually prevented by the soft-tissue, whereas in the unconstrained device rotation does occur but in so doing friction plus ploughing generates a significant torque on the tibial components.

When it is stated that the roller-in-trough geometry is relatively constrained, it is important to appreciate that the degree of constraint which it provides has been studied experimentally in the cadaver [4]. If the femoral roller is articulated with the tibial trough and rotated while an axial compressive load of three times the bodyweight is applied, the femur eventually "climbs" out of the tibial trough, transmitting to the latter a certain torque which reaches a maximum (in much the same way as would that transmitted by a torque wrench) the magnitude of which is dependent on the depth of the trough. The rotational torque generated by the Freeman-Samuelson geometry can easily be resisted (in the cadaver) by a number of methods of tibial fixation [4]. Of course, in clinical practice the tendency of the femoral component to rotate and climb is resisted not simply by the tibiofemoral geometry but mainly by the tibiofemoral soft tissues, thus further reducing the torque which is actually transmitted to the tibial component interface.

Isolated femoral component loosening has not represented a major problem [8]. This is presumably because (a) the femoral component is of a shape which makes it intrinsically more stable on the lower femur than is the tibial component on the proximal tibia, and (b) the bone of the femur is stronger point-for-point than that of the tibia. We have not demonstrated statistically that cement improves femoral fixation, although there has been a trend in this direction (a recent unpublished review showing an incidence of femoral loosening in none of 225 in cemented devices as against 3 of 180 uncemented press-fits).

Wear

The third problem identified in 1978 [12] was that of wear of the tibial component produced by impacted fragments of polymethylmethacrylate. Initially, the posterior flange of the femoral component was not split centrally, so as to increase the tibiofemoral contact area. This made it difficult to extract excess cement from the back of the tibial and femoral components. Furthermore, it was not appreciated that the tibia could be fully subluxed forwards when the tibial component was implanted, a feature of modern techniques which makes the extraction of posterior cement more reliable. To facilitate the removal of posterior cement we followed Insall and Walker in dividing the posterior flange of the femoral component so that the posterior compartment could be reached through the intercondylar notch, the posterior cruciate ligament having been removed. A disadvantage of this step was that it reduced the contact area and thus increased the contact stresses in the tibiofemoral joint. Two other features aimed at reducing wear have already been mentioned. Firstly, the component was fixed without the use of cement with the object of eliminating cement debris as an abrasive. Secondly, a conforming tibiofemoral articulation has been used from the outset to reduce the contact stresses on the polyethylene, a feature peculiar to this series of prostheses and to some implants of the meniscal type.

A tibial component having been fixed without cement retrieved at postmortem 11 years postoperatively is shown in Fig. 6. In this figure the machining marks on the original polythene surface can be seen, and the imprint made by the femoral component is evident. This imprint is due partly to creep and partly to wear. Were this the only pattern to be seen, the wear problem might be viewed with some equanimity. Unfortunately, some polyethylene components demon-

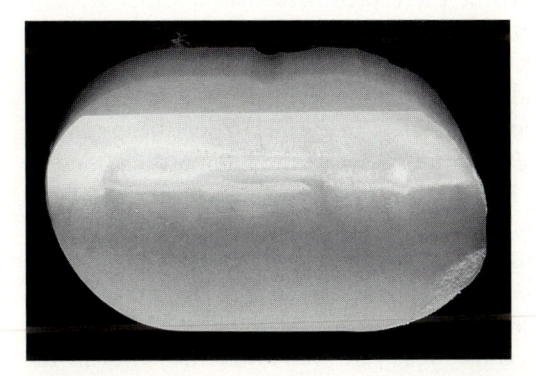

Fig. 6. A tibial component retrieved at postmortem examination 11 years postoperatively showing polishing but no other material wear

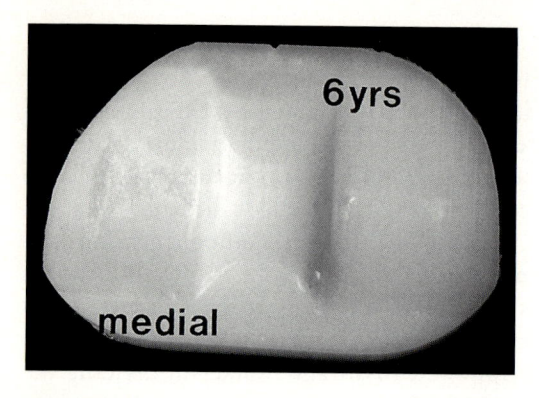

Fig. 7. A second polyethylene tibial component removed 6 years after operation, at revision for infection showing significant wear in the medial compartment

strate subsurface fatique leading to the separation of flakes of polyethylene from the flat surface auterior to the articular area (Fig. 7). At the present time it is not clear why there is this variation in the behaviour of an apparently similar articulation. It is, however, worth noting that similar variation, also unexplained, occurs with regard to wear at the acetabulum.

In the early 1980s Tuke (confirmed by McKellop et al. [19]) showed that Delrin could be used as a bearing material against polyethylene. Polyethylene wear against Delrin was 62 % less than against CoCr and the combined wear rates of the two materials was 10 % less. In view of this an experimental series of Freeman-Samuelson prostheses were implanted in 1981 and 1982 in which the femoral component was made of Delrin and not CoCr (Fig. 8). To date, one postmortem specimen has been retrieved at 8 years: no visible wear was present. These findings are clearly encouraging but await further study and publication.

In 1993 Plante-Bordeneuve et al. [20] published a study of 27 tibial components retrieved from Freeman-Samuelson knee arthroplasties between 1 and 9 years after operation. Twenty two of these prostheses had a CoCr femoral component and in five the femoral component was polyacetal. The design of the Freeman-Samuelson knee provides a nominal contact area of 320 mm^2 on each condyle. In every component studied the tibial polyethylene was at least 6 mm thick, and no component had been heat treated. In the metal/polythene components the average wear rate was 0,025 mm per year, the rate on each condyle being related to the postoperative knee axis: if the axis was less than 5° of valgus, the medial side wore more rapidly whereas the lateral side wore more rapidly if the knee had been aligned in more than 5° of valgus. No prosthesis showed severe disruption of the surface, but some degree of wear similar to that shown in Fig. 7 was seen in 5 of the 22 knees.

In the polyacetal knees the average wear rate was lower than that in the metal/high-density polyethylene prostheses, but this difference did not reach statistical significance. No knee showed surface damage.

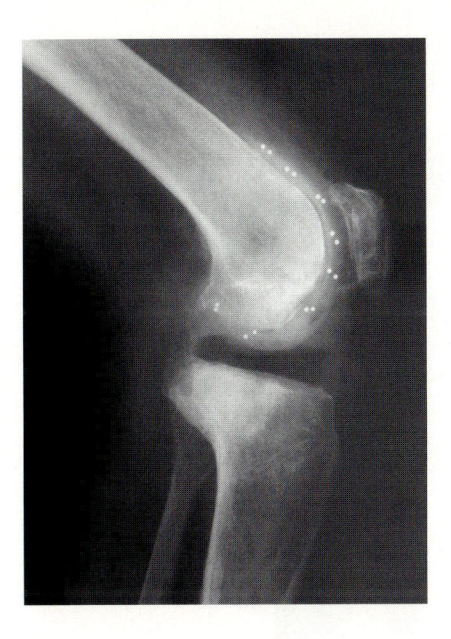

Fig. 8. The postoperative radiograph of a knee in which the femoral component was made of Delrin

These wear rates are similar to those reported for a fully conforming meniscal knee (the Oxford prosthesis) by Argenson and O'Connor (1992) [3] and about one-tenth of those reported for the linear wear rate of the Charnley prosthesis (Wroblewski 1985 [23]). It may be concluded that the provision of conforming bearing surfaces and thus area contact, combined with sufficiently thick polythene (at least 6 mm) which has not been heat treated, provides acceptable wear rates even though the components are fixed in a conventional fashion. There would therefore appear to be no argument based on wear for the use of meniscal arthroplasties.

One further aspect of wear should be considered: the problem of wear of a polyethylene surface when it is articulating against bone at the fixation surface. In practice wear of this kind is not a clinical problem unless (a) the component loosens, and (b) the interface is under a compressive load sufficient to crush the soft tissue which otherwise separates polyethylene from bone. This combination of loosening and direct polyethylene-bone contact certainly produces unacceptable polyethylene abrasion (and it was partly for this reason that a metal back was placed on the undersurface of the tibial component). In contrast to the tibial component, this problem has never been seen at the patella (Fig. 4) where fixation with an uncemented, purely polyethylene device has proved satisfactory (see above). (It is interesting to note that the purely polyethylene device appears to have functioned better than similar metal-backed devices: perhaps the adverse effect of rigidity noted at the tibia is equally applicable to the patella.) The appearance of the prosthesis as it had evolved in the light of these findings by 1990 is shown in Fig. 9.

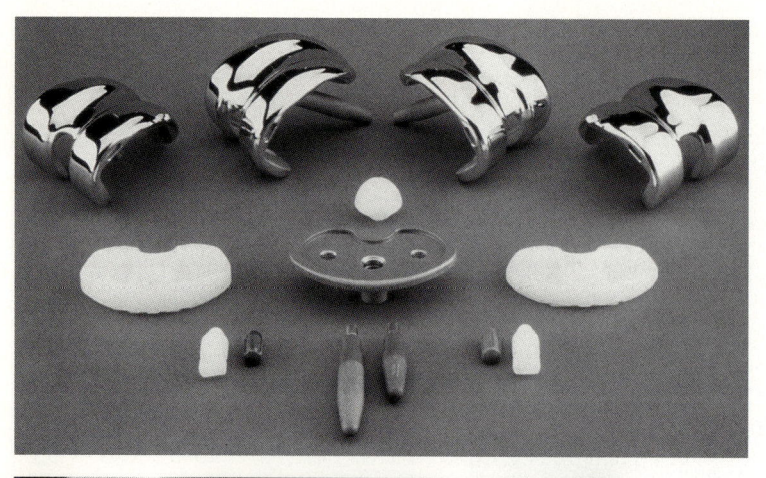

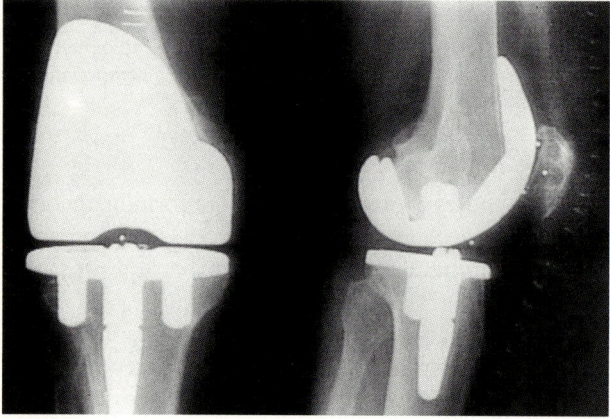

Fig. 9a. Freeman-Samuelson modular prosthesis showing the separated components, and **b** a postoperative radiograph.

Surgical Technique

The discussion to this point has concerned itself with the evolution of the prosthesis. It should be emphasized, however, that the results of knee arthroplasty today do not depend on the remaining small differences between one condylar prosthesis and another. On the contrary, they do depend, critically, upon the quality of the surgical technique. This in its turn is dependent on the surgeon and upon the concepts and instruments being used. Unfortunately, space does not allow a detailed description of the evolution and present concepts underlying the surgical technique, which are fully dealt with elsewhere (manufacturer's literature). Certain points are, however, worth making in summary form.

Firstly, it is essential that the knee should be appropriately aligned and stabilized in extension: failure to do this reliably was an important cause of early failure [12]. The ideal alignment should result in a resultant load acting through the centre of the tibial component. This in turn means that the knee should be aligned in about 7° of valgus (i. e. 7°±3° valgus) or, to put the same anatomical fact another way, with the centres of the hip, knee and ankle in straight alignment. To achieve this in a knee with preoperative fixed varus or valgus deformity, it is necessary to understand how to release the soft-tissue contractures which produce the deformity. At the start of the author's experience in 1969, the concept of medial and lateral soft-tissue release procedures was not understood, and it has been a critical part of the evolution of knee arthroplasty in the ensuing years that now the required techniques are fully appreciated.

Not only must the soft tissues be released to produce the requisite alignment, but at the same time they must be placed under balanced and appropriate tension in extension so as to result in a stable knee. In the early days of unlinked condylar arthroplasty it was thought to be impossible to achieve this, and thus linkages of various kinds were proposed. It is now known that by appropriately adjusting the relationship between the thickness of the prosthesis and the separation of the proximal tibial and distal femoral osteotomies, the knee can be satisfactorily stabilized. This concept was first introduced to surgical practies in the Freeman-Swanson arthroplasty in the early 1970s. The results were reported in 1978 [12], the first report so far as the author is aware of soft-tissue release applied to total knee arthroplasty (Fig. 10).

Stability at 90° flexion has not been as widely discussed as stability in extension. However, the knee must be stabilized in this (and intermediate) positions if it is to wear and function satisfactorily, particularly in activities such as stairclimbing. It is of course possible to rely on both the cruciate ligaments to provide stability. However, if the tibial component has a stem, the anterior cruciate ligament must be resected (and of course it is often absent). With the authorts present prosthesis, the posterior cruciate ligament can be left in place but no special advantage for this has as yet been demonstrated in the authors' view [11]. If one or both of the cruciate ligaments are to be resected, anteroposterior stability depends upon the relationship between the height of the gap between the posterior femoral osteotomy and the proximal tibial osteotomy, on the one hand, and the thickness of the prosthesis, on the other. If the prosthesis is thicker than the gap, the knee will not flex. If the prosthesis is thinner than the gap, the femoral roller can move over the anterior (or rarely the posterior) lip of the tibial component to produce an unstable knee. Thus, the requirement is to

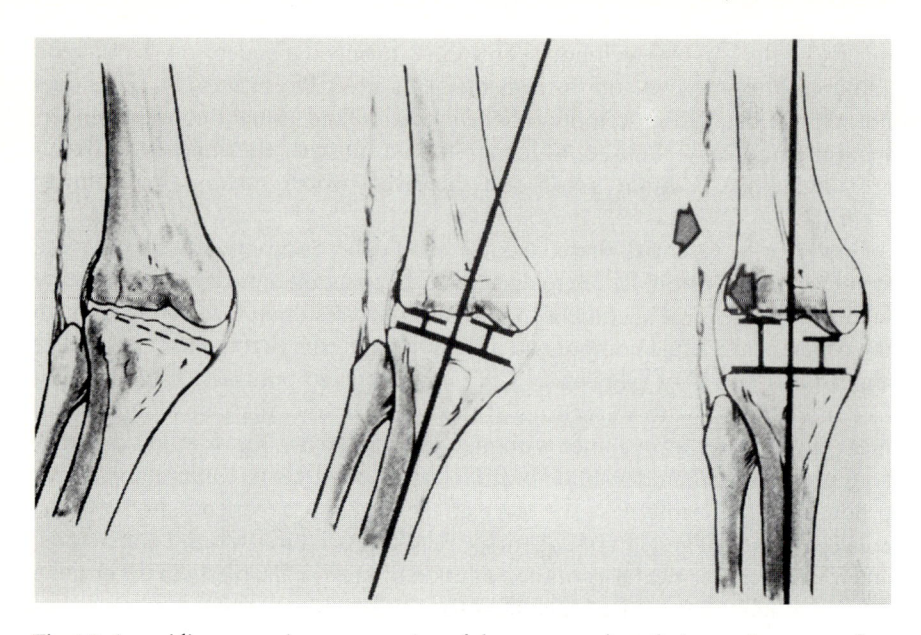

Fig. 10. A semidiagrammatic representation of the concept of a soft tissue release procedure (here shown for a valgus deformity) and the use of the "tensor". (From [4]; reproduced with the kind permission of the Editor of the *Journal of Bone and Joint Surgery* [Br])

produce an appropriate relationship between the thickness of the prosthesis and the gap both in flexion and in extension and at the same time correctly to align the knee in extension.

As has been mentioned, in 1978 the author described an instrument, the tensor, with which these objectives could be achieved in extension [12]. The instrument has since been modified to enable the flexion objective to be met with the same device as follows. The posterior femur and proximal tibia are resected. The tensor is introduced into the gap in flexion and the femur is tensed away from the tibia. The instrument automatically measures the height of the gap. The knee is now extended and the two compartments (medial and lateral) are tensed open separately (accompanied by whatever soft tissue release is needed) until the knee is both stable and correctly aligned. The tensor now transfers the gap measured in flexion into the extended knee, referencing from the already cut tibia to indicate the correct level and valgus/varus attitude of distal femoral section. This technique can be used with both extramedullary or intramedullary alignment. The difference between these two is a matter of convenience provided that the hip is found radiologically if extramedullary alignment is used. If intramedullary alignment is to be accurate, the femoral shaft must be neither obstructed nor deformed.

Anteriorly, the femur must be resected so as to enable the anterior flange of the femoral component to be placed on the anterior femoral cortex. Posteriorly, the femur must be resected so that the resected femur will fit one of the available sizes of femoral component.

The proximal tibia should be resected perpendicular to the long axis of the tibia, and for this an extramedullary technique is the authors' preference. Resection should be as high as practicable provided that an adequate thickness of polyethylene can be inserted.

In view of these consideration the sequence of bone resections preferred by the senior author is as follows:
1. The anterior femur is cut flush with the anterior cortex.
2. The posterior cortex is cut so as to provide an adequate posterior fixation surface to fit one of the three sizes of femoral component.
3. The proximal tibia is cut as high as possible and perpendicular to the long axis of the bone.
4. The tensor is used to determine what thickness of prosthesis is appropriate, to control the alignment of the knee in extension, and to determine the valgus/varus attitude and proximal/distal position of the distal femoral cut.
5. The distal femur is then cut perpendicular to the anterior femoral osteotomy as viewed from the side.
6. A single chamfer cut is made anterodistally to fit the femoral component. It is important that this cut be sufficiently deep to enable the patella to track anatomically.
7. The patella is drilled, not transected, to receive a prosthesis. The femur and tibia are similarly drilled to receive fixation pegs and stems.

Results

The results of condylar arthroplasty in general are well known and are no different (so far as the author is aware) using the author's prosthesis and techniques from those achieved with other well-known devices. In round terms, 95 % of replaced knees should not require analgesia postoperatively [7]. Some 2 %–3 % of patients require analgesia for undetermined reasons. The remainder develop pain as a consequence of aseptic loosening in the first 10 years.

The average range of motion obtained is about 110°, but this depends mainly upon the preoperative arc. Knees starting with a preoperative arc of less than 90° gain 30°, with maximum in the authors' experience (operating on a knee preoperatively stiff) of 110°. (At operation the tibiofemoral joint always flexes fully: it is indeed impossible to implant the tibial component unless this is done. The postoperative arc thus depends upon the elasticity of the extensor mechanism and the patellofemoral reconstruction.)

Patients are able to walk essentially unlimited distances postoperatively, although it is the authors' view that they should be encouraged to conserve their prosthesis mechanically because of the long-term danger of wear. Unless patients are over 70 years of age or have rheumatoid arthritis, virtually all can walk 30 min. or more at any one time and can join in such activities as golf (although, again, it is probably wise to recommend the avoidance of this activity postoperatively). They should be able to rise from a chair without the use of their hands and ascend and descend stairs of ordinary steepness, again, without using their hands and in a natural fashion. Wear does not appear to occur to an important extent, at least within the first 10 years.

Revision for aseptic loosening is now a routine procedure using techniques referred to briefly above. The early results using these techniques were reported by Bertin et al. [5]. A recent review [12] or 99 consecutive revisions for aseptic loosening with a maximum follow-up of 9 years revealed no case of recurrent loosening and only one re-revision for infection.

Infection remains an important hazard. Débridement and antibiotics may be tried initially for well-fixed implants [13]. We have employed single-stage revision using gentamicin-impregnated Palacos cement as a fixative, for infected loose prostheses: in a recent study of 18 loose, infected prostheses, 16 appear to have been cured [10]. Two other cases developed further infections, but it was felt that these did not represent true recurrence (one was secondary to an infected leg ulcer and one occurred in an immunosuppressed patient who suffered multiple infections elsewhere).

Conclusions

Knee replacement of the condylar variety started at the London Hospital in 1968 and has since undergone a process of continuous evolution. The operation can now be said to have come of age. The essential features of the operative technique and (less importantly) of the prosthesis are clear. The operation appears to be as reliable as hip replacement and provides results of a similar symptomatic kind at a slightly lower functional level. Revision is possible in the event of aseptic loosening or in the event of sepsis. Today, therefore, it is possible to say that any knee can if necessary be replaced. Fortunately, most knees do not need it.

References

1. Albrektsson BEJ, Ryd L, Carlsson LV et al. (1990) The effect of a stem on the tibial component of knee arthroplasty: a roentgen-stereophotogrammetric study of uncemented tibial components in the Freeman-Samuelson knee arthroplasty. J Bone Joint Surg [Br] 72: 252–258
2. Albrektsson BEJ, Freeman MAR, Carlsson LV et al. (1992) Proximally cemented versus uncemented Freeman-Samuelson knee arthroplasty: a prospective randomised study. J Bone Joint Surg [Br] 74: 233–238

3. Argenson JN, O'Connor JJ (1992) Polyethylene wear in meniscal knee replacement: a one to nine-year retrieval analysis of the Oxford knee. J Bone Joint Surg [Br] 74: 228-232
4. Bargren JH, Day WH, Freemann MAR et al. (1978) Mechanical test on the tibial components on non-hinged knee prostheses. J Bone Joint Surg [Br] 60: 256-261
5. Bertin KC, Freeman MAR, Samuelson KM et al. (1985) Stemmed revision arthroplasty for aseptic loosening of total knee replacement. J Bone Joint Surg [Br] 67: 242-248
6. Blaha JH, Day WH, Freeman MAR et al. (1982) The fixation of a proximal tibial polyethylene prosthesis without cement. J Bone Joint Surg [Br] 64: 326-335
7. Brach Del Prever EM, MacPherson IS, Freeman MAR et. al. (1988) Esperienza clinica con la protesi di ginocchio Freeman-Samuelson (1980-1985). G Ital Orthop Traumatol XIII(4): 423
8. Colley J, Cameron HU, Freemann MAR et al. (1978) Loosening of the femoral component in surface replacement of the knee. Arch Orthop Trauma Surg 92: 31-34
9. Elias SG, Freeman MAR, Gokcay EI (1990) A correlative study of the geometry and anatomy of the distal femur. Clin Orthop 260: 98-103
10. Freeman MAR, Goksan SG (1992) One-stage reimplantation for infected total knee arthoplasty. J Bone Joint Surg [Br] 74: 78-82
11. Freeman MAR, Railton GT (1988) The current status of total replacement of the knee with special reference to prostheses of the condylar variety. In: Galasko CSB, Noble J (eds). Current trends in orthopaedic surgery. Manchester University Press, Manchester, p 221
12. Freeman MAR, Todd RC, Bamert P et al. (1978) ICLH arthroplasty of the knee: 1968-1977. J Bone Joint Surg [Br] 60: 339-344
13. Freeman MAR, Sudlow RA, Casewell MW et al. (1985) The management of infected total knee replacements. J Bone Joint Surg [Br] 67: 764-768
14. Freeman MAR, Samuelson KM, Elias SG et al. (1989) The patellofemoral joint in total knee prostheses: design considerations. J Arthroplasty (Suppl) 4: S69-S74
15. Grewal R, Rimmer M, Freeman MAR, (1992) Early migration of prostheses related to long-term survivorship: comparison of tibial components in knee replacement. J Bone Joint Surg [Br] 74: 239-242
16. Kujala UN, Osterman K, Kormano M et al. (1989) Patellofemoral relationships in recurrent patellar dislocation. J Bone Joint Surg [Br] 71: 788-792
17. Levai JP, Freeman MAR (1984) Les complications patellaires de la prothèse du genou ICLH. Rev Chir Orthop 70: 41
18. Levai JP, McLeod HC, Freeman MAR (1983) Why not resurface the patella? J Bone Joint Surg [Br] 65: 448-451
19. McKellop H, Hossenian A, Tuke M et al. (1985) Superior wear properties of an all-polymer hip prostheses. Trans Orthop Res Soc 10: 322
20. Plante-Bordeneuve P, Freeman MAR (1993) Tibial high-density polyethylene wear in conforming tibiofemoral prostheses. J Bone Joint Surg [Br] 75: 630-636
21. Rostocker W, Galante JO (1979) Contact pressure dependence of wear rates of ultra high molecular weight polyethylene. J Biomed Mater Res 13: 957-964
22. Ryd L (1986) Micromotion in knee arthroplasty. A roentgen-stereophotogrammetric analysis of tibial component fixation. Acta Orthop Scand Supply 220: 857
23. Wroblewski BM (1985) Direction and rate of socket wear in Charnley low-friction arthroplasty. J Bone Joint Surg [Br] 67: 757-761

The APS Cement-Free Knee Joint Prosthesis in Varus Osteoarthritis: Treatment and Results

W. Schwägerl, P. Zenz

Introduction

A gliding knee joint prosthesis, developed in our Department has been in use here since 1984 (Fig. 1). It was designed for: Cementless fixation with immediate and stable anchorage, osseous integration to obtain long-term fixation, and easily reproducible surgical technique.

Immediate fixation is achieved by means of dowel anchorage of all three parts of the implant, tapered shaping of the femur component, and a concave bearing surface of the patellar shield. Immediate stabilization of the tibial implant is also achieved by means of dowel anchorage on a flat osseous surface. On the back of the patella a symmetrical truncated cone is prepared, in which the gliding surface of the patella component is inserted through dowel anchorage. The dowel effect on the patella and the tibia is achieved by the introduction of polyethylene pegs into the titanium flanges. The mechanism on the femur is

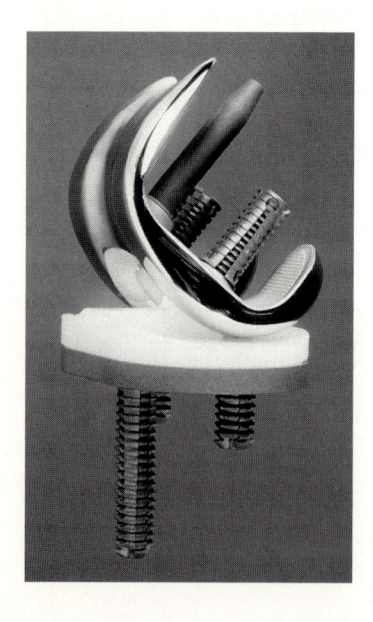

Fig. 1. APS knee joint prosthesis

reached by the introduction of the titanium flanges over the introduced primary polyethylene pegs.

The implant is available in four sizes (60, 65, 70, 75). Different materials with proven body adaptability are used for the femur, tibia, and patella components. This favors long-term stabilization.

Femur Component

The femur component consists basically of frictionless 28CoCr/6Mo Protasul alloy. The gliding part is polished technologically. The back part laid on the bone is structured and covered with 3–5 mm titanium nitrite ("coatasul"). The metal pegs screwed onto the back of the implant base are composed of a titanium alloy (Ti 6 Al 4V Protasul 64 VF ISO 5832/3 ASTNF 136, i. e., Ti 6 Al 7 Nb Protasul-100 SN 056512). The dowels introduced into the metal pegs are composed of polyethylene-chirulen 5261 Z. Their microstructured surface is coated with pure titanium "coatasul" Tl.

Tibia Component

The disc with its fixed metal pegs consists of a titanium alloy (Ti 6 Al 4V Protasul 64 WF, i. e. Ti 6 Al 7 Nb Protasul 100). The tibia part as well as the dowel is composed of polyethylene RCH-1000 chirulen (ISO 5834/2 DIN 58836). The microstructured surface of the dowels is coated with pure titanium "coatasul" Tl.

Patella Component

The concave bearing surface and the pegs fixed onto it consist of a titanium alloy (see above), the inlay and the dowels are composed of polyethylene (Chirulen), and the microstructured surface of the dowels is coated with pure titanium "coatasul" Tl.

Implantation Technique

The femur component is implanted on the femur condyles by an anatomical design. This is the basis of the implantation, which is determined by the upright position of the femoral implant on the anatomical weight-bearing axis. It is therefore important to evaluate the anteroposterior full-leg standing position of the patient on a preoperative radiograph to determine the angle between the axis of the femoral shaft and the weight-bearing axis. The angle is situated at 7° or tends more towards 5°. According to this measurement, the right angle is chosen intraoperatively. The upright structure of the bearing surface indicates the correct position of the intramedullary guide rod during operation. The resection plane at the tibia is in an upright position on the longitudinal tibia axis. When it is on the correct axis, it is situated on the weight-bearing axis of the leg.

The upright structure of the bearing surface running through the tibial head produces the relationship between the resection of the medial and the lateral part of the tibial head. An optimal and absolutely plain base area of the femoral condyles is achieved using a round reamer. The concave bearing surface ot the patellar shield is also achieved by means of a rounder reamer, which also improves the immediate stabilization of the femoral implant anchorage. Optimal positioning and setting of the femur component is attained thanks to a round reamer. Built on this, the resection plane at the tibial head is fixed in an upright position onto the longitudinal tibia axis. Slight resection on the back of the femoral condyles favors stability of the implant.

As varus knee joint arthrosis often represents an indication for a gliding knee joint replacement and often causes correction and treatment difficulties, a group of patients underwent a clinical and radiographical examination after a knee joint operation.

Patients

Between 1984 and 1988, 185 patients were operated on. Indications were arthrosis (120 patients) and rheumatoid arthritis (65 patients). In 14 % the patients were provided with a knee joint prosthesis implanted with cement, and the rest one without cement. Of these, 64 arthrosis patients receiving a cement-free prosthesis had varus deformities (of 63 patients, plus one operated on both legs, 15 were male and 48 were female). The average age of the patients was 70 years (54–86 years). There were 97 % of the patients available for follow-up (one patient died, one patient did not appear), and the average follow-up period was 40 months (36–60 months).
Conditions for cement-free implant include adequate bone quality, which is a prerequisite for this operation. This can be verified both radiographically and intraoperatively. In patients with rheumatoid arthritis and receiving long-term cortisone treatment or age over 70 years among female patients the surgery is contraindicated. There is no age limit for among men; but they must have excellent bone quality.

Clinical Results

The clinical and radiographical results concern only joints followed up and not reoperated ($n = 59$). In Table 1 are the results for postoperative pain, postoperative walking ability, which was significantly improved, and knee flexion. Average postoperative knee flexion is 94°. A slight improvement in extension was achieved through a decrease in flexion contracture (see Tables 1, 2).

Average preoperative varus deformity was 11° (Table 3), and the corrections achieved are shown in Table 4. In most cases it was possible for the preoperative deformity to be clinically aligned in the anatomical axis of the leg. In one case after an intraoperative femur fracture, the deformity was 18° valgus malposition, and in six cases alignment was slightly varus. The radiographically verified implant position indicated more than 2° implant varus alignment on the tibia for

Table 1. Clinical results of joints followed up and not reoperated (n=59)

	Preoperative	Postoperative
Pain		
severe	21	0
moderate	37	8
slight	1	18
none	0	33
Ability to walk		
at home only	5	0
0–10 min	17	2
30–60 min	33	23
> 60 min	4	34
Knee flexion		
> 90°	34	31
90°	11	19
60°–89°	12	7
< 60°	2	2

Table 2. Average knee flexion, contracture, and range of movement

	Preoperative	Postoperative
Flexion	99°	94°
Contracture	7°	2°
Range of movement	89°	90°

Table 3. Preoperative varus deformity (n=62; mean=11°)

< 5°	6
5°– 9°	18
10°–14°	17
15°–19°	14
20°	7

Table 4. Postoperative positioning

Normal	55
Varus	6 (3–6, diameter 4°)
Valgus	1 (18°)

Table 5. Positon of the femur and tibia implants

	Femur	Tibia
Valgus > 2°	12	2
Normal	47	39
Varus > 2°	0	18

18 patients and more than 2° valgus alignment on the femur for 12 patients (see Table 5). This results in an incorrect implant position. The surgical technique with regard to the positioning of the tibial plateau has been modified, and since then correct positioning of the implant has been achieved.

Radiographic Follow-Up Examination

Radiographic check-up is divided into five states of examination. These indicate that in group 1 (full osseointegration) and group 2 (good osseointegration) implants were 80 % successful at tibia level and nearly 100 % successful at femur level (Table 6). The remaining 20 % of group 3 (lucent lines > 1 mm) on the tibia are followed up continuously. The radiographic follow-up examination over a period of 5 years is shown in Fig. 2a, b, which indicate that better implant stabilization was achieved at the femur. Gaps and radiolucencies around the dowel system of the tibia were seen after a period of 2 years. No changes were observed afterwards. Improvement in the fifth year was due to osseointegration of several implants.

Table 6. Result of the radiographic examination by group

Group (n=59)	Femoral	Tibial
1	41	28
2	17	19
1+2 (firm)	58 (98,3 %)	47 (79,6 %)
3	1	11
4	0	1
5	0	0

Group 1, full osseointegration; group 2, good osseointegratiOn; group 3, lucent lines ›1 mm; group 4, lucent lines, complete; group 5, loosened

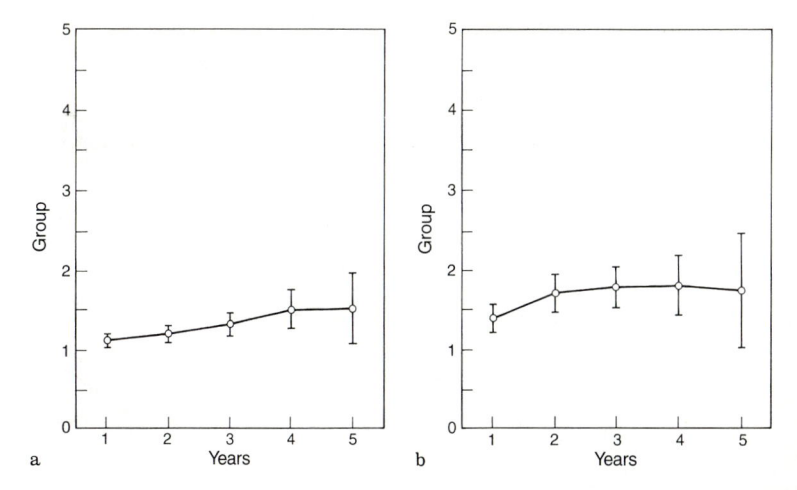

Fig. 2a, b. Radiographic follow-up results over the first 5 years (mean, standard deviation) of implant by group. a Femur. b Tibia

Complications

Intraoperatively one femur fractured distally during impacting of the femur component. Even an osteosynthesis with screws and wires and a fixation in a plaster spica resulted in 18 % valgus deformity. It was necessary to reoperate three times because of aseptic loosening (4.7 %) of the tibial implant. Twice the tibia component had to be replaced by a cemented tibial implant APS, and once it was necessary to substitute this with a Gschwend-Scheier-Bähler constraint prosthesis. Twice varus implant position and inadequate medial release were the reasons for this aseptic loosening, which resulted in a varus malposition and medial overloading of the bone area. In the third case the implant of a undersized tibia component caused the plateau to subside. Twice we had to perform the tuberositas transposition of *Elmslie* and a patellectomy because of a patella luxation, and a loose patella implant hat to be changed.

Discussion

Providing varus deformities with cementless implantation of a gliding knee joint prosthesis showed satisfying results during the 3- to 5-year follow-up period. Difficulties resulted from the anatomical positioning of the implant, which led to a too valgus implantation on the femur and a too varus implantation on the tibia. Essential improvements were achieved by the introduction of an extended intraosseous guiding rod into the femur and by attention to the preoperatively

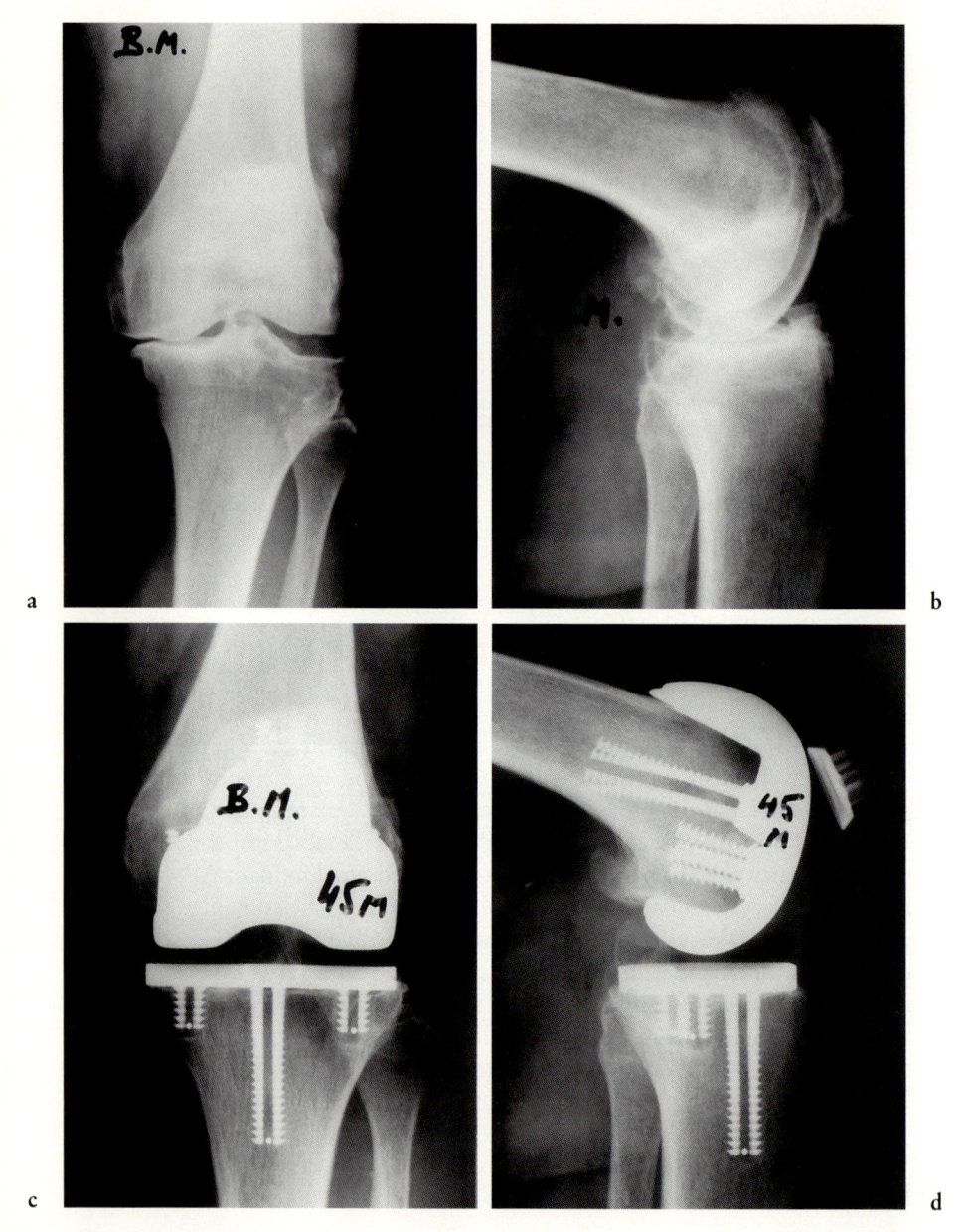

Fig. 3a–d. A 73-year-old female patient with varus osteoarthritis. a, b Preoperative: anteroposterior a and lateral b. c, d Postoperative: 45 months after surgery. Osseointegration of the implant at the femoral c and d tibial levels

measured angle between the longitudinal axis of the femur and the weight-bearing axis.

At the tibia it is extremely important to pay attention to external rotation when introducing the extramedullary guiding pin for positioning of the resection guide. Balance between medial and collateral ligaments in the knee-joint area is another factor. Medial release should be carried out carefully until ligamentous balance has been achieved. For this reason it is important to perform a scaled-down dissection of the superficial medial collateral ligament, the pes anserinus insertion, and possibly the deep portion of the medial collateral ligament. This is achieved by osseous detachment of the medial epicondyle, which remains with the periosteum in a sleevelike connection.

Preoperative varus deformity of more than 20° represents a limit to the application of the gliding knee joint system. The resulting ligamentous imbalance is problematic and influences the prognosis of the method. Further ligament transpositions can be carried out, but these require careful indication.

Osseous deficiency at the medial femur could be compensated with autologous bone filling. Cavities at the tibia could also be autologically filled. Complete deficiency with osseous destruction of the tibial head is compensated by a hight cutting level of the tibial resection and the use of a higher tibia implant. If this cannot be carried out, a more constraint implant is provided.

So far the follow-up period for varus osteoathritis has shown that APS gliding knee joint with cement-free implantation to be successful. Nevertheless, age limit, adequate bone quality, and no long-term cortisone medication are prerequisites for this operation. Correct anatomical positioning of the implant components are extremely important (Fig. 3).

References

1. Edwards E, Miller J, Chan KH (1988) The effect of postoperative collateral ligament laxity in total knee arthroplasty. Clin Orthop 236: 44
2. Jonnson B, Aström J (1988) Alignment and long-term clinical results of a semiconstrained knee prothesis. Clin Orthop 236: 124
3. Schwägerl W, Zenz P (1990) The APS knee joint prothesis. A review of 32 patients. Arch Orthop Trauma Surg 109: 252
4. Schwägerl W, Zenz P (1994) Die Behandlung der Varusgonarthrose mit dem zementfreien „APS"-Kniegelenk. Orthop Prax 30/2: 113
5. Smith JL, Tullos HS, Davidson JP (1989) Alignment of total knee arthroplasty. J Arthroplasty Suppl
6. Windsor RE, Scuderi GR, Moran MC, Insall JN (1989) Mechanisms of failure of the femoral and tibial components in total knee arthroplasty. Clin Orthop 248: 15

Uncemented Unicompartmental Knee Arthroplasty

N. Böhler, K. Pastl, A. Infanger

History of Unicompartmental Knee Arthroplasty

Unicompartmental knee arthroplasty (UKA) was one of the first orthopedic implants used succesfully in joint replacement. MacIntosh published his first results in 1958 [9]. Marmor carried out most of the scientific work on UKA; created his own implant, spent substantial investigations working out the right indications, and began publishing studies in 1977 with a minimum of 2 years' follow-up to publish [11–13]. In 1988 Marmor published 10– 13-year results reviewing 60 patients, with 70 % good results and 86 % pain relief [14, 15].

In the middle of the 1980s the subject of UKA was controversial. In addition to very good results reportet by Larsson et al. in 1988 [7] (102 knees, 4 % loosening) and others [1, 6, 9, 16, 17, 19], unsatisfactory results were published by Insall and Aglietti [4]. The reasons for the failures at that time were:
(a) erroneous indication, choice of unstable or contract knees, degenerative changes especially at the patella; (b) inadequate operation technique, since at this time insufficient instrumentation was used, and a correct position of the implant was generally not achieved; and (c) wrong implant design: the femoral implants were large with anterior contact to the patella, and the tibia implant had very thin plateaus leading to polyethylene deterioration.

Even under these conditions here, however, unicompartmental implants were more successful than total knees implants in osteoarthritis patients. This one sees in the swedish arthroplasty project, a multicenter study following 8000 cases [6], which showed similar results between UKA and total knee arthroplasty afer 1 year: after 6 years, however, the UKA survival rate was still 90 %, compared with 87 % with total knee arthroplasty. On the other hand, these researchers found that UKA is not successful in rheumatoid patients, since this desease destroys the whole joint.

Indication for Unicompartmental Knee Arthroplasty

Finding the right indication is very important for achieving good results. The Osteonecrosis of the femoral condyl (Ahlbaeck's disease) is the classic indication. In knees with degenerative arthritis several criteria must be controlled. These are detailed below.

Soft Tissue Related Criteria

Ligamentous stability is a very important criteria, not only at the collateral ligament site but also at the cruciate ligament site. There must be an intact anterior and posterior cruciate ligament. Minor grades of medial collateral ligamentous laxity in varus knee deformity can be corrected by the implant. In cases of severe medial laxity or combined laxity of medial and lateral collateral ligamant the destruction of the lateral femoral condyle has to be expected. This is due to the so-called kissing leson, resulting from a bony contact between eminentia intercondylica and the femoral condyle. In such a case UKA should not be used. Flexion contractures of more than 10°–15° are also a contraindication for UKA since they cannot be corrected.

Osteocartilagineous Related Criteria

Osteoarthritis of the second compartment is a strict contraindication to UKA. Osteoarthritis of the patella may constitute a contraindication, especially in patients with pain in this region or with a larger amount of cartilage loss. We do not consider pain-free osteoarthritis with osteophytes at the patella to be a necessary contraindication for UKA.

Criteria Related to Patients, General Circumstances

Very heavy patients (exceeding 80 kg) and patients engaged in heavy sport activities are poor candidates for UKA. Patients under the age of 60 years should be operated on with UKA only under special circumstances, such as inactive patients or those with multiple joint involvement. In younger, heavy, and very active patients a high tibial osteotomy should be carried out. Even in the age group aged under 60, however, we should keep in mind that the results in the optimal candidate group for UKA are more predictable, and early results are much more satisfying and postoperative rehabilitation remains shorter than following osteotomy [5]. On the other hand, total knee replacement must be used for total joint destruction and knees with contractures or cruciate ligament instability. The post-operative management is somewhat more difficult than with UKA, the range of movement is less, and in cases of complication such as infection or loosening a reoperation is more difficult after the total knee implantation [8]. The patella also presents an yet unsolved problem. Patella replacement – yes or no – is still the question. For all these reasons we consider a large group of patients to be excellent candidates for UKA since results with the implants and modern technology have been very satisfying.

Implant Design

Cementless fixation has proven advantageous in total hip and total knee arthroplasty. We therefore also tried to provide cementless fixation in UKA. Press fitting together with a special dowel system gives optimal primary stability and the possibility of cementless fixation (Fig. 1).

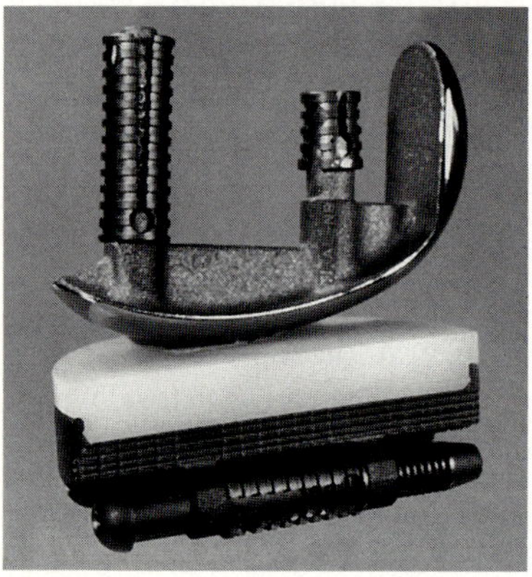

Fig. 1. The APB Unicondylar knee implant fixed with dowels and press-fit without cement

The design of the implant using a more or less constrained type of movement has been controversial. The main problem is polyethylene wear.

Constrained prostheses offer the advantage of reducing pressure on the polyethylene of the tibial implant due to a larger contact area. However, this advantage is found only with optimal conditions; since the UKA must follow the biomechanics of the intact ligaments, a correct position in the rotational plane is neccesary.

If one cannot achieve the correct position of a constrained implant – which is hard to define – the sharing forces produced by the nonreplaced compartment lead to a loosening of the implant and to even greater stress on the polyethylene compared with unconstrained prostheses. Hodge demonstrated this in 1992 [2]. Clinical long-term results are good in 98 % of nonconstrained UKA cases compared with 70 % in constrained types. To avoid sharing forces and early implant loosening we use a nonconstrained type of implant with a flat tibial plateau.

Implant Material

Cementless fixation requires materials that allow complete bony ingrowth. Titanium is presently the best candidate for intimate bone interlocking. Since the flat plateau, which is needed to avoid sharing forces, is exposed to high contact stress with single-point contact, numerous investigations have been performed to optimize the articulating joint materials [18]. Ultrahigh molecular weight polyethylene (UHMWPE) was optimized by using sterilization and irradiation with 60 Co and nitrogen (N 2). This procedure reduces the wear rate to one-half that of the standard sterilized UHMWPE using gamma-irradiation and air.

Furthermore, oxygen diffusion hardening (ODH) is used to increase the surface hardness of the titanium femoral surface component. Compaired with CoCrMo components or titanium N+ion hardening, another 30 % of polyethylene wear reduction was achieved [18]. This technique has been used for all implants since 1991.

Clinical Results

The Allo-Pro-Böhler monocondylar implant has been used at the Orthopedic Department of the Allgemeines Krankenhaus Linz since 1988. We conducted a prospective study on the first 100 prostheses between April 1988 and October 1990 (Table 1). The mean age of patients at operation was 69 years (range 51–81). Seven patients have died, two reoperations have been performed, and the remai-

Table 1. Clinical results in uncemented unicompartmental knee arthroplasty ($n = 91$)

	Preoperative	Follow-up
Flexion		
≤ 90	20	5
91–100	16	19
101–110	31	20
111–120	13	30
> 121	11	17
Pain (Hungerford)		
Grades 0 + 1	0	71
Grade 2	0	11
Grade 3	0	7
Grades 4+5	91	2

	6 month postop.	Follow-up
Femur (on radiology)		
Full contact	88	91
Zone 6	3	0
Tibia (on radiology)		
Full contact	31	30
Zone 5	40	48
Zones 3+5	15	10
No contact	5	2

ning 91 knees were studied over a mean follow-up period of 44 months (range 36–60). Cementless fixation was achieved in all cases. The indication for this operation was osteoarthritis in 91 cases, aseptic femoral necrosis in 8, and posttraumatic destruction in 1.

Range of Movement

Good **range of movement** is one of the great advantages of UKA. The preoperative range of movement of 2.5°–107.6° was increased to 1.8°–112.8° postoperatively. Only five patients had joint movement of less than 90° (Table 1).

Stability and Alignment

Stability and **alignment** the of tibio-femoral axis is not a problem in UKA. Only seven patients had collateral ligament laxity of more than 6°, and only five had more than 5° of valgus deformity in the case of medial compartment replacement. Since there is always the danger of deterioration of the second compartment, we prefer to create a slight varus position to keep the weight on the implant.

Walking Capacity

There were 79 patients who could walk up to 1 h., 8 up to only 30 min., and 4 were restricted to their home because of osteoarthritis of the hips and the other knee. Of the 91 patients, 66 could walk without a cane, 21 used a cane, and 3 relied on crutches. Again, the reason was osteoarthritis of other joints.

Pain

Pain was examined using the Hungerford [3] score (six grades). Postoperatively, 82 patients had no or slight pain (grades 1, 2), 4 reported moderate pain (grade 3) in the patellofemoral joint due to osteoarthritis in this region, 3 (grade 3) in the lateral compartment, and only 2 patients had severe pain (Table 1). In one of these two, X-ray and technetium scan in the region of the operated knee showed normal results, and we think that it might be sciatic nerve pain unrelated to the implant. The other patient complained of pain in the lateral compartment due to degenerative changes. The total Hungerford score for the overall situation was 93, which was very good.

X-Ray Results

For X-ray controls we examined the femoral and the tibial implant using image intensifier to guarantee the orthograde view to the bone-implant interface (Fig. 2). At the femoral site we found complete bony ingrowth without resorption or sclerosis in all the 91 cases. Only three patients showed an unchanged gap in the very dorsal area due to incorrect resection.

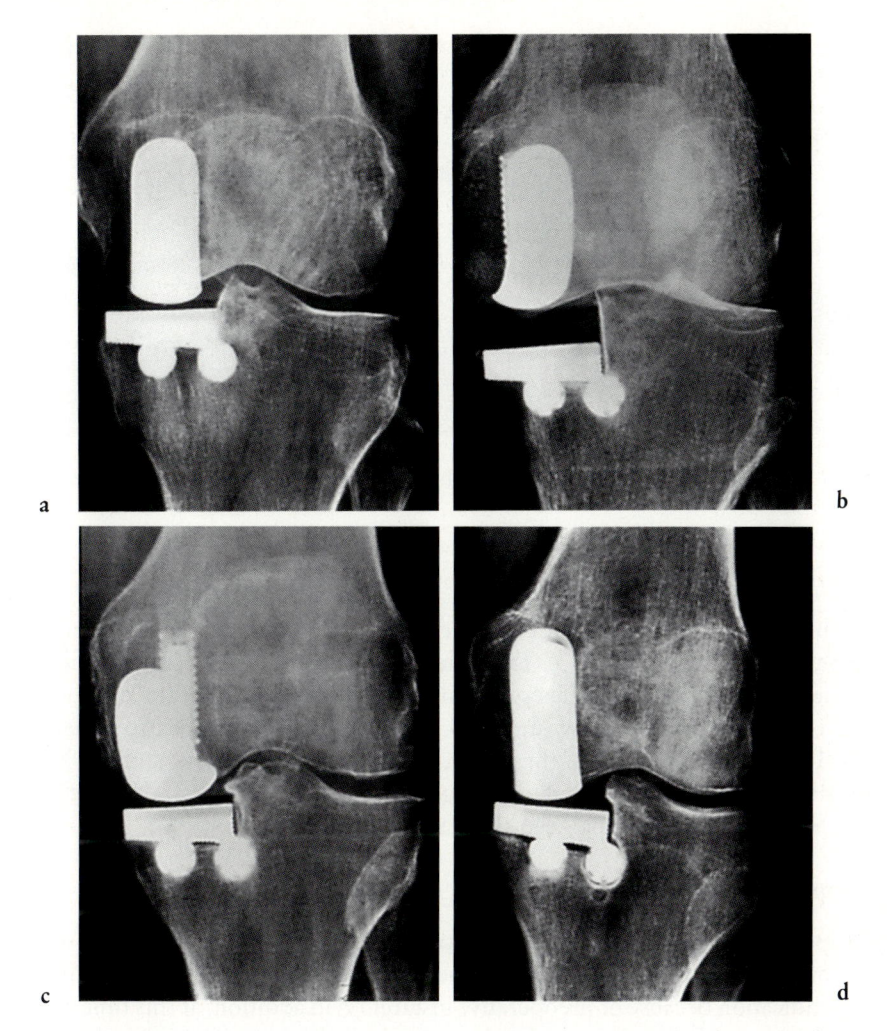

Fig. 2a–d. Four types of bony integration. Types 1–3 (**a–c**, respectively) show complete or partial bony implant integration; type 4 (**d**) is fixed only by the dowels

On the tibial side we found four types of bony integration:
Type one, complete ingrowth in all areas (Fig. 2a).
Type two, central gap at the eminentia (Fig. 2b).
Type three, central gap and gap between the dowels (Fig. 2c).
Type four, complete gap except the dowel area (Fig. 2d).
  Since the central gap at the eminentia is due to the polyethylene inlay exceeding the metal cage, this gap is not a sign of any instability.

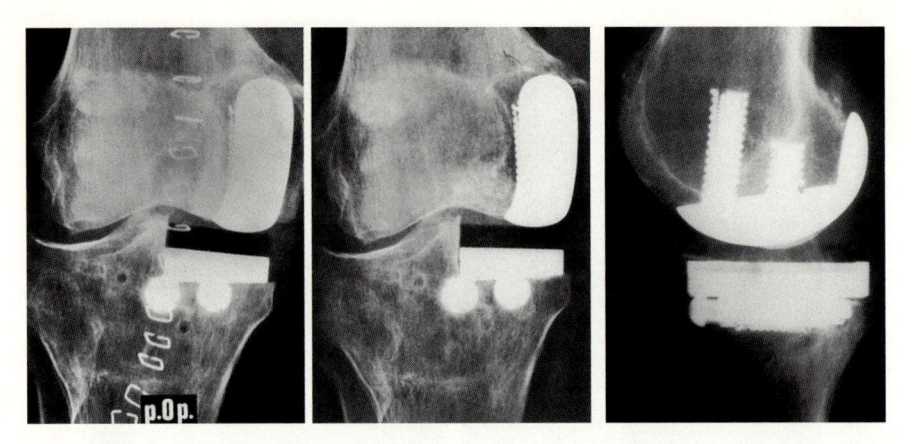

Fig. 3 APB Unicondylar implant 5 years after operation, showing complete bony integration

There were 79 patients with complete bony ingrowth of the tibial implant (types 1 and 2; Table 1; Fig. 3). Ten patients had a partial gap filled with fibrous tissue between the dowels. These remained unchanged for 2 years and showed no relation to pain at follow-up. Two patients had a complete gap under the tibial surface except around the dowel. Since they had no pain, and the X-ray remained unchanged, we think that, together with the fibrous fixation, the bone dowel fixation in the bone keep them stable.

Reoperations

Reoperations had to be carried out in two knees. In one knee a luxation of the femoral implant on the tibial plateau occurred. In the other there was in incorrect indication because of preoperative instability; in addition, at this time (1988) we lacked an adequate size of implants to cover the complete tibial plateau in this case. During reoperation and change to a total knee we found even in this knee – despite high shearing forces – complete bone ingrowth at the femoral and tibial site showing the high primary stability of this implant. The second reoperation was due to loosening of the cementless implanted tibial plateau in a woman with osteoporosis. Since the femoral implant was stable, we reimplanted only the the tibia implant, using cement for refixation.

Polyethylene Wear

Five patients had polyethylene wear exceeding 2 mm. We found this wear after 2 years, without deterioration thereafter. The reason may be the high local pressure at the time when we were not using an ODH surface. Since the implant contact is increased by building a groove in the tibia, polyethylene wear did not deteriorate during the following 3 years and does not constitute a real problem in this type of arthroplasty (Table 1).

Summary

In summary, the results of the cementless monocondylar implants have been very satisfying. A study of 100 implants showed a survival rate of 98 % after 5 years. The indication for this implant must be made very accurately and must follow the rules described above [3, 4]. Selecting patients brings very good results with shorter rehabilitation compared with high tibial osteotomy and total knee arthroplasty. Monocondylar knee replacement should be a technique in the operative repertoire of every orthopedic surgeon.

References

1. Bernasek TL, Rand JA, Bryan RS (1988) Unicomparmental porous coated anatomic total knee arthroplasty.
Orthop Trans 12: 654
2. Hodge WA, Chandlery HP (1992) Unicompartmental knee replacement: comparison of constrained and unconstrained designs. J Bone Joint Surg Am 74: 877
3. Hungerford DS, Kenna RV (1983) Preliminary experience with a total knee prosthesis with porous coating used without cement. Clin Orthop 176:95–107
4. Insall JN, Agliettit P (1980) A five to seven-year follow-up of unicondylar arthroplasty. J Bone Joint Surg Am 62: 1329
5. Ivarsson I, Giliquist J (1989) Rehabilitation after high tibial osteotomy and unicompartmental arthroplasty. Clin Orthop 266:139
6. Knutson K, Lindstrand A, Lidgren L (1986) Survival of knee arthroplasties. A nation-wide multicentre investigation of 8 000 cases. J Bone Joint Surg Br 68: 795
7. Larsson SE, Larsson S, Lundkvist S (1988) Unicompartmental knee arthroplasty. A prospective consecutive series followed for six to 11 years. Clin Orthop 232: 174
8. Laurencin CT, Zelicof SB, Scott RD, Ewald FC (1991) Unicompartmental versus total knee arthroplasty in the same patient: a Comparative study. Clin Orthop 273: 151
9. MacIntosh, DL (1958) Hemiarthroplasty of the knee using a space occupying prosthesis for painful varus and valgus deformities. J Bone Joint Surg Am 40: 1431
10. Mackinnon J, Young S, Baily RAJ (1988) The St. George sledge for unicompartmental replacement of the knee. J Bone Joint Surg Br 70: 217
11. Marmor L (1977) Result of single compartment arthroplasty with acrylic cement fixation. A minimum follow-up of two years. Clin Orthop 122: 181
12. Marmor L (1979) Marmor modular knee in unicompartmental disease. J Bone Joint Surg Am 61: 347
13. Marmor L (1984) Lateral compartment arthroplasty of the knee. Clin Orthop 186: 115
14. Marmor L (1988) Unicompartmental knee arthroplasty. Ten- to 13-year follow up study. Clin Orthop 226: 14
15. Marmor L (1988) Unicompartmental arthroplasty of the knee with a minimum ten-year follow-up period. Clin Orthop 228: 171
16. Scotts RD, Santore RF (1981) Unicondylar unicompartmental replacement for osteoarthritis of the knee. J Bone Joint Surg Am 63: 536

17. Scott RD, Cobb AG, Mc Queary FGI, Thornhill TS (1991) Unicompartmental knee arthroplasty. Eight to 12 years follow up evaluation with survivorship analysis. Clin Orthop 271: 96
18. Streicher RM, Weber H, Schoen R, Semlitsch MF (1992) Wear resistant couplings for longer lasting articulating total joint replacements. Adv 10/179: 186
19. Thornhill, TS (1986) Unicompartmental knee arthroplasty. Clin Orthop 205: 121

Part VIII

Arthroplasty of the Upper Extremities

Part VII

Elbow Arthroplasty, with Particular Regard to the Gschwend-Scheier-Bähler III Elbow Joint Prosthesis

N. Gschwend, B. Simmen, H. Bloch

Introduction

A total of 774 implantations of artificial joints were performed at the Wilhelm Schulthess Clinic during 1992 (Table 1).

Table 1. Arthroplasties Clinic W. Schulthess 1992

Hip	455
Knee	241
Shoulder	51
Elbow	27
Total	774

There are several reasons why elbow joint replacement was significantly less frequent than that of analogous joints of the lower extremities. The main reason is probably that only one useless joint of the lower extremity (e.g. the knee) makes walking virtually impossible, but impairment of one elbow joint, because of the integrity of its – sometimes more skilled – counterpart, still leaves a large degree of independence in daily activities.

Furthermore, in rheumatoid arthritis (RA), the main indication for elbow arthroplasty, one observes a conservation of elbow flexion in the range of at least 110° for 80 %–90 % of the substantially destroyed joints. This allows patients to lead the hand to the mouth and to use it in performing number of other tasks essential for moderate independence. In contrast, equally serious destruction of the shoulder joint quickly leads to a significant loss of function, which strongly impairs the ability for self-help. A third reason for the relatively low frequency of elbow arthroplasties is the availability of quite effective alternative surgery, particularly in the case of RA lesions. Synovectomy may reduce or eliminate pain even in advanced stages (e.g., in Larsen stage IV) [17]. Simple resection arthroplasty, as still practiced in other clinics, leads to a relatively high percentage of acceptable results, quite in contrast to resection arthroplasty of other joints.

Resection Arthroplasty of the Elbow Joint

Practiced first by Moreau [23] and, in the last two decades of the nineteenth century, by Ollier [26], simple resection arthroplasty may be counted among the most successful and simple modes of arthroplasty. We used it according to the modified technique of Hass [14] into the early 1970s. Careful analysis of the results found for a closed series of 25 cases observed over 6 years [6] revealed disturbing signs of progressive, troublesome instability in at least one-third of the patients, the majority of which were, because of their underlying disease, either forced to use crutches or had developed a pronounced tendency for bone

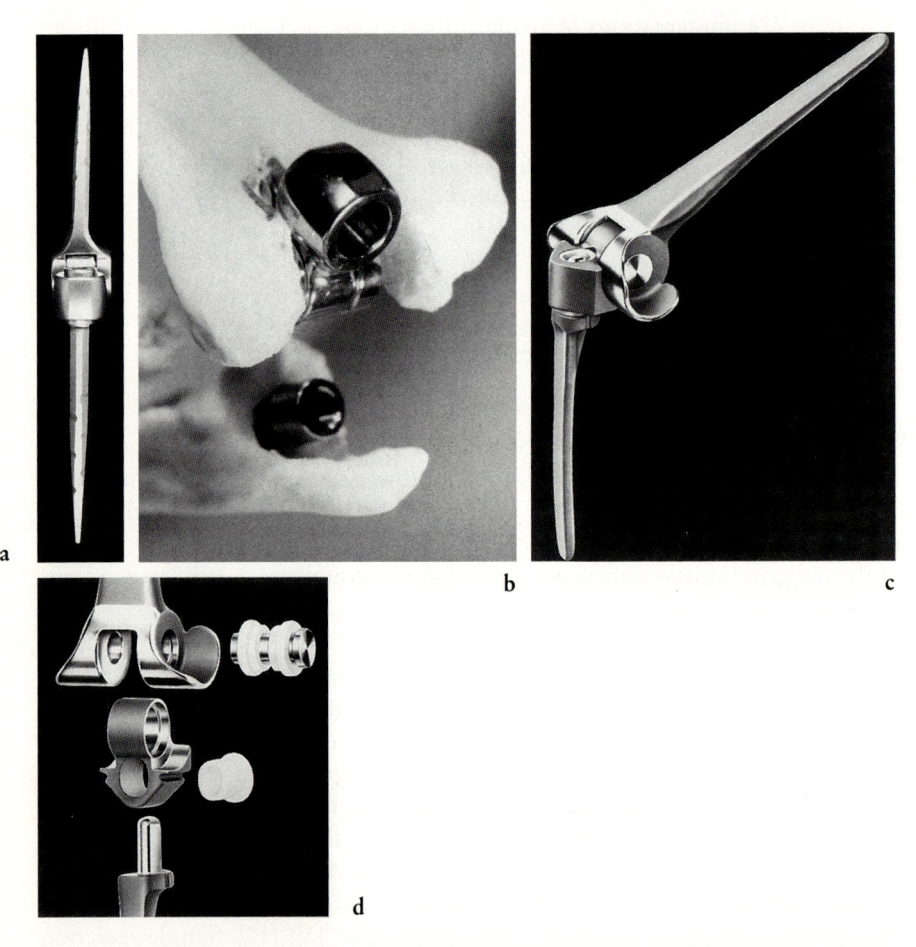

Fig. 1a, b. The GSB I prosthesis had rigid hinges, but this limited the amount of bone resection, hence leaving open a safe retreat possibility in cases of loosening. **c,d** GSB III prosthesis with high-density polyethylene bushes on the axle and the coupling mechanism linking the two components

resorption, often in connection with cortisone medication. The main problem presented by resection arthroplasty is the inverse relationship between the amount of resection and stability. To ensure ample mobility one is forced to resect a large amount of bone. This leads to a greater chance of instability followed by progressive bone resorption, which in turn further decreases stability. Similar experiences have also induced other authors to develop prostheses for the elbow joint, which – drawing on the positive results of Charnley [1] with the hip joint – were cemented into the intramedullary canal. The first prostheses of this type (Dee [2], McKee [22], Shiers, Mazas [21]) were, as a result of the initial optimism, implanted after a generous resection of the humerus condyles together with the origin of ligaments and muscles. As a consequence, loosening of the prosthesis was often observed after a rather short period. If the prosthesis had to be removed, serious instability usually led to a useless limb.

Such observations induced our group [10] (in collaboration with Sulzer) to develop the GSB I elbow prosthesis (Fig. 1a). As with those mentioned above, this prosthesis consisted of a rigid metal-on-metal hinge but was constructed in such a manner that made easy its conversion to a sine-sine resection arthroplasty [6, 11]. The GSB I prosthesis necessitated the resection of only a small, intercondylar piece of bone, thus leaving intact a great part of the humeral condyles and with it the origins of the ligaments and muscles. The intended easy conversion to a sine-sine resection arthroplasty soon proved its worth, as a considerable number of GSB I prostheses came loose and were then readily converted to a comparatively stable sine-sine arthroplasty [7].

Newer Models of Elbow Prostheses

The more recent models of elbow joint prostheses can be divided into three categories.
Nonlinked elbow prostheses either have smooth surfaces, consisting of a metal alloy at the humerus and of polyethylene at the ulna, or they reproduce the configuration of the natural elbow joint as closely as possible to achieve a relatively stable situation. The first group, the nonconstrained prostheses, encompasses those of Roper et al. [28], Lowe [20], Ishizuki [16], and Kudo [17] (Fig. 2a), whereas the prostheses developed by Souter [30], Ewald [4] (Fig. 2b) and others belong to the semiconstrained prostheses.

Since fixation of the nonconstrained prostheses (Roper, Lowe, Kudo) is often rather difficult because of a progressive destruction of the distal humerus and the proximal ulna, the developers of the *semiconstrained* surface prostheses (Souter, Ewald, and others) immediately sought a means of intramedullary fixation.

There are two types of *linked prostheses*.
Because of the above-average rate of loosening of the fully constrained metal-to-metal hinge prostheses, several authors developed *modern hinge prostheses* on

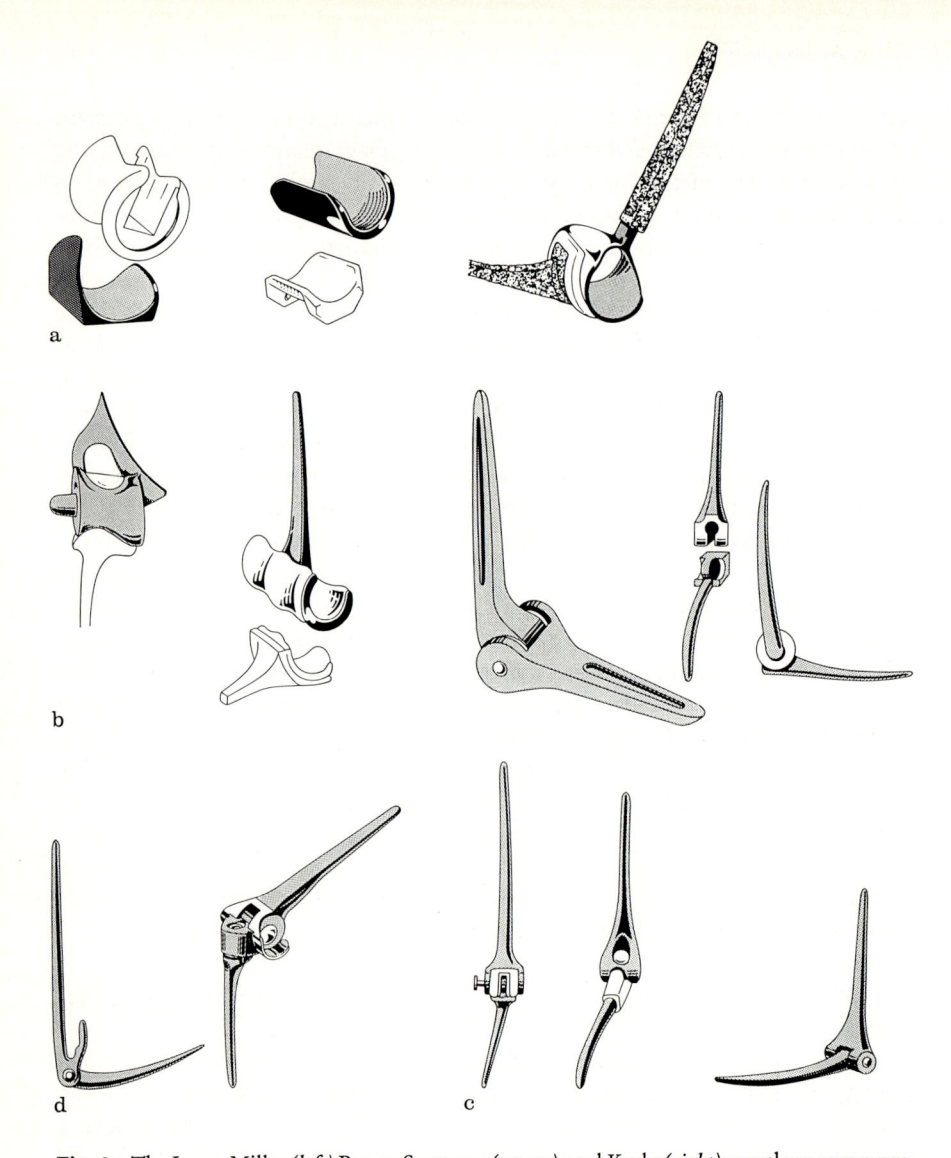

Fig. 2a. The Lowe-Miller *(left)* Roper-Swanson *(center)*, and Kudo *(right)* prostheses are examples of nonlinked nonconstrained metal-on-polyethylene prostheses with smooth surfaces. The Lowe-Miller prosthesis is also available with stems. The more recent Kudo prosthesis is used as a noncemented prosthesis. **b** The Souter-Strathclyde *(left)* and capitello-condylar (Ewald; *right*) are examples of nonlinked, semiconstrained prostheses imitating the natural anatomy as far as possible (particularly the Souter-Strathclyde prosthesis). These use an intramedullary fixation, the Souter-Strathclyde prosthesis having a modification with a longer humeral stem. **c** The Schlein *(above, left)*, Inglis *(above, right)*, Pritchard-Walker 2 *(below, left)* Dee 2 *(below, center)*, and Coonrad *(below, left)* prostheses are examples of floppy hinges using an axel for the linkage or a snap-fit mechanism. **d** The Mayo modification of the Coonrad 2 *(left)* and GSB III *(right)* prosthesis are examples of floppy hinges using flanges resting on the carefully preserved humeral condyles. The GSB III prosthesis flanges also have a larger radioulnar extension of the flanges resting on the distal ulnar und radial humeral condyles in addition to the anterior part of each

the two principles of clearance between the two components (floppy hinges) and low friction (metal on polyethylene). This construction was designed to use the conserved ligamentous system as an element of stabilization and thus to minimize the strain at the prosthesis-cement interface. This type of prosthesis encompasses, among others, those of Schlein [29], Dee [3], Pritchard and Walker [7], and the triaxial prosthesis of Inglis [15] (Fig. 2c).

A somewhat special status is taken by *floppy hinges* (Fig. 2 d), which seek additional support on the conserved humeral condyles. This is the case particularly for the GSB III prosthesis [8, 9, 12], in which this principle was realized for the first time. Later Morrey and Bryan [25] at the Mayo Clinic modified the Coonrad 2 prosthesis along similar lines, adding to the original Coonrad prosthesis an anterior flange.

Goldberg et al. [5] in their article concluded that the "less constrained" prostheses exhibiting kinematics close to those of the physiologic elbow should provide better results than others. However, this type of prosthesis depends on an almost complete integrity of the bone in the metaphysial region and of the collateral ligaments. The same authors also concluded that hinged prostheses with some clearance between the components (floppy hinges) give better results for the posttraumatic cases because they allow ample release of the soft tissue. Pain relief and mobility can be achieved more reliably with this type of prosthesis than with those of nonconstrained or semiconstrained nonlinked prostheses. In the same review article Goldberg et al. concluded that the results of the surface-replacement and the semiconstrained hinge-type prostheses are quite similar in RA. However, they recommend a prosthesis that rests broadly on the humeral condyles in order to better transmit the stresses, particularly those of torsion and compression, to the metaphysial bone. Physicians should in the future aim at the construction of this type of prosthesis.

The GSB III Prosthesis

Ten years prior to the article of Goldberg et al. [5] our group developed the postulated floppy hinge, based on the principles of low friction and broad support on the condyles [9]. We have been using this GSB III elbow prosthesis for 16 years (Fig. 1b). It works on the low-friction principle with no metal gliding on metal and has a clearance of a few degrees between the humeral and ulnar components.

The operative technique has been described on several occasions: here we mention only a few points that seem to us essential for success. The surgery is carried out with the patient lying on his side and his arm supported above the elbow. The use of a tourniquet is recommended. As approach we use a dorsal skin incision slightly convex in the radial direction. With the transtricipital approach that we have previously described [12], the integrity of the entire extensor mechanism is retained, since we detach the latter from the posterior surface of the olecranon and the proximal ulna together with thinnest bone slivers using an Ombredanne chisel. This measure allows reliable transosseous fixation of the extensor mechanism at the end of the operation. Before the detachment, however, the ulnar nerve must be laid free and mobilized as far as the first muscle branch for the extensor carpi ulnaris. Damage to the ulnar nerve, described unusually often in the literature, is in our opinion caused particularly by a bony spur on the lower ulnar border of the articular surface. At this point one usually finds, particularly in patients suffering from RA, an edge of the bone protruding as sharp as a knife directly adjacent (about 1–2 mm) to the ulnar nerve, perforating the deeper muscular structures. Any manipulation of the forearm, such as is necessary for the implantation of the prosthetic components, increases the risk of a direct lesion of the nerve by this sharp edge. We therefore remove it before proceeding with the mobilization of the elbow articulation. Only after this step do we prepare the radial part of the articulation and then perform the resection of the radial head distal of the radioulnar articulation. After resection of the proximal end of the olecranon we gain by our approach an excellent overview of the whole articulation. There follows a radical synovectomy, then, removal of the coronoid process, and – in the case of an established contracture of the flexor mechanism – the partial detachment of the brachialis insertion. This allows a comparatively safe performance of the specific steps necessary for the GSB III implantation, i. e., bone resection and preparation of the medullary cavity for the implant. Our transtricipital approach is probably one of the main reasons for the small number of cases with an important extensor lag in our casuistics compared with the numbers reported by others.

Results with GSB III Arthroplasty

Between 1978 and March 1992 we treated 144 elbows with the GSB III prostheses. Of these patients 109 suffered from RA, 7 from juvenile arthritis, and 2 from psoriatic arthritis, or Reiter's disease. In 26 cases osteoarthritic lesions (OA) of posttraumatic nature were diagnosed. The number of female patients with secondary osteoarthritic lesions equaled that of the male patients, but their number was much greater among the cases of RA (4:1). The abolishment of pain, or its significant mitigation, is the main indication for the implantation of a prosthesis. Figure 3 shows the pre- and the postoperative pain level in two groups of patients, one suffering from RA and the other from posttraumatic OA. We observe that in both groups, particularly that of RA patients, pain was virtually abolished to a small residual. An excellent effect is also seen among the posttraumatic patients. In the posttraumatic cases still experiencing moderate pain the pain appeared to be caused by the soft tissues.

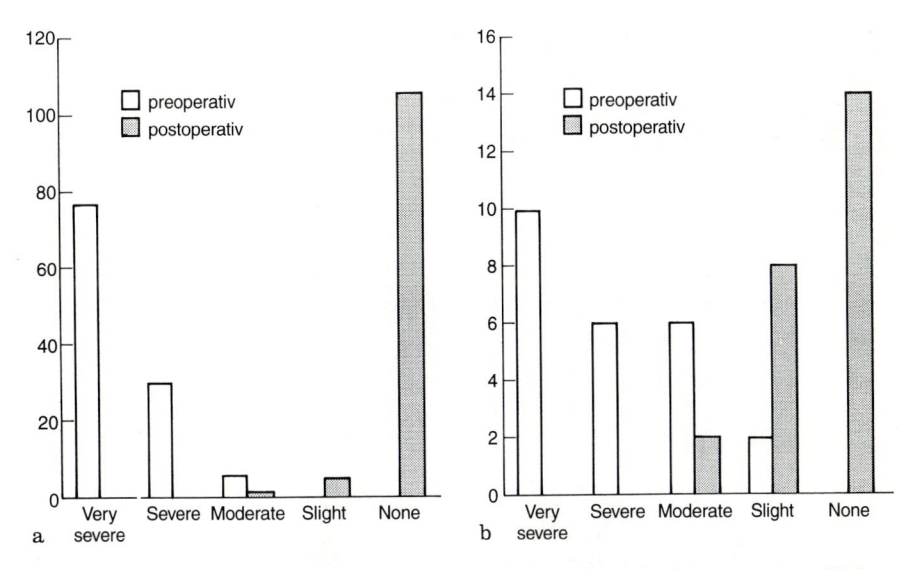

Fig. 3a, b. GSB III elbow pain. **a** RA (n = 118). **b** Posttraumatic OA (n = 26). *Solid bars*, preoperative; *shaded bars*, postoperative

Table 2. Range of motion in RA and OA

RA	Preoperative	Postoperative	Gain
Flexion	118°	134°	28°
Extension	−38°	−26°	
Pronation	54°	67°	25°
Supination	50°	62°	

OA	Preoperative	Postoperative	Gain
Flexion	95°	126°	37°
Extension	−40°	−34°	
Pronation	55°	73°	36°
Supination	49°	67°	

The preoperative range of motion was greater in the group of RA patients than in that of the postttraumatic patients. It was therefore possible to achieve a greater postoperative mobility in the first group, both with respect to flexion and lack of extension (Table 2). On the other hand, the relative increase in mobility was greater for the posttraumatic group. Figure 4 demonstrates in two cases one of RA the other of posttraumatic OA what can be expected for mobility and function from arthroplasty with the GSB III prosthesis.

a

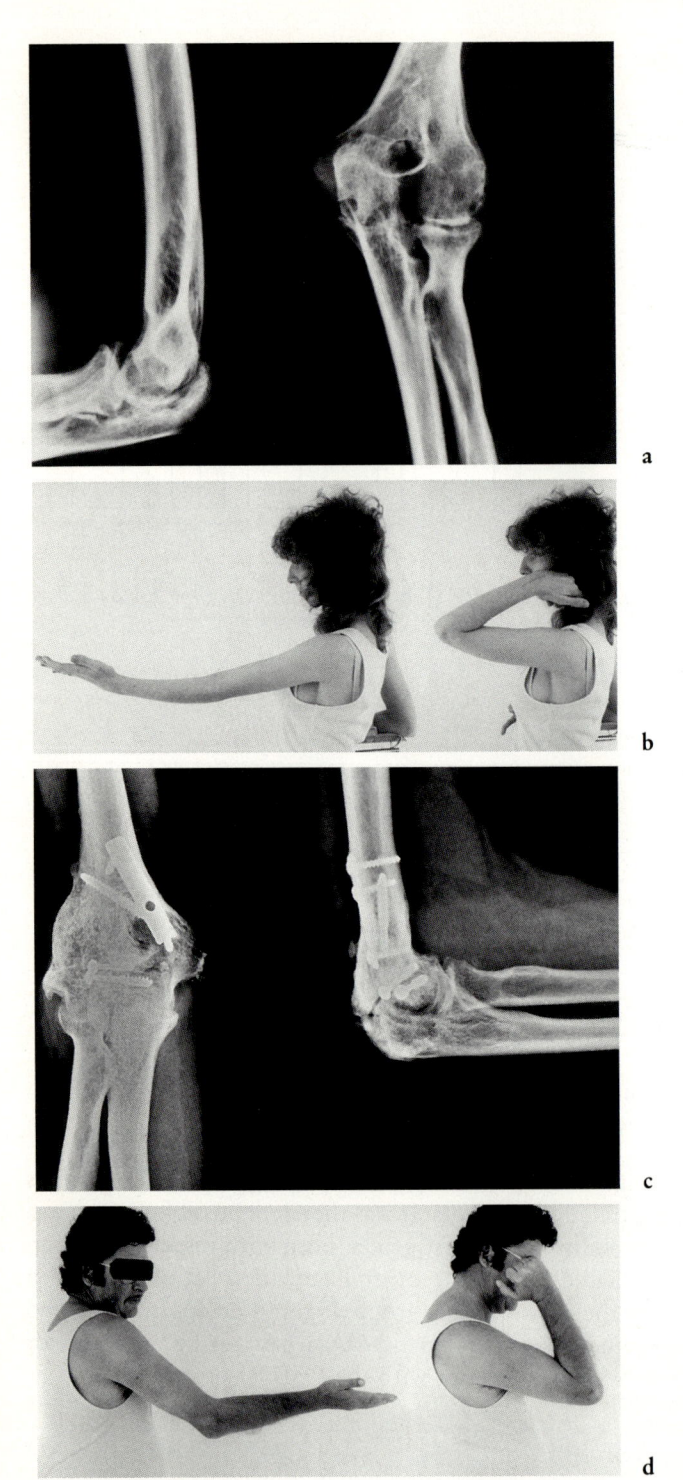

b

c

d

Results with Elbow Joint Arthroplasty in the World Literature

An inspection of the recent international literature [13] has demonstrated the extraordinarily high percentage of complications reported, sometimes even exceeding 50 % as Morrey indicated in 1991 [23]. Our analysis of the international literature between 1986 and 1992 gives the following picture: In 828 cases, 357 complications were observed (43); 23 % were designated as late complications. There were revisions in 151/828 (18 %). In 121/828 (15 %) there were permanent complications. With a mean follow-up period of only 55 month (3–12 years) this was a quite considerable number. The complications in terms of decreasing frequency were:

Radiological loosening   17.2 % (humerus 12.1 %, ulna 5.1 %)
Clinical loosening   6.4 % (humerus 3.4 %, ulna 2.7 %
Neuropathy of the n. ulnaris 10.4 %
Infections   8.1 % (superficial 3.5 %, deep 4.6 %)
Instability   7.1 %
Dislocation   4.3 %
Subluxation   2.2 %; (total 6.5 %)

Further complications are 3.2 % bone fractures, 0.6 % fractures of the implant.

No wonder that elbow joint arthroplasty is, on a worldwide scale, regarded with reserve. We were further impressed by the important lack of extension (30°–50°) reported in the international literature, particularly since the majority of reports deal with the results of arthroplasty performed on patients with RA, a group usually having less problems with mobility than the second largest group, those with posttraumatic OA.

Complications with the GSB III Prosthesis

Comparison of the complications in our own 144 cases with those reported in the world literature between 1986 and 1992 shows the following: Since 1978 we have had to make only one revision (0.7 %) because of loosing in a posttraumatic OA and none in RA. In only three og 48 cases which had been operated on more than 10 years earlier, and which we had followed by clinical and radiological

◄
Fig. 4a, b. This patient with juvenile arthritis had a severely limited preoperative range of motion, corresponding to the severe radiological destruction of the articular surfaces. **c,d** Posttraumatic OA which had been operated several times before coming for a GSB III replacement. We do not expect a normal range of motion due to extensive scarring around the joint. Pain relief and useful flexion is the main goal, whereas a rather remarkable however functionally not relevant lack of extension is to be expected

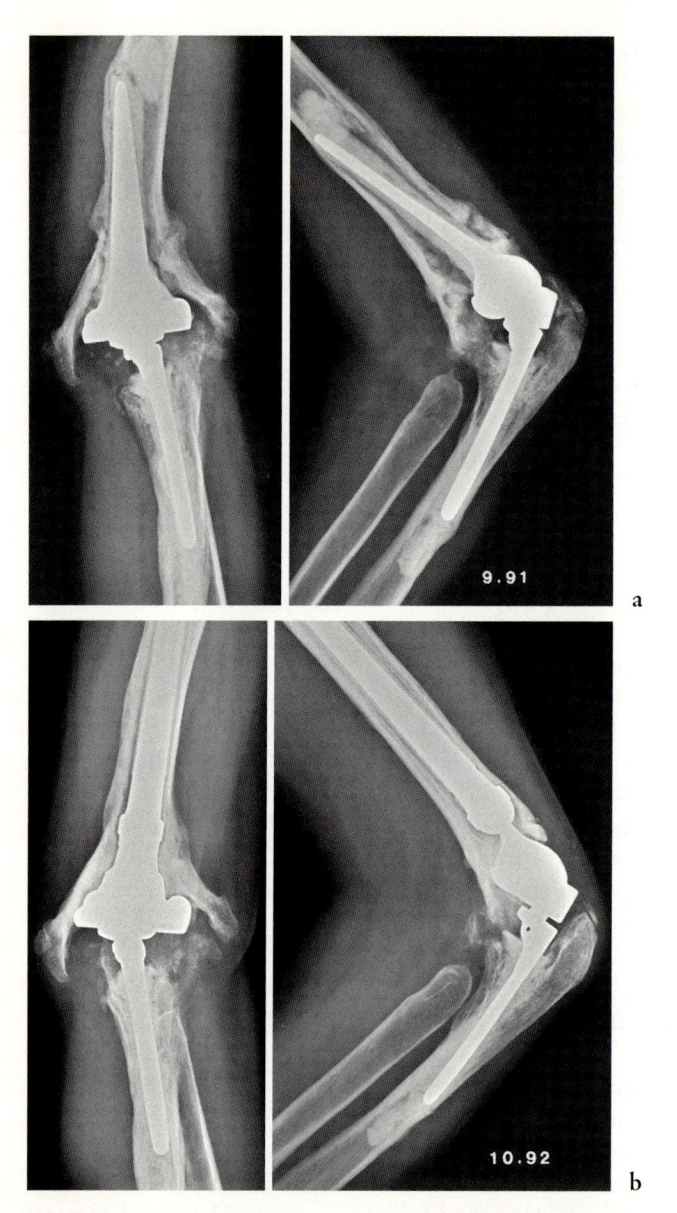

Fig. 5a, b. Posttraumatic OA in a relatively young man working as a painter and paper hanger, who developed painful loosening of the GSB III prosthesis with spontaneous fractures of the thinned cortical bone of the humerus. The implantation of a new cementfree GSB III humeral component with custom-made, conically shaped, longer titanium stem similar to that of the Wagner prosthesis for hip revision led to spontaneous regeneration of the bone

examination did we find a complete or progressive radiolucent line with bone resorption. The only revision with exchange of the prosthesis because of aseptic loosening was in a patient who had suffered a comminuted fracture and had years ago twice undergone operations for it and then, because of the persisting pseudoarthrosis of a condyle with severe OA of the articulations, obtained a GSB III prosthesis. This male patient's occupation was painter and paperhanger, which obviously put excessive demand on the operated arm. In his case we replaced the cemented GSB III prosthesis by a modified version of the GSB III prosthesis in which the intramedullary stem was replaced by a longer, conical, cementless stem of titanium shaped according to the principle used by Wagner for hip joint revisions. Astonishing is the comparison of the X-ray prior to, shortly after, and 6 months after the implantation of this modified GSB III prosthesis, which was implanted without cement (Fig. 5); the ultrathin and spontaneously fractured cortical bone of the humeral shaft has increased manyfold in thickness, and the prosthesis appears to have become solidly fixed.

Lesions of the ulnar nerve have been reported in the world literature (1986–1992) as having a rate of 10.5 %. Morrey's statistics reveal 7 % [23] and Souter's even 14 % [31]. Our own statistics indicate only 3/144 (2 %) of the cases operated in our clinic. Our opinion of how best to avoid this type of lesion is given above.

The *infection rate* of elbow joint arthroplasty is, according to the recent world literature, 8.1 %, and on the average significantly greater than for prostheses in other locations. In our opinion, one must distinguish infections in the wake of primary implantations from those after secondary implantations that were preceeded by one or more other operations. With this in mind, we would expect a higher rate of infections in posttraumatic cases in which difficulties with osteosynthesis had been experienced. Our own statistics appear to support this notion. Whereas the rate was only 2/118 (1.7 %) in cases with RA, we found 1/26 (3.8 %) in posttraumatic cases. In all of these infection cases, which had occurred in the early stages of our casuistics, we removed the prosthesis and converted the endoprosthesis arthroplasty into a sine-sine resection arthroplasty – with moderate functional results. Today, as in other articulations, we replace the prosthesis in either one or two stages, depending on the type of infectious agent and the condition of the soft tissue, thereby practicing as a matter of course extensive debridement and the local and general application of specific antibiotics.

Dislocations and subluxations of floppy hinge prostheses are not to be expected, however, an uncoupling of the two parts. The literature reports an uncoupling rate of 5%–10 %. Abrasion of the polyethylene in a snapfit mechanism is described as the major cause of uncoupling. We have also observed such a disassembling of the two components as the major complication, particularly during the early years of our experience. This was observed in 5/118 (4.2 %) of RA cases and in 4/26 (15.3 %) of posttraumatic cases. As the main causes, we diagnosed a too extensive release of the soft tissues and a position of the center of rotation of the prosthesis that did not quite correspond to the normal anatomy. As it is often difficult, if not impossible, to determine the exact position of the original center of rotation, particularly for posttraumatic cases, we have since developed an easily applicable elongation of the ulnar component that should prohibit a disassembling in future cases.

For an appraisal of our own method, we may consider the percentage of *permanent or lasting complications*, i. e., remaining complications after revision. This percentage was 3.4 % in our RA cases and 15.3 % in our posttraumatic ones. Table 3 indicates which type of complication is involved. These were mainly irritations of the ulnar nerve, and in one case a carpal tunnel syndrome in which the usual operation might well be able to achieve permanent relief. However, even if we include the patients for whom the prosthesis was removed and the elbow articulation converted to a sine-sine arthroplasty, there remain only two who were not pleased with the result, whereas the other two indicate no pain and are able to use their arm with reasonable force.

Table 3. Lasting complications in RA = 3,4 %

9 None
2 Residuel symtoms ulnar nerve
2 Sine-sine arthroplasty

Lasting complications in OA = 15,3 %

5 None
2 Sine-sine arthroplasty
1 Irritation of the ulnar nerve
1 Carpal tunnel syndrom

Discussion

Although a comparison of the kinematics of the elbow joint with those of a hinge joint appears unjustified, London [199] and Sorbie et al. [32] have shown that the elbow articulation has practically a single center of rotation. Only during the last degrees of extension does a mechanism of simultaneous rotation and sliding come into effect. This observation justifies the construction of an artificial elbow articulation as a hinge. Our GSB III prosthesis is such a hinge, constructed along the principle of low friction and exhibiting a certain amount of clearance between the humeral and the ulnar components. This clearance, essentially constituting a floppy hinge, is intended to relieve excessive forces at the bone-cement interface with the help of the intact capsular-ligamentous mechanism. In addition, the broad founding of the humeral part of the prosthesis on the humeral condyles, purposely left intact, should counter the forces that arise during the most frequent daily tasks such as lifting weights with the bent arm or supporting the body weight with the stretched arm. With other prostheses these forces lead to an extraordinary physical stress on the dorsal wall of the humerus, which the prosthesis may sink into the humerus, as we observed in our GSB I prosthesis. However, with the present type of prosthesis (GSB III) we have observed no indications of such detrimental behavior. The transtricipital approach that we recommend not only allows a perfect view of the operation field but especially the prevention of ulnar nerve lesions and a smaller lack of extension by preserving the continuity of the triceps. The results obtained with the GSB III prosthesis are quite comparable to the very best results described in the international literature, both with respect to functional improvement and (particularly) low percentage of complications. The low rates of loosening, of ulnar nerve lesion, and of infections are truly impressive. Special significance concerning the extraordinary quality of the prosthesis is attached to the results obtained in patients of posttraumatic OA, most of whom had undergone several other operations previous to our final arthroplasty.

We pay particular attention to the reconstruction of the humeral condyles where they are missing because of resorption (mutilans RA) or preoperative removal after comminuted fracture. We have reported our method of reconstruction using autologous full thickness pelvic grafts elsewhere [7]. The approximate reconstruction of the anatomy of the distal humerus in this manner allows us to take advantage of a firm support of the prosthesis on the humeral component and also, in the infrequent case of a necessary removal of the prosthesis, of easy conversion to a relatively stable sine-sine arthroplasty.

In summary, the GSB III elbow prosthesis has provided us good results in over 90 % of the cases in the last 16 years, a rate of long-term success of elbow arthroplasty that is by all means comparable to that of hip and knee arthroplasty.

References

1. Charnley J (1962) The long-term results of low-friction arthroplasty of the hip as primary intervention. J Bone Surg Joint [Br] 54: 61
2. Dee R (1969) Elbow arthroplasty. Proc R Soc Med 61: 1031
3. Dee R (1992) Revision surgery after failed elbow endoprosthesis. In: Juglis AE (ed) Symposium on total joint Replacement of the upper extremity, Mosby, St. Louis, pp 126-140
4. Ewald FC, Scheinberg RD, Poss R, Thomas WH, Scott RD, Sledge CB (1980) Capitellocondylar total elbow arthroplasty. Two to five year follow-up in rheumatoid arthritis. J Bone Surg Joint 62 [Am]: 1259–1263
5. Goldberg VM, Figgie HE III, Inglis AE, Figgie MP (1988) Current concepts review, total elbow arthroplasty. J Bone Joint Surg [Am] 70: 778–783
6. Gschwend N (1980) Surgical treatment of rheumatoid arthritis. Thieme, Stuttgart
7. Gschwend N (1983) Salvage procedure in failed elbow prosthesis. Arch Orthop Traume Surg 102: 95–99

8. Gschwend N (1991) The case for a linked elbow prosthesis. In: Hämäläinen MJ, Hagena FW (eds) Rheumatoid arthritis surgery of the elbow. Rheumatology 15: 98–112
9. Gschwend N, Loehr J (1980) Ellbogenarthroplastik. Orthopädie 9: 158–168
10. Gschwend N, Scheier H, Bähler A (1972) Die GSB-Ellbogen-Endoprothese. Arch Orthop Unfall-Chir 73: 316–326
11. Gschwend N, Scheier H, Bähler A (1977) GSB elbow-, wrist- and PIP-joints. In: Joint replacement in the upper limb. Mechanical Engineering Publications, London, pp 107–116
12. Gschwend N, Loehr J, Ivosevic-Radovanovic D (1988) Die Ellbogen-Arthroplastik. Orthopädie 17: 366–373
13. Gschwend N, Schwyzer H, Simmen B, Bloch H (to be published) Late complications in elbow arthroplasty. Presented in Aarhus, Dänemark
14. Hass J (1930) Die Mobilisierung ankylotischer Ellbogen- und Kniegelenke mittels Arthroplastik. Langenbecks Arch Chir 160: 693
15. Inglis AE (1982) Tri-axial total elbow replacement: indications, surgical technique and results. In: Symposium on total joint replacement of the upper extremity. Mosby, St. Louis, pp 100–110
16. Ishizuki M (1981) Quoted by Ewald reconstructive surgery and rehabilitation of the elbow. In: Kelley WN, Harris ED, Ruddy S, Sledge CB (eds) Textbook of rheumatology. Saunders Philadelphia, pp 1921–1943
17. Kudo H (1985) Long term follow-up study of total elbow arthroplasty with nonconstrained prosthesis. In: Kashiwagi D (ed) Elbow joint. Proceedings of the International Seminar Kobe, Japan. Excerpta Medica, Amsterdam (International Congress Series 678: 269–276)
18. Larsen A, Dahle K, Eek M (1977) Radiographic evaluation of rheumatoid arthritis and related conditions by standard reference films. Acta Radiol Diagn 18: 481
19. London JT (1981) Kinematics of the elbow. J Bone Joint Surg [Am] 63: 529–535
20. Lowe LW (1978) The development of an elbow prosthesis at Northwick Park Hospital. J Roy Soc Med 72: 117–120
21. Mazas F (1975) Prothèses totales du coude. Acta Orthop Belg 41: 462
22. McKee (1973) Total replacement of the elbow joint. Proceedings of the 12th SICOT Congress, 1972. Excerpta Medica, Amsterdam, pp 891–893
23. Moreau PF (1805) Observations pratiques relative à la résection des articulations affectées de carie. Paris
24. Morrey BF, Admas RA (1991) Semiconstrained devices: techniques and results. In: Morrey BF (ed) Joint replacement arthroplasty. Churchill Livingstone, New York, pp 311–329
25. Morrey BF, Bryan RS (1985) Total joint replacement. In: Morrey BF (ed) The elbow an its disorders. Saunders, Philadelphia, p. 546
26. Ollier LX (1878) De la résection du coude dans les cas d'ankylose. Rev Med Chir 6: 12
27. Pritchard RW (1981) Long-term follow-up study: semiconstrained elbow. Orthopedics 4: 151–155
28. Roper BA, Tuke M, O'Riordan SM, Bulstrode CJ (1986) A new unconstrained elbow. A prospective review of 60 replacements. J Bone Joint Surg [Br] 68: 566–569
29. Schlein AP (1976) Semiconstrained total elbow arthroplasty. Clin Orthop 121: 222–229
30. Sorbie CH, Shiba R, Sin D, Saunders G, Wevers P (1986) The development of a surface arthroplasty for the elbow. Clin Orthop 208: 100
31. Souter WA (1985) The Evolution of total replacement arthroplasty of the elbow. In: Kashiwagi D (ed) Elbow joint. Proceedings of the International Seminar Kobe, Japan. Excerpta Medica, Amsterdam, International Congress Series 678: 255–268
32. Souter WA (1987) Le traitement chirurgical du coude rhumatoide. Cahiers d'enseignement de la SOFCOT. Conférences d'enseignement, pp 159–172

Total Wrist Arthroplasty

H. C. Meuli

Design and Development of Total Wrist Prostheses

Total wrist prostheses appeared relatively late in the history of articular prostheses, mainly because arthrodesis is a reliable procedure for the treatment of advanced painful destruction of the wrist. However, for the management of rheumatoid arthritis, in which both wrists are commonly involved, arthroplasty is becoming increasingly popular.

In 1967 Swanson [19, 20] developed a silicone rubber flexible hinge implant for the radiocarpal joint. Our first total wrist prosthesis was designed in 1970. It was introduced clinically in 1971. A preliminary review was published in 1973 [11]. Until that time the Silastic spacer by Swanson was the only implant available. In the design and development of the total wrist prosthesis we were guided by following criteria: (a) the prosthesis must imitate as closely as possible the function of a normal wrist, (b) the materials used must be those with proven worth as components of other joint arthroplasties, and (c) the operative technique must be reproducible and performed in such a way that in case of failure acceptable salvage procedures are possible.

It became clear in the early stages of the design that the very complex joint kinematics of the wrist could not be simply copied, and we had to find a compromise. The fact that the center of motion is located within the head of the capitate bone inspired the design of a ball-and-socket joint, the simplest approach possible. A ball joint is easily made and presents no material problems. It is unconstrained, permitting motion in all planes as well as a slight distraction. The unconstrained design greatly reduces any unfavorable stresses on the anchorage of the parts in bone because impingement occurs only at the very limits of motion. It is also advantageous that the use of a ball joint compensates for technical rotational failures of implantation.

During the past two decades descriptions of numerous wrist prostheses have been reported, which demonstrates the interest and the need for such implants [1, 2–4, 6–10, 16, 21–23]. Better understanding of the functional anatomy and kinematics of the carpus were decisive for this evolution. In the course of the time our original prosthesis has been continuously improved. The range of motion was considerably increased by making the socket shallower, without sacrificing stability. In the final design the anchoring prongs were located eccentrically to simplify the precise centering of the prosthesis. The refinements of the surgical technique, careful selection of the patients, and strict observation of the indications and contraindications have substantially reduced the failure rate and therefore the need of subsequent revision surgery [12–14].

However, some problems still had to be solved, such as centering of the prosthesis, fixation of the prosthesis in the carpus, the use of cement and the problems associated with polyethylene wear. Exact positioning of the center of rotation is extremely important for the prosthesis to function well, and a prerequisite for adequate tendon balance. Fixation of current prostheses in the carpus is difficult because, instead of one solid bone, only an assemblage of several small bones with joint spaces between them is present. Cementing is therefore difficult and often insufficient. In case of instability the wear products of cement leads to granulomatous soft-tissue reactions resulting in local osteolysis with severe subsequent reduction of the bone stock. Furthermore, the polyethylene ball in our former prosthesis was considered inadequate because of increased wear rate, deformation and the inherent consequences of polyethylene debris. To reduce these problems a new prosthesis was developed in 1986. It is the result of a completely new technology and manufacturing process and is made from state-of-the-art materials.

The Meuli Wrist Prosthesis III

The third revised implant Meuli Wrist Prosthesis (MWP III) is composed of titanium 6-aluminium 7-niobium wrought alloy Protasul 100. The surface is corundum rough blasted. The ball head is coated with titanium nitride, which is exceptionally hard and therefore has excellent wear resistance. The cup inset is made of ultrahigh molecular weight Polyethylene Chirulen. The prosthesis consists of two components: the proximal ball (radius part) and the distal socket (carpal part). There are two sizes in right- and left-hand versions. The radius part can be used for both the right- and left-hand prosthesis, the head being offset to the ulnar side. The anchoring prongs of the carpal part are inclined at an angle of 15° dorsally to the median axis. Both anchoring prongs are straight, the stem for the second metacarpal bone is in a radial offset position helping to center and balance the prosthesis (Fig. 1).

Although the prosthesis can be alternatively cemented into the bone with methylmethacrylate, it is designed for use without cement. The prongs, which can be contoured to adapt to the position of the metacarpals, the anchorage flanges, and the accurate fit provide excellent primary stability in the previously prepared bone stock. Secondary fixation is expected as a result of bony ongrowth to the titanium implant [18]. The ball joint remains unchanged. Its fixed base at the radiolunate junction guarantees stability of the system and maintains carpal height. Ligamentous support is therefore no longer necessary. The mobility of the system is ensured by free movement within the ball and socket joint.

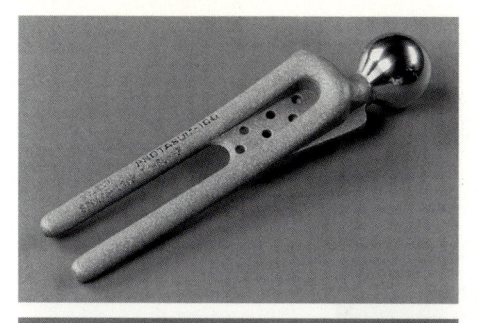

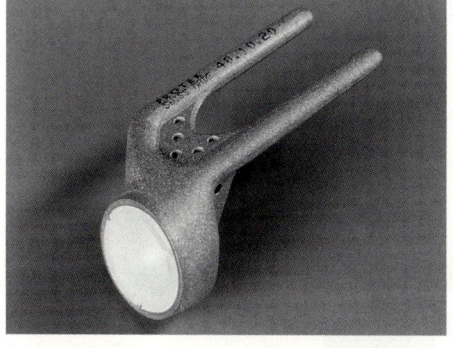

Fig. 1a, b. The MWP III total wrist prosthesis. (a) Radial component (ball head). (b) Carpal component (socket)

The rotational axis has no adverse effects. On the contrary, the rotational movements of the ball joint reproduce intercarpal rotation, which in the normal wrist is the result of intercalary motion of the proximal carpal row.

Obviously it is more difficult to balance such a nonconstrained ball and socket joint than a semiconstrained prosthesis or a prosthesis with an ellipsoid head. The prosthetic parts require precise placement, the center of motion being within the head of the capitate bone. For this reason intraoperative X-ray control and adequate tendon balancing are important steps of the operative procedure. Indeed, these are absolute prerequisites for a successful outcome with this prosthesis (Fig. 2).

Indications and Contraindications

Indications for a total wrist prosthesis must take into account pain, disability, and the local findings. Patient motivation is decisive. Total wrist replacement may be indicated when there is severe painful destruction and instability of the wrist due to rheumatoid arthritis or posttraumatic arthritis. However, it should be undertaken only if a reconstructive, motion-preserving procedure such as limited carpal fusions or proximal row carpectomy are no longer feasible and wrist arthrodesis is being considered. Contrary to wrist fusion, total wrist arthroplasty is a motion-preserving operation designed to prolong wrist func-

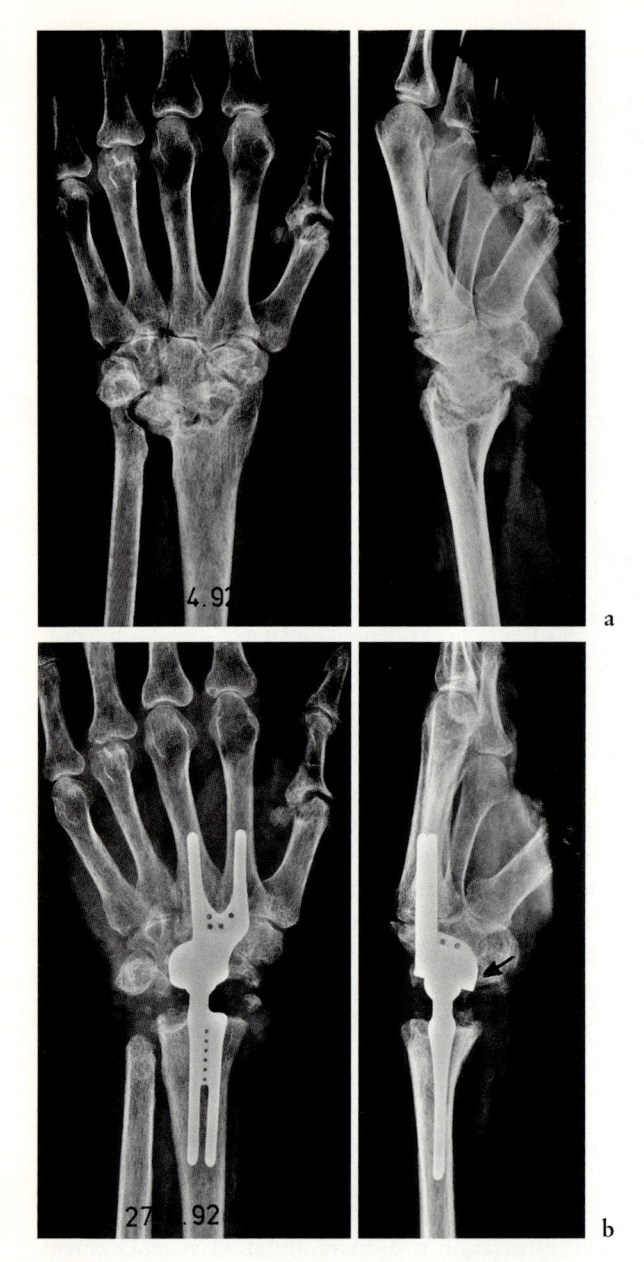

Fig. 2a, b. MWP III prosthesis in a 74-year-old woman with rheumatoid arthritis. (**a**) X-ray before surgery. (**b**) X-ray after surgery. Note reconstruction of the carpus and axial alignment. Prosthesis firmly fixed in the carpal bone stock (*arrow*)

tion in time. Loosening of the implant can always be salvaged with arthrodesis at a later date.

Wrist arthrodesis is still the preferred procedure if there are definite contraindications for a total wrist replacement, for example in workers engaged in heavy manual labor and in patients who must rely on walking aids. In the presence of insufficient bone stock, severe extensor tendon deficiencies, or malposition of the metacarpophalangeal joints with hyperflexion, a total wrist prosthesis is also contraindicated.

Surgical Technique and Postoperative Treatment

A very careful surgical technique must be observed to offer the patient the best possible result. Complications directly related to incorrect surgical technique may be avoided by following exactly the given guidelines [15].

The most important step is the correct placement of the prosthesis. Bone resection must be minimal. It is absolutely necessary to preserve solid bone support at the palmar side of the carpus to guarantee a solid anchorage of the carpal component of the prosthesis. Intraoperative fluoroscopic X-ray control is routinely performed before and after reduction of the prosthetic parts. The reconstruction of the extensor retinaculum is mandatory to avoid bow stringing of the extensor tendons.

Active exercises are started 1 week after the operation. The wrist is maintained in a neutral position for up to 2 weeks as the wound is healed. Then the flexion-extension exercises are gradually increased, but the resting splint should be worn for 6 weeks, especially during the night. Excessive range of motion exercise should be avoided in favor of maximum stability. Sometimes when the position is incorrector there is a tendency to contract a dynamic splint is used.

Discussion

The preliminary results of a first series of 50 prostheses with an average follow-up of 4.5 years have been carefully analyzed [15]. It could be clearly demonstrated that a solid fixation of the wrist prosthesis is possible without the need of bone cement.

Between 1986 and 1991, 50 prostheses were implanted in 45 patients, 33 of whom had rheumatoid arthritis and 12 posttraumatic arthritis. One patient died and 44 could be followed up 2–6 years after surgery. Evaluation included questioning of the patient on pain, satisfaction, and ability to perform daily activities, motion and grip strength measurements, and X-ray findings. The final result was rated as excellent in 24 wrists, good in 12, fair in 5, and poor in 8. The most common cause of unsatisfactory results was incorrect alignment of the carpal component in our early cases. The importance of absolutely correct positioning with the help of intraoperative X-ray control was underestimated and occurred in 11 instances. This palmarly directed tilt of the prosthesis was associated with progressive loosening in eight patients, six of which required removal of the prosthesis and arthrodesis with iliac bone grafting and plate

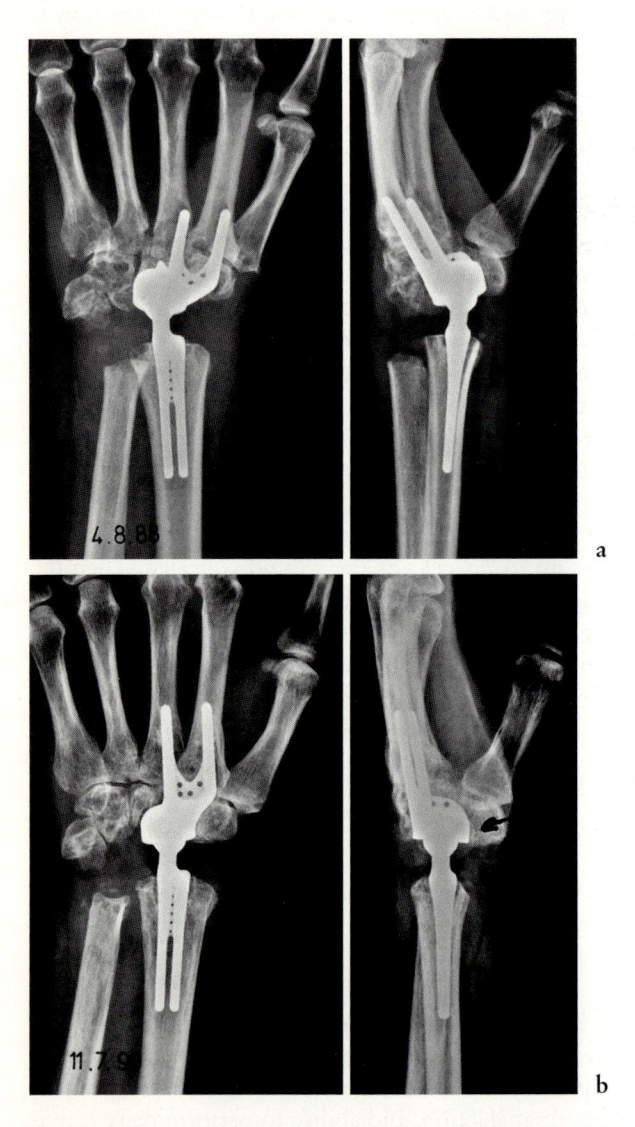

Fig. 3a, b. A 52-year-old woman with rheumatoid arthritis. (a) Incorrect placement of carpal prosthesis, no bony support within the carpus, loosening, and migration with palmar tilting of the prosthesis. (b) Revision: prosthesis correctly implanted. Bone graft to provide palmar buttress on the carpal part of the prosthesis (*arrow*)

fixation. One other prosthesis was removed (resection arthroplasty) and had an adequate functional result. The other case had removal of the carpal prosthesis and reimplantation and had an acceptable final outcome.

It is absolutely necessary to preserve sufficient carpal bone reserve to provide palmar buttress on the carpal part of the prosthesis. Since long-lasting fixation of the prosthesis depends solely on bony ongrowth on the implant surface, maximal coverage of the socket during implantation is imperative. This principle of osseointegration of the prosthesis is also valid for the radial side. Therefore, whenever the local bone stock is insufficient as in revision surgery or severe rheumatoid destruction, bone grafting (autologous iliac bone) is strongly recommended to provide the best possible mechanical and biological environment for bony ongrowth.

This observation of reducing bone resection to a minimum may well serve as a general principle for any type of wrist prosthesis, since loosening and migration of the carpal component appears to be the most common complication associated with total wrist replacement, and has been repeatedly emphasized by several other authors [3–7, 9, 17, 21] (Fig. 3). This is particularly true for voluminous carpal implants that are not solidly fixed within the carpus, and in which ultimate stability depends entirely on the metacarpal anchorage with bone cement. Even the use of longer prongs may result in late loosening due to the absence of bony support of the prosthesis proximally [17]. Functional loading in these instances may be responsible for bending and torsional stresses of the implant, micromotion, and progressive loosening of the metacarpal bone cement interface.

Our current philosophy is to reduce the size of the prosthesis to maintain the maximum of bony support within the carpus, so that a balanced biological fixation without cement can be guaranteed both at the carpus and at the metacarpals. Bone resection should therefore be minimal to allow fixation of a not too voluminous prosthesis with solid bone stock. The new MWP III total wrist prosthesis meets these prerequisites, and the midterm results are encouraging.

References

1. Alnot JY, Guepar (1982) Les arthroplasties du poignet. In: Razemon JP, Fisk GR (eds) Le poignet. GEM Exp Scientifique France. Paris
2. Alnot JY, Aubriot JH, Condamine JL et al.(1988) L'arthroplastie totale GUEPAR de poignet dans la polyarthrite rhumatoide. Rev Chir Orthop (Suppl II) 74: 340–345
3. Beckenbaugh RD (1991) Arthroplasty of the wrist. In: Morrey BF (ed.) Joint replacement arthroplasty. Churchill Livingstone, New York, pp 195–215
4. Beckenbaugh RD, Linscheid RL (1982) Arthroplasty in the hand and wrist. In: Green DP (ed) Operative hand surgery. Churchill Livingstone, New York
5. Cooney III WP, Beckenbaugh RD, Linscheid RL (1984) Total wrist arthroplasty. Problems with implant failures. Clin Orthop 187: 121–128

6. Ferlic DC (1992) Management of the rheumatoid wrist. In: Clayton ML, Smythe CJ (eds) Surgery for rheumatoid arthritis. Churchill Livingstone, New York, pp 155–187
7. Figgie MP, Ranawat CS, Inglis AE, Sobel M, Figgie III HE (1990) Trispherical total wrist arthroplasty in rheumatoid arthritis. J Hand Surg 15A. 2: 217–223
8. Gagey O, Lanoy JF, Mazas Y, Mazas F (1986) Prothèse totale radiocarpienne. Etude préalable. Rev Chir Orthop 72: 165–171
9. Hamas RS (1979) A quantitative approach of total wrist arthroplasty. Development of a „precentered" total wrist prosthesis. Orthop Clin North Am 3: 245-255
10. Kapandji IA (1982) Principes d'expérimentations d'une nouvelle famille de prothèses de poignet de Type Cardan. Ann Chir Main Memb Super 2: 155–167
11. Meuli H C (1973) Arthroplastie du poignet. Ann Chir 27: 527–530
12. Meuli H C (1980) Arthroplasty of the wrist. Clin Orthop 149: 118–125
13. Meuli H C (1984) Meuli total wrist arthroplasty. Clin Orthop 187: 107–111
14. Meuli H C (1992) Total wrist arthroplasty. In: Simmen BR, Hagena FW (eds) The wrist in rheumatoid arthritis. Basel, Karger Rheumatology, vol 17 pp 198–204
15. Meuli H C, Fernandez DL (1995) Uncemented total wrist arthroplasty. J Hand Surg 1995; 20 A: 115–122
16. Ranawat CS, Green NA, Inglis AE, Straub LR (1982) Special tri- axial total wrist replacement. In: Inglis AE (ed) American academy of orthopedic surgeons. Symposium on total joint replacement of the upper extremity. Mosby, St. Louis
17. Rettig ME, Beckenbaugh RD (1993) Revision total wrist arthroplasty. J Hand Surg Am 18: 798–804
18. Spotorno L, Schenk RK, Dietschi C, Romagnoli S, Mumenthaler A (1987) Unsere Erfahrungen mit nicht zementierten Prothesen. Orthopäde 16: 225–238
19. Swanson AB (1968) Silicone rubber implants for replacement of arthritic or destroyed joints in the hand. Surg Clin North Am 48: 1113–1127
20. Swanson AB (1973) Flexible implant resection arthroplasty of the hand and extremities. Mosby, St. Louis
21. Taleisnik J (1985) The wrist. Churchill Livingstone, New York
22. Volz RG (1976) The development of a total wrist arthroplasty. Clin Orthop 116: 209
23. Volz RG (1984) Total wrist arthroplasty. Clin Orthop 187: 112–120

Printing: Saladruck, Berlin
Binding: Buchbinderei Lüderitz & Bauer, Berlin